TREATMENT WITH GnRH ANALOGS: CONTROVERSIES AND PERSPECTIVES

TREATMENT WITH GnRH ANALOGS:

CONTROVERSIES AND PERSPECTIVES

The Proceedings of a Satellite Symposium
of the 15th World Congress on Fertility and Sterility
held in Bologna, Italy, 15-16 September 1995

Edited by

MARCO FILICORI
AND
CARLO FLAMIGNI

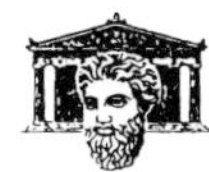

The Parthenon Publishing Group
International Publishers in Medicine, Science & Technology

NEW YORK   LONDON

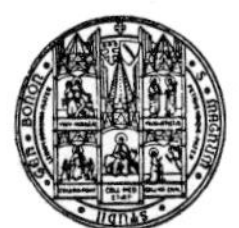

Reproductive Endocrinology Center
Department of Obstetrics and Gynecology
University of Bologna

Published in the UK by
The Parthenon Publishing Group Ltd.
Casterton Hall, Carnforth,
Lancs. LA6 2LA, UK

Published in the USA by
The Parthenon Publishing Group Inc.
One Blue Hill Plaza, PO Box 1564,
Pearl River, New York 10965, USA

Copyright © 1996 Parthenon Publishing Group Ltd.

British Library Cataloguing in Publication Data
Treatment with GnRH analogs: controversies and
  perspectives
  1. Luteinizing hormone releasing hormone 2. Luteinizing hormone
  releasing hormone – Derivatives 3. Pituitary hormone
  releasing factors
  I. Filicori, Marco II. Flamigni, Carlo
  615.7'04

ISBN 1-85070-690-5

**A Library of Congress Cataloging-in-Publication record is
available from the Library of Congress – LC96-33672**

First published 1996

Typeset by H&H Graphics, Blackburn, UK
Printed and bound in Great Britain by
Butler & Tanner Ltd., Frome and London

Contents

Section 4: Steroid replacement during GnRH analog treatment

Section 5: Cancer

Section 6:   Ovulation induction

Section 7:   Preparation for surgery in leiomyoma patients

Section 8:   Other applications

List of principal contributors

K. H. Baumann
Medizinische Klinik
Klinikum Innenstadt der LMU
Ziemsserstraße 1
D–80336 München
Germany

C. M. R. Bax
Department of Medical Oncology
St Bartholomew's Hospital
London EC1A 7BE
UK

P. Bouchard
Service d'Endocrinologie
Hôpital Saint Antoine
184, rue du Faubourg Saint Antoine
75012 Paris
France

W. J. Bremner
Chief Medicine Service (111)
Seattle VA Medical Center
1660 South Columbian Way
Seattle, WA 98108
USA

N. A. Bridges
The London Centre for Paediatric
    Endocrinology and Metabolism
The Middlesex Hospital
Mortimer Street
London W1N 8AA
UK

C. G. Brook
The London Centre for Paediatric
    Endocrinology and Metabolism
The Middlesex Hospital
Mortimer Street
London W1N 8AA
UK

C. Bulletti
Department of Obstetrics and Gynecology
University of Bologna
via Massarenti 13
40138 Bologna
Italy

E. Carmina
Department of Obstetrics and Gynecology
Columbia University College of Physicians
    and Surgeons
PH16 Room 16
630 West 168th Street
New York, NY 10032
USA

H. J. T. Coelingh Bennink
Medical Research and Development Unit
Organon International bv
PO Box 20
5340 BH Oss
The Netherlands

P. M. Conn
Oregon Primate Research Center
505 NW 18th Avenue
Beaverton, OR 97006
USA

L. Cusan
Clinique Cancers Hormonaux Dependants
Research Center
Le Centre Hospitalier de L'Universite Laval
2705 Laurier Boulevard
Quebec C1V 4G2
Canada

R. Deghenghi
Europeptides (GEIE)
Bt. Aristote-9
Avenue du Marais
95100 Argenteuil Cedex
France

J. Donnez
Service de Gynecologie et d'Andrologie
Clinique Universitarie Saint-Luc
Universite Catholique de Louvain
Avenue Hippocrate 10
1200 Bruxelles
Belgium

G. Emons
Department of Obstetrics and Gynecology
Philipps University
Pilgrimstein 3
D-35033 Marburg
Germany

J. Engel
ASTA Medica
Weissmüllerstraße 45
D-80314 Frankfurt am Main
Germany

L. Fedele
Centre for the Study and Therapy of
   Endometriosis
Università di Milano
via Commenda 12
20122 Milano
Italy

M. Filicori
Reproductive Endocrinology Center
University of Bologna
via Massarenti 13
40138 Bologna
Italy

C. Flamigni
Department of Obstetrics and Gynecology
University of Bologna
via Massarenti 13
40138 Bologna
Italy

A. J. Friedman
Boston Regional Fertility Center
Suite 321
3 Woodland Road
Stoneham, MA 02180
USA

D. Gonzàlez-Bàrcena
Department of Clinical Endocrinology
C. M. La Raza-IMMS
Hospital de Especialidades
Seris Y Zaachila, Col. La Raza
Mexico D. F. 02990
Mexico

W. Jäger
Universitäts-Frauenklinik
Labor Tumor-Marker
Universitätsstraße 21
91054 Eriangen
Germany

L. Kiesel
Eberhard-Karls Universität
Tübingen Frauenklinik
Schleichstraße 4
D-720076 Tübingen
Germany

R. A. Lobo
Department of Obstetrics and Gynecology
Columbia University College of Physicians
   and Surgeons
PH 16 Room 16
630 West 168th Street
New York, NY 10032
USA

E. Loumaye
Obstetrics and Gynecology
Ares Serono
15 bis Chemin des Mines
Case Postale 54
CH-1211 Geneva 20
Switzerland

A. Manni
Division of Endocrinology
Hershey Medical Center
500 University Drive
Hershey, PA 17033
USA

M. Motta
Instituto di Endocrinologia
Cattedra di Fisiologia Generale
Universita' di Milano
via Balzaretti
9-20133 Milano
Italy

E. Nieschlag
Institut für Reproduktionsmedizin
Westfälische Wilhelms-Universtät
Steinfurter Straße 107
D-48149 Münster
Germany

Y. Ogawa
DDS Research Laboratoires
Pharmaceutical Research Division
Takeda Chemical Industries Ltd
17–85, Jusohonmachi 2-chome
Yodogawa-ku
Osaka 532
Japan

E. Porcu
Department of Obstetrics and Gynecology
University of Bologna
via Massarenti 13
40138 Bologna
Italy

Th. Reissmann
ASTA Medica
Weissmüllerstraße 45
D-60314 Frankfurt am Main
Germany

J. E. Rivier
Clayton Foundation Laboratories for Peptide
    Biology
The Salk Institute
PO Box 85800
San Diego, CA 92186-5800
USA

J. Sandow
Pharma Research
Pharmacology H821
Hoechst AG
D-65926 Frankfurt am Main
Germany

A. V. Schally
VA Medical Center
Research Building F
VA Medical Center
1601 Perdido Street
New Orleans, LA 70146
USA

G. A. Shangold
Gynecology and Reproductive Research
The R. W. Johnson Pharmaceutical Research
    Institute
Route 202
PO Box 3000
Raritan, NJ 08869-0602
USA

D. J. Stanislaus
Oregon Health Sciences University
6181 SW Sam Jackson Park Road
Portland, OR 97201
USA

E. S. Surrey
Department of Obstetrics and Gynecology
Centre for Reproductive Medicine and Surgery
9675 Brighton Way
Beverly Hills, CA 90210
USA

Foreword

This book contains the proceedings of the conference 'Treatment with GnRH Analogs: Controversies and Perspectives' held in Bologna (Italy), on 15–16 September 1995. The conference was attended by 270 scientists from 22 different countries and permitted a timely update in this important area of reproductive endocrinology.

A quarter of a century has passed since the pioneering studies of Dr Andrew Schally and Dr Roger Guillemin that resulted in the characterization and synthesis of the gonadotropin-releasing hormone GnRH; the Nobel prize was awarded in 1977 to these investigators for their breakthrough in reproductive endocrine physiology. Few, however, could have anticipated the widespread impact that this compound and its derivatives (GnRH analogs) would have had on the clinical treatment of such diverse conditions as precocious puberty, prostate cancer and anovulatory infertility. GnRH and its analogs have become the primary mode of treatment for several of these disorders worldwide.

Nevertheless, like with every important drug, GnRH analogs continue to stir a fair amount of controversy. In addition, new applications of GnRH analogs are being proposed as attested by the numerous scientific publications that appear monthly in the international literature. Finally, a new family of compounds, GnRH antagonists, are beginning to emerge as valuable treatment tools and their clinical availability to practicing physicians is probably close.

For all these reasons, we felt that a high-level update in the area of GnRH analogs was important. We strived to gather in Bologna world experts in this field to understand the present status of these drugs and its clinical perspectives. We are grateful for their high-level presentations and timely manuscript submission. We also wish to thank CSR Congressi and Mrs Silvia Batani for providing excellent organizational skills and Ms Samantha Oliver of Parthenon Publishing for assistance in the preparation of this volume.

Marco Filicori
Carlo Flamigni

Section 1

Basic aspects

GGH₃ cells: a model for GnRH mechanism of action

D. J. Stanislaus, D. A. Kuphal and P. M. Conn

UNDERSTANDING THE MECHANISM OF GnRH ACTION HAS LED TO THERAPEUTIC APPLICATIONS FOR GnRH AND ITS ANALOGS

Gonadotropin releasing hormone (GnRH) is synthesized and released by the arcuate nucleus of the brain, then transported via the hypothalamic–hypophyseal portal system to the pituitary. In the mammalian pituitary, GnRH stimulates gonadotropes to release the gonadotropins, luteinizing hormone (LH) and follicle stimulating hormone (FSH)[1]. In addition, GnRH evokes other cellular responses such as target cell sensitization and desensitization, up- and down-regulation of GnRH receptors and synthesis of gonadotropins[1].

Understanding the molecular and physiological mechanisms of action of GnRH and its analogs has made possible the design of therapeutic applications which regulate the hypothalamic–pituitary–gonadal axis[2]. For example, administration of low, pulsatile doses of GnRH or its agonists via portable infusion pumps is an appropriate therapy for some types of infertility[2]. Alternatively, continuous administration of metabolically stable GnRH agonists can provoke desensitization of the gonadotrope, leading to decreased production of gonadotropins and a state of biochemical castration. This induced desensitization relieves the gonadal steroid influence from a variety of diseases such as endometriosis and uterine fibroids in females, prostate cancer in males and precocious puberty in both sexes[2].

GGH₃ AND αT3-1 CELLS SERVE AS MODELS FOR STUDYING THE MECHANISM OF GnRH ACTION

When GnRH binds and activates its membrane receptor, intracellular signaling leads to gonadotropin release and synthesis, gonadotrope desensitization and other cellular events. Details of signal transduction systems involved in the mechanism of GnRH action are not precisely understood. In order to study signal transduction mechanisms, primary gonadotrope cell cultures prepared from immature female rats are often treated with pharmacological agents that target second messenger molecules (e.g. inositol phosphate, cyclic adenosine-3',5'-monophosphate and calcium) and intracellular effector molecules (e.g. protein kinases and phosphatases, transcription factors and proteins involved in hormone synthesis and release).

Frequently, agents such as cholera toxin (CTX), pertussis toxin (PTX) and methylisobutylxanthine influence signaling cascades in a number of pituitary cell types. Since gonadotropes constitute only 20% of the cell population in primary pituitary cultures and other pituitary cell types may utilize second messengers common to the gonadotrope, it can be difficult to assess the source of second messenger molecules being influenced. Therefore, a continuous and homogeneous source of gonadotrope cells or other adequate model is useful in studying the intracellular events following activation of the GnRH receptor. Two such continuous cell lines, the gonadotropic αT3-1[3] and the lactotrope derived GGH₃ (GH₃ cells altered genetically to express the GnRH receptor[4]), offer alternative approaches to studying intracellular signaling mechanisms activated via the GnRH receptor.

The αT3-1 cell line was established by directing the expression of simian virus-40 T-antigen oncogene linked to the human glycoprotein α-subunit promoter/enhancer in transgenic mouse pituitaries[3]. These clonally derived cells release α-subunit (but not β-subunit or intact

Table 1 Comparison of primary pituitary cells, αT3-1 and GGH$_3$ cells

	Primary cells	*αT3-1 cells*	*GGH$_3$ cells*
Secretory product	LH and FSH	glycoprotein α-subunit[3]	prolactin[6]
Efficiency of transactions	low	high	high
Detectable release of secretory product (time)	15–20 min	4 hours[36]	3–6 hours[6]
Maximal release of secretory product	9 hours	> 48 hours[36]	> 120 hours*[7]
Secretory granules	present	present[36]	not present[7]
Acute dependence on protein synthesis for release of sensory product	no[6]	no[36]	yes[6]
Receptor down-regulation and recovery	1–5 hours	**	3–7 hours[7]

*Maximal release from GGH$_3$6' cells is 24 hours; **data not available

gonadotropin) of mouse pituitary glycoprotein hormones (LH, FSH and thyroid stimulating hormone) in response to GnRH[3]. When stimulated with physiological concentrations of GnRH, αT3-1 cells produce a transient increase in inositol-1,4,5-triphosphate and a biphasic rise of intracellular Ca^{2+} [5], which is an activation of second messengers similar to that observed in primary pituitary cultures.

The GGH$_3$ cell line was established by stable transfection of an immortalized lactotrope-derived cell line (GH$_3$ cells) with the rat GnRH receptor complementary deoxyribonucleic acid (cDNA)[4]. Characterizing the signaling mechanisms activated by the GnRH receptor in GGH$_3$ cells has been the focus of current investigation in the author's and other laboratories[4,6–10]. This chapter reviews our understanding of GnRH receptor–effector coupling in GGH$_3$ cells and focuses on their utility as a model of GnRH action.

For studies on the mechanisms of GnRH action, the GGH$_3$ cells have a number of advantages compared to primary pituitary cells and αT3-1 cells. For example, GGH$_3$ cells are clonally derived and homogeneous; these, then, have desired characteristics for studying intracellular signaling mechanisms (noted earlier in the chapter). Gonadotrope cells in primary pituitary culture are not homogeneous and it is a technical achievement to obtain gonadotrope cultures even at 50% homogeneity. Also, the ease of transfecting GGH$_3$ cells (compared to gonadotropes in primary culture) enables the manipulation of GnRH receptor number and expression of other peptide molecules significant for studying signaling processes. Moreover, unlike αT3-1 cells, which release only glycoprotein α-subunit, GGH$_3$ cells release an authentic hormone (prolactin) as a measurable end-point to GnRH stimulation. Table 1 shows a comparison of primary pituitary cells, αT3-1 and GGH$_3$ cells.

Unlike αT3-1 and primary gonadotrope cells, GGH$_3$ cells synthesize hormone immediately prior to release; there is no apparent intracellular storage of the hormone. Accordingly, the GGH$_3$ cells provide a model to study desensitization without the influence of either depletion of stored hormone or enhancement of storage. In addition to regulation of stored hormone, GnRH-stimulated gonadotrope desensitization involves receptor down-regulation. This event occurs in GGH$_3$ cells, which are not derived from gonadotropes. Also, the process of homologous desensitization can be studied in GGH$_3$ cells since, after GnRH receptor number recovers to control levels, both gonadotropes and one GGH$_3$ cell line become refractory to sustained GnRH stimulation.

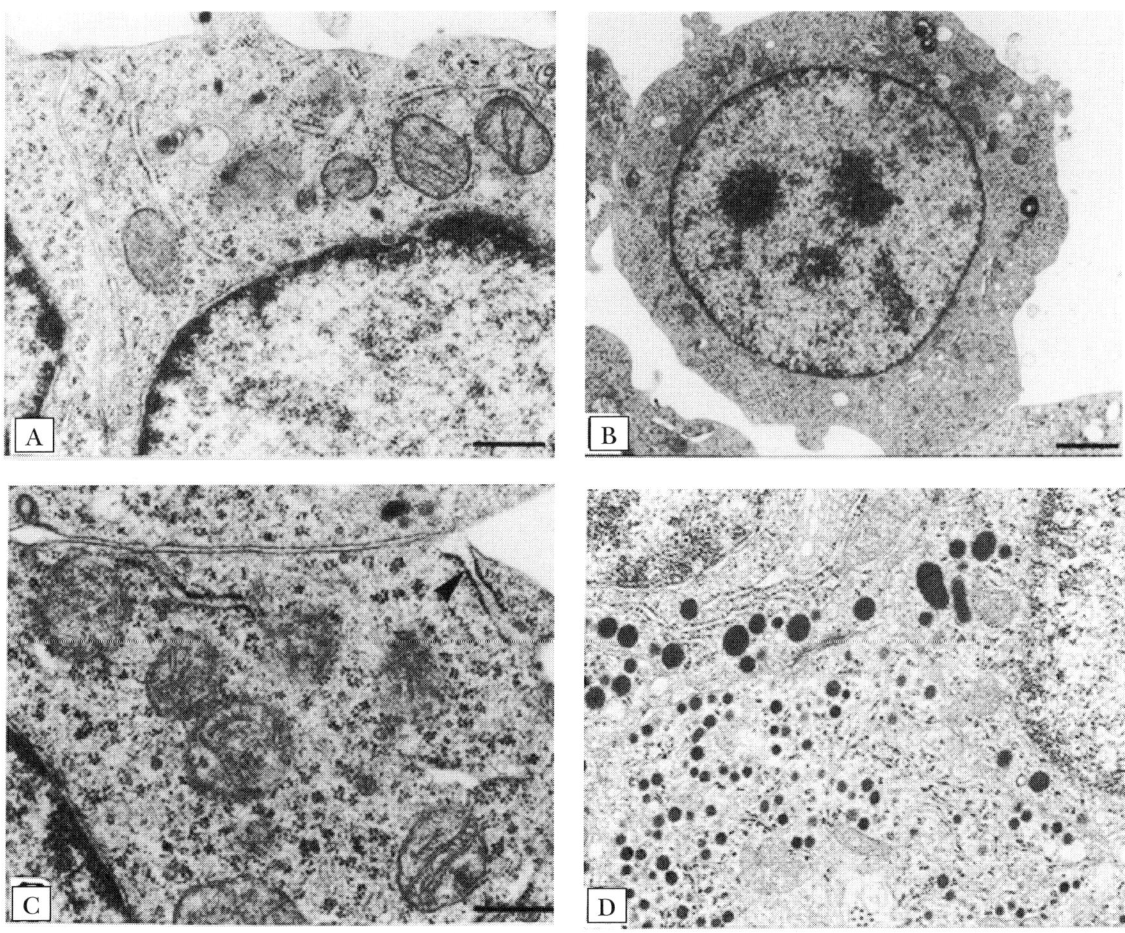

Figure 1 Electron micrographs of GGH₃ (A, B and C) and gonadotrope (D, lower half) cells showing vector-transfected (A), and vector and insert transfected GGH₃ cells (B and C). No differences are apparent in the morphological features of the different GGH₃ cell lines as judged by the appearances of the nuclei, Golgi apparatus, mitochondria, smooth and rough endoplasmic reticula, polysomes and occasional small secretory granules. Note the close proximity of a rough endoplasmic reticulum cisterna to the plasma membrane (C, arrow head). Scale bars: B = 2 μm; A and C = 0.5 μm. From Stanislaus, D., Janovick, J. A., Jennes, L. *et al.* (1994). Functional and morphological characterisation of four cells derived from GH₃ cells stably transfected with rat GnRH receptor cDNA. *Endocrinology*, **135**, 2220–7[7]. Reproduced with permission of the Endocrine Society

GGH₃ CELLS SHOW MORPHOLOGY CONSISTENT WITH HIGH SYNTHETIC ACTIVITY

Four GGH₃ clonal cell lines expressing the rat GnRH receptor were prepared by electroporating the parent cell line (GH₃) in the presence of a pcDNA1–GnRHR expression vector containing a neomycin resistance gene[4]. The four cell lines (GGH₃1', GGH₃2', GGH₃6' and GGH₃12') are morphologically indistinguishable from of either the vector-transfected cells or the parent GH₃ cells (Figure 1)[7].

The presence of enlarged nuclei with a marginal heterochromatin display and large numbers of rosettes of circular polyribosomes suggest high protein synthetic activity. Lack of secretory vesicles and the close proximity of rough endoplasmic reticulum with the plasma membrane suggest that a potential pathway for prolactin release may occur independently of secretory vesicles and may be regulated at the level of protein synthesis[7].

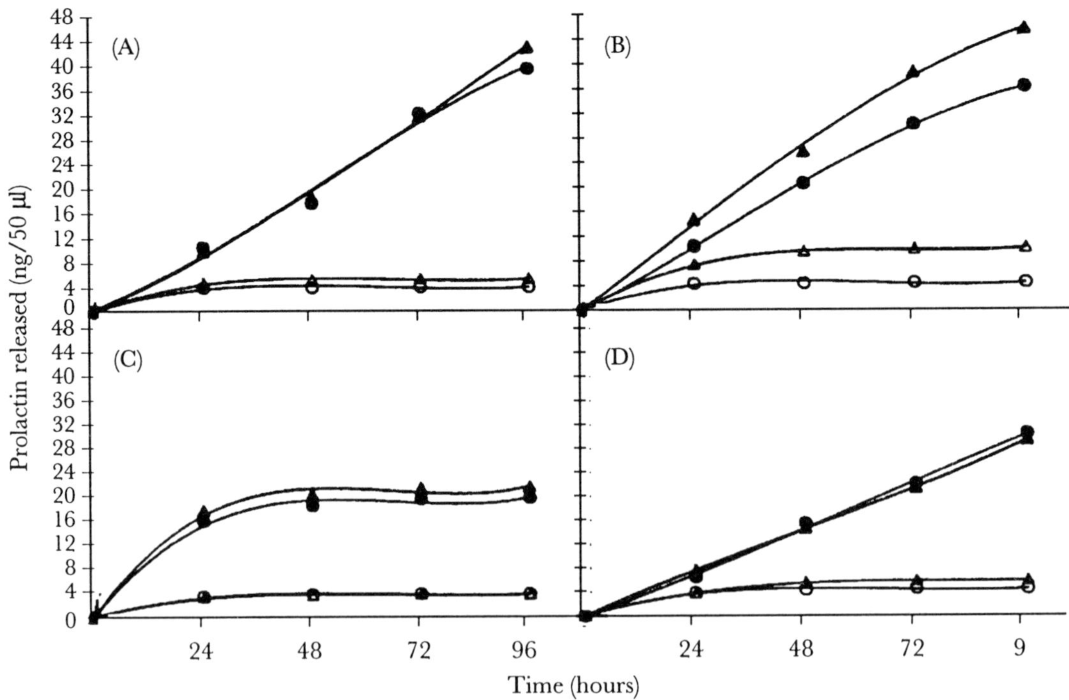

Figure 2 Time–course of prolactin release in response to various secretogogues in GGH$_3$1' (A), GGH$_3$2' (B), GGH$_3$6' (C) and GGH$_3$12' (D) cells respectively. GGH$_3$ cells were incubated with the vehicle buserelin (0.01 mg/ml), TRH (1 µg/ml) or buserelin (0.01 µg/ml) and TRH (1 µg/ml) for 24, 48, 72 and 96 hours. ○, Control; ●, buserelin 0.01 µg/ml; △, TRH 1 µg/ml; ▲, buserelin+TRH. Reproduced with the permission of the Endocrine Society from reference 7. Full copyright information is given in Figure 1

GnRH STIMULATES PROLACTIN RELEASE FROM GGH$_3$ CELLS

The metabolically stable GnRH analog buserelin stimulates prolactin production from GGH$_3$ cells in a time- and dose-dependent manner (Figure 2)[7]. GnRH-stimulated prolactin release is measurable at 3–6 hours in GGH$_3$ cells. Thyrotropin releasing hormone (TRH), which stimulates prolactin release from lactotropes, does not stimulate prolactin production in all GGH$_3$ cells even though the presence of TRH receptors have been demonstrated in all four GGH$_3$ cell lines[4]. Agonist binding to the GnRH receptor in GGH$_3$ cells stimulates increased inositol phosphate (IP) production, cyclic AMP release and prolactin synthesis and release. Since more than one type of signal transduction mechanism is activated by GnRH, the GnRH receptor expressed by GGH$_3$ cells must couple to multiple types of G-proteins, probably G$_s$ and G$_q$. As described later in this chapter, the signal transduction mechanism coupled to the GnRH receptor in the GGH$_3$ cell line differs from the mechanism involved in primary gonadotrope cultures.

Morphological and physiological studies show that GnRH-stimulated prolactin release from GGH$_3$ cells is regulated at the level of protein synthesis. In primary pituitary cells gonadotropin is stored and then released from secretory granules, suggesting that GnRH-stimulated gonadotropin release is not regulated at the level of synthesis. Furthermore, the protein synthesis inhibitor cycloheximide (in millimolar concentrations) has no effect on GnRH-stimulated LH release from gonadotrope cells, even after 24 hours administration of the agent[6]. GGH$_3$ cells, however, do not have secretory granules and GnRH-stimulated prolactin release is immediately sensitive to micromolar concentrations of cycloheximide[6,7]. Also, the time course for prolactin release is slower (measurable at 3 to 6 hours) than that observed for GnRH-stimulated LH release in primary cultures of rat pituitaries (measurable at 15 to 20 min)[6].

Further evidence that GnRH-stimulated prolactin release from GGH$_3$ cells is regulated at the level of synthesis comes from a time–course study of intra- and extracellular prolactin concentrations during incubation in medium alone or medium containing either a GnRH agonist or antagonist. At times from 15 to 87 hours the percentage of prolactin released, regardless of the contents of the incubation, was 94–98%[6]. GGH$_3$ cells incubated with agonist have a higher total prolactin content (intra- and extracellular) which, at a fixed percentage of release, means that a higher total amount of release occurs in response to agonist.

GGH$_3$ CELLS RELEASE SECRETOGRANIN II THROUGH A CONSTITUTIVE PATHWAY AFTER GNRH ANALOG STIMULATION

The regulated pathway of release, which is under the control of external signals, is typically associated with cells containing secretory granules. Secretogranin II (SII) is a molecule believed to be a component of secretory granules and, as such, a marker for the regulated pathway of release. SII is released in a dose- and time-dependent manner in GGH$_3$ cells in response to buserelin[9]. The release of SII is constitutive due to the lack of secretory granules and is probably a synthesis-dependent event in GGH$_3$ cells (in contrast to other cells with secretory granules containing SII[11]). These observations suggest that in GGH$_3$ cells, proteins associated with regulated pathways of release do not have sorting domains to preclude release via constitutive routes or which require processing through secretory granules[9].

GGH$_3$ CELLS EXPRESSING THE GnRH RECEPTOR SPECIFICALLY BIND GnRH AND REGULATE GnRH RECEPTOR NUMBER

All four GGH$_3$ cell lines show down-regulation of the GnRH receptor followed by recovery (but not

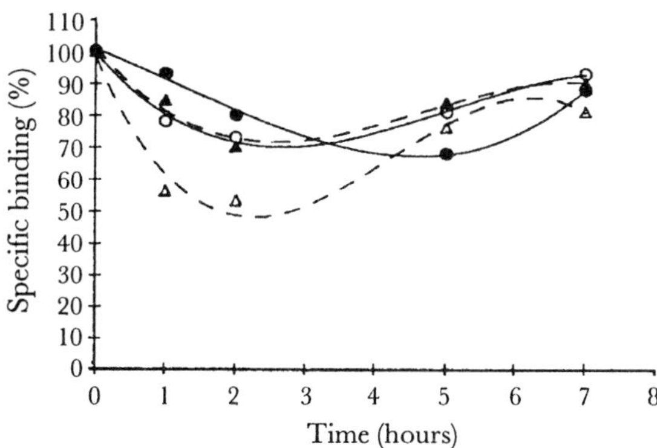

Figure 3 Down-regulation and up-regulation of the GnRH receptor in GGH$_3$1', GGH$_3$2', GGH$_3$6' and GGH$_3$12' cells. GGH$_3$1' cells recover from down-regulation by 5 hours whereas the other cell lines recover by 2 hours. Specific binding is that of the GnRH analog buserelin. ●, GGH$_3$1'; ○, GGH$_3$2'; ▲, GGH$_3$6'; △, GGH$_3$12'. Reproduced with the permission of the Endocrine Society from reference 7. Full copyright information is given in Figure 1

up-regulation) to control numbers[7]. When stimulating GGH$_3$ cells with a desensitizing dose of GnRH (10 nM), GGH$_3$1' cell receptor number recovers after a 5-hour treatment. Receptor number for the other three GGH$_3$ cells recovers in approximately 2 hours which is reminiscent of the receptor regulation pattern observed for the gonadotrope in primary pituitary culture (Figure 3)[12]. The binding affinity of buserelin to the GnRH receptor, as assessed by saturation binding experiments (Figure 4) or Scatchard analysis (Figure 4, inset), is slightly lower in GGH$_3$ cells ($K_d = 4.1 \pm 1 \times 10^{-8}$ M) than in primary cells[6]. This is consistent with the rightward shift of the dose–response curve for GnRH-stimulated prolactin release in GGH$_3$ cells compared to the dose–response of GnRH-stimulated LH release in primary cell cultures[6]. The lower binding affinity for the expressed receptor and slow rate of prolactin release in response to GnRH analogs may reflect intrinsic differences in GGH$_3$ cells or irregular positioning or post-translational modification of the receptor.

In β_2/β_3 adrenergic receptors, as well as many other G-protein coupled receptors (GPCRs), a long carboxyl terminal cytoplasmic tail mediates receptor down-regulation and desensitization[13].

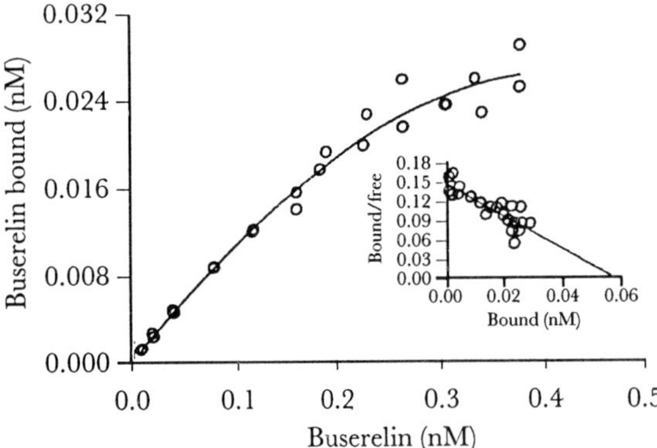

Figure 4 Saturation plot and Scatchard plot (inset) for binding of radio-iodinated GnRH agonist buserelin to GGH$_3$1' cells. The Scatchard plot indicated a specific affinity (K$_d$=4.1 ± 1 × 10^{-8} M) of buserelin for the GnRH receptor expressed in GGH$_3$1' cells. The affinity is similar to that observed in binding studies of gonadotrope cells. From Kuphal, D. A., Janovick, J. A., Jennes, L. *et al.* (1994). Stable transfection of GH$_3$ cells with rat GnRH receptor which is coupled to cyclic AMP-dependent prolactin release via G-protein. *Endocrinology*, **135**, 315–20[6]. Reproduced with permission of the Endocrine Soceity

Although the GnRH receptor does not have a long carboxyl terminal tail in any species sequenced to date[14], the receptor can be down-regulated by GnRH in GGH$_3$ cells. The ability of agonist-stimulated GGH$_3$ cells to down-regulate the GnRH receptor shows that receptor down-regulation does not require a long carboxyl terminus.

GGH$_3$ CELLS CAN BECOME REFRACTORY TO GnRH STIMULATION

After 24 hours exposure to buserelin (0.01 µg/ml), GGH$_3$6' cells return to a basal rate of prolactin release, reflecting refractoriness to agonist induced hormone release (Figure 2, panel C)[7]. In contrast, neither GGH$_3$1', GGH$_3$2' nor GGH$_3$12' cells show any such desensitization, even at the longest time examined (96 hours)[7]. Desensitization in GGH$_3$6' cells does not appear to be due to receptor down-regulation, because the receptors recover from down-regulation within 2 hours. Thus, the ability

of GGH$_3$6' cells to undergo agonist-induced desensitization (apart from receptor down-regulation) demonstrates that the GnRH receptor as cloned (a GPCR lacking the long intracellular tail) does not require a long intracellular tail for such a function.

An unexplored mechanism of desensitization may involve a decreased ability of the GnRH receptor to couple G-proteins. In β$_2$/β$_3$ adrenergic receptors as well as other G-protein-coupled receptors, phosphorylation leads to decreased coupling to G-proteins and subsequent desensitization[13]. Since the GnRH receptor couples to multiple G-proteins, the desensitization which develops upon prolonged GnRH stimulation in one GGH$_3$ cell line may occur through a similar mechanism. For this aspect of receptor–effector coupling, GGH$_3$ cells can serve as useful models for exploring GnRH receptor coupling to G-proteins.

GnRH-STIMULATED SIGNALING MECHANISMS ARE DISTINCT IN GGH$_3$ AND IN GONADOTROPE CELLS

Preincubation of GGH$_3$1' cells with cholera toxin, which activates α-subunit of G-protein leading to increased production of cyclic adenosine-3',5'-monophosphate (cAMP), potentiates GnRH-stimulated prolactin release. Also, GnRH directly stimulates increased release of cAMP from GGH$_3$1' cells in a dose-dependent manner. These observations suggest that the α$_s$-type G-protein subunit as well as its effector, adenylyl cyclase, are involved in GnRH-stimulated prolactin release from GGH$_3$ cells. Furthermore, two inhibitors of phosphodiesterases, methylisobutyl-xanthine and theophylline, promote prolactin release from GGH$_3$ cells in response to low concentrations of GnRH (10^{-12} M to 10^{-9} M), but are non-additive at higher concentrations of GnRH (10^{-8} M to 10^{-6} M). This suggests that both phosphodiesterase inhibitors increase prolactin release by enhancing the accumulation of cAMP. Treatment of GGH$_3$1' cells with active analogs of cAMP, 5 mM dibutyryl cAMP or 5 mM 8-bromo-cAMP, effectively stimulates prolactin release above basal levels. Therefore, it appears that one role of cAMP in GGH$_3$ cells is that of a second messenger which couples ligand binding to release of prolactin.

As mentioned earlier, events other than hormone release, such as desensitization of GGH$_3$6' cells, are also stimulated by treatment with GnRH agonists, and cAMP is probably not the only regulatory second messenger in GGH$_3$ cells. It is not clear whether desensitization in GGH$_3$6' cells is regulated through a cAMP pathway. Increasing cAMP levels alone with cholera toxin (CTX) treatment or the addition of cAMP analogs is coincident with a decrease in prolactin synthesis in all GGH$_3$ cell lines (unpublished). It seems possible that cAMP could, therefore, be involved in regulating desensitization. However, GGH$_3$6' cells do not produce cAMP per cell at a greater rate than any other GGH$_3$ cell line (unpublished data), yet GGH$_3$6' cells solely demonstrate desensitization to GnRH agonists[7].

Inositol phosphate (IP) production is the earliest measurable response of GGH$_3$ cells to a GnRH agonist, although this event does not appear coupled to buserelin-stimulated prolactin release. Production of IPs in GGH$_3$ cells is measurable at 15 to 30 min and maximal at 60 min after treatment with buserelin. In contrast, prolactin release, which is dependent upon protein synthesis, is not measurable until 3 to 6 hours and total cAMP production is not measurable until about 24 hours[7]. Measurable expression of the prolactin gene also requires a minimum of 24 hours[4]. All four GGH$_3$ cell lines produce IPs robustly after treatment with buserelin, although TRH-induced IP production is minimal in all lines, being the best in the GGH$_3$2' cell line. Pretreatment of cells with CTX or pertussis toxin (PTX) attenuates TRH-induced IP production in GGH$_3$1', GGH$_3$2', and GGH$_3$12' cells. Neither CTX nor PTX have a measurable effect on GGH$_3$6' cells in terms of TRH-stimulated IP production. In contrast, both toxins augment buserelin-stimulated IP production in GGH$_3$1' and GGH$_3$6' cells but have no action in either GGH$_3$2' or GGH$_3$12' cells. These studies suggest that buserelin and TRH regulate IP production by different mechanisms.

It appears that Ca^{2+} plays a role as a second messenger in GGH$_3$ cells, as it does in the gonadotrope. Three major classes of Ca^{2+} channel antagonists, methoxyverapamil (D600), nifedipine and diltiazem, blocked buserelin-stimulated prolactin release from GGH$_3$ cells. However, LH release from pituitary cells in response to either GnRH, veratridine or maitotoxin is only blocked by D600[15]. In primary lactotropes and clonal GH$_3$ cell lines, Ca^{2+} plays an important role in the biphasic release of prolactin[16]. In these cells both internal (for the transient peak) and external (for the plateau phase in a time course for prolactin release) Ca^{2+} are used in regulating the release of prolactin, and Ca^{2+} channel blockers can inhibit the plateau phase of prolactin release[17].

THE GnRH RECEPTOR EXPRESSED BY GGH₃ CELLS COUPLES TO MULTIPLE G-PROTEINS AND EFFECTORS

As mentioned earlier, GnRH-stimulated prolactin release and cAMP production in GGH$_3$1' cells is a CTX-sensitive event, supporting the view that GnRH action in GGH$_3$ cells involves a G-protein (Gα_s) coupled to adenylyl cyclase. The mechanism observed here is different fundamentally from that by which GnRH regulates gonadotropin release from primary cultures[17], although other observations[18–20] indicate that the GnRH receptor and other receptors[21] can be coupled to multiple G-proteins. This 'promiscuous' coupling presents the possibility that ultimate expression of receptor function may reflect the availability and accessibility of G-proteins within a particular cell. The role of Gα_s and cAMP in the lactotrope and lactotrope-derived tumor cells can vary widely and has been reviewed[16]. Recent studies in cell lines[22,23] have shown that both the TRH receptor and the GnRH receptor couple to the PTX-insensitive G-proteins, G$_q$/G$_{11}$.

It is well known that ligand binding to G-protein-coupled receptors results in the dissociation of the heterotrimeric G-protein into α and β/γ moieties. These two distinct moieties enable the regulation of two potential signaling pathways via a single extracellular signal. The binary complex of β/γ-subunits are tightly coupled and were believed initially to play only a minor role in signal transduction by regulating the amount of available activated α-subunits. Recent findings suggest that the β/γ-subunits alone regulate effector molecules which include certain types of adenylyl cyclase and phospholipase C (PLC), cardiac muscarinic K[+] channels and phospholipase A2[24–29].

The ability of a β-adrenergic receptor kinase peptide to bind and inhibit β/γ-subunits was exploited to determine whether β/γ-subunits played an important role in the molecular mechanism of GnRH. The β-adrenergic receptor kinase 1 (βARK1) is one member of the recently described G-protein-coupled receptor kinases[30] that are responsible for phosphorylation of activated receptors and attenuating receptor responsiveness to further stimulation. The membrane anchored β/γ complex specifically mediates the translocation of cytosolic βARK1 to the plasma membrane by directly binding the C-terminal pleckstrin homology domain of βARK1. βARK1 binding to β/γ complexes inhibits signal transduction via these moieties[25]. The co-expression of a peptide representing the βARK1 C-terminus (amino acids 495–689) with the GnRH receptor in GGH₃ cells was used as an approach to distinguish between α- and β/γ-mediated signal transduction pathways via the GnRH receptor.

Transient expression of βARK1 C-terminus inhibits prolactin and cAMP release as well as IP production in GGH₃1' cells[10]. Among various isoforms of adenylyl cyclase, type II and IV (which are widely distributed in various tissues) are reported to be activated by β/γ in the presence of G_s α-subunit, although type I cyclase can be inhibited by β/γ[31,32]. There is no evidence to show which isoform of adenylyl cyclase is involved in the GnRH-stimulated cAMP production in GGH₃ cells, but these studies suggest that β/γ-dependent adenylyl cyclase isoforms play an important role in the regulation of cAMP release in GnRH action.

There are three major families of PLC comprised of β-, γ- and δ-isoforms, of which β-isoforms are responsible for the IP production regulated by G-proteins G_q/G_{11}[33]. It is known that receptors activate PLC via two signaling pathways which include PTX-sensitive and PTX-insensitive G-proteins[22,23,27,34]. The α-subunit of the G_q family is presumed to mediate the toxin-insensitive pathway; PTX-sensitive activation of PLC is mediated by β/γ-subunits of G-proteins. Previous studies in the pituitary gonadotropes and GGH₃1' cells indicate that GnRH-stimulated IP production is also sensitive to pretreatment with PTX. This supports the view that the β/γ moiety of G-proteins plays an important part in this process[8,20]. These data indicate that β/γ-subunits participate in the regulation of PLC-β in GnRH-stimulated IP production with G_q/G_{11} family G-proteins.

SUMMARY

Four GGH₃ clonal cell lines were prepared by stably transfecting a lactotrope derived GH₃ cell line with the rat sequence GnRH receptor cDNA. These cells, when stimulated with GnRH, can regulate GnRH receptor number and, on recovery of receptor numbers, homologous desensitization occurs in one GGH₃ cell line. In response to GnRH, GGH₃ cells produce prolactin in a protein synthesis-dependent manner. GnRH also stimulates time- and dose-dependent production of inositol phosphate and cAMP in GGH₃ cells. The β/γ-subunit of the trimeric G-protein also plays a role in the GnRH receptor-coupled signal transduction cascade. Multiple G-protein-coupled pathways are activated by GnRH agonist binding to its receptor. The activation of G-proteins can lead to a multitude of intracellular events, making GnRH mechanism of action a complex process.

In GGH₃ cells, signal transduction mechanisms necessary for release of an authentic hormone are present and activated by GnRH agonist binding to its receptor. With these features, GGH₃ cells are notably operative in screening potential GnRH analogs. In addition to providing valuable information about the regulated pathway of secretory protein release, GGH₃ cells are useful in the study of the mechanisms of GnRH receptor-effector coupling and homologous desensitization.

ACKNOWLEDGEMENTS

The authors thank Jody Janovick, Vivek Arora and Chuan-hai Guo for commenting on the manuscript. They are also grateful to Linda Wolf for her help in preparing the manuscript.

References

1. Braden, T. and Conn, P. M. (1992). Gonadotropin releasing hormone and its actions. In Crowley, W. F. Jr and Conn, P. M. (eds.) *Modes of Action of GnRH and GnRH Analogs,* pp. 26–54. (New York: Springer-Verlag)

2. Conn, P. M. and Crowley, W. F. Jr (1994). Gonadotropin-releasing hormone and its analogs. *Annu. Rev. Med.,* **45**, 391–405

3. Windle, J. J., Weiner, R. I. and Mellon, P. L. (1990). Cell lines of the pituitary gonadotrope lineage derived by targeted oncogenesis in transgenic mice. *Mol. Endocrinol.,* **4**, 597-603

4. Kaiser, U. B., Katzenellenbogen, R., Conn, P. M. and Chin, W. W. (1994). Evidence that signalling pathways by which thyrotropin-releasing hormone and gonadotropin-releasing hormone act are both common and distinct. *Mol. Endocrinol.,* **8**, 1038–48

5. Anderson, L., Milligan, G. and Eidne, K. A. (1993). Characterization of the gonadotropin-releasing hormone receptor in αT3-1 pituitary gonadotroph cells. *J. Endocrinol.,* **136**, 51–8

6. Kuphal, D. A., Janovick, J. A., Kaiser, U. B., Chin, W. W. and Conn, P. M. (1994). Stable transfection of GH$_3$ cells with rat GnRH receptor which is coupled to cyclic AMP-dependent prolactin release via G-protein. *Endocrinology,* **135**, 315–20

7. Stanislaus, D., Janovick, J. A., Jennes, L., Kaiser, U. B., Chin, W. W. and Conn, P. M. (1994). Functional and morphological characterization of four cell lines derived from GH$_3$ cells stably transfected with GnRH receptor cDNA. *Endocrinology,* **135**, 2220–7

8. Janovick, J. A. and Conn, P. M. (1994). GnRH receptor coupling to inositol phosphate and prolactin production in GH$_3$ cells stably transfected with rat GnRH receptor cDNA. *Endocrinology,* **135**, 2214–19

9. Janovick, J. A., Jennes, L. and Conn, P. M. (1995). GH$_3$ cells transfected with gonadotropin-releasing hormone (GnRH) receptor complementary deoxyribonucleic acid release secretogranin-II through a constitutive pathway after GnRH analog-regulated synthesis: evidence that secretory proteins do not contain a sequence that obligates processing through a secretory granule or by regulated secretion. *Endocrinology,* **136**, 202–8

10. Guo, C.-H., Janovick, J. A., Kuphal, D. and Conn, P. M. (1995). Transient transfection of GGH$_3$1' cells (GH$_3$ cells stably transfected with the GnRH receptor cDNA) with the carboxyl terminal of β-adrenergic receptor kinase 1 blocks PRL release: evidence for a role of the G-protein $\beta\gamma$ subunit complex in GnRH signal transduction. *Endocrinology,* **136**, 3031–6

11. Conn, P. M., Janovick, J. A., Braden, T. D., Maurer, R. A. and Jennes, L. (1992). SIIp: a unique secretogranin/chromogranin of the pituitary released in response to GnRH. *Endocrinology,* **130**, 3033–40

12. Conn, P. M., Rogers, D. C. and Seay, S. (1984). Biphasic regulation of the gonadotropin-releasing hormone receptor by the receptor micro-aggregation and intracellular Ca^{2+} levels. *Mol. Pharmacol.,* **25**, 51–5

13. Liggett, S. B., Freedman, N. J., Schwinn, D. A. and Lefkowitz, R. J. (1993). Structural basis for receptor sub-type-specific regulation revealed by a chimeric β_2/β_3-adrenergic receptor. *Proc. Natl. Acad. Sci. USA,* **90**, 3665–9

14. Davidson, J. S., Flanagan, C. A., Becker, I. I., Illing, N., Sealfon, S. C. and Millar, R. P. (1994). Molecular function of the gonadotropin-releasing hormone receptor: insights from site-directed mutagenesis. *Mol. Cell. Endocrinol.,* **100**, 9–14

15. Conn, P. M., Staley, D. D., Yasumoto, T., Huckle, W. and Janovick, J. (1987). Homologous desensitization with gonadotropin-releasing hormone (GnRH) also diminishes gonadotrope responsiveness to maitotoxin: a role for the GnRH receptor-regulated calcium ion channel in mediation of cellular desensitization. *Mol. Endocrinol.,* **1**, 154–9

16. Lamberts, S. W. J. and Macleod, R. M. (1990). Regulation of prolactin secretion at the level of the lactotroph. *Physiol. Rev.,* **70**, 279–318

17. Conn, P. M., Morrell, D. V., Dufau, M. L. and

Catt, K. J. (1979). Gonadotropin-releasing hormone action in cultured pituicytes: independence of luteinizing hormone release and adenosine 3',5'-monophosphate production. *Endocrinology*, **104**, 448–53

18. Barnes, S. J. and Conn, P. M. (1993). Cholera toxin and dibutyryl cyclic AMP sensitize GnRH-stimulated inositol phosphate production to inhibition in PKC depleted cells: evidence for cross talk between a cholera toxin sensitive G-protein and PKC. *Endocrinology*, **133**, 2756–60

19. Hawes, B. E. and Conn, P. M. (1992). Sodium fluoride provokes gonadotrope desensitization to GnRH and gonadotrope sensitization to A23187: evidence for multiple G-proteins in GnRH action. *Endocrinology*, **130**, 2465–75

20. Hawes, B. E., Barnes, S. and Conn, P. M. (1993). Cholera toxin and pertussis toxin provoke differential effects on luteinizing hormone release, inositol phosphate production, and gonadotropin-releasing hormone (GnRH) receptor binding in the gonadotrope: evidence for multiple guanyl nucleotide binding proteins in GnRH action. *Endocrinology*, **132**, 2124–30

21. Milligan, G. (1993). Mechanisms of multifunctional signalling by G-protein-linked receptors. *Trend. Pharmacol. Sci.*, **14**, 239–44

22. Hsieh, K.-P. and Martin, T. F. J. (1992). Thyrotropin-releasing hormone and gonadotropin-releasing hormone receptors activate phospholipase C by coupling to the guanosine triphosphate-binding proteins G_q and G_{11}. *Mol. Endocrinol.*, **6**, 1673–81

23. Aragay, A. M., Katz, A. and Simon, M. I. (1992). The $G\alpha_q$ and $G\alpha_{11}$ proteins couple the thyrotropin-releasing hormone receptor to phospholipase C in GH_3 rat pituitary cells. *J. Biol. Chem.*, **267**, 24983–8

24. Taussig, R., Quarmby, L. M. and Gilman, A. G. (1993). Regulation of purified type I and type II adenylyl cyclases by G-protein βγ subunits. *J. Biol. Chem.*, **268**, 9–12

25. Koch, W. J., Hawes, B. E., Inglese, J., Luttrell, L. M. and Lefkowitz, R. J. (1994). Cellular expression of the carboxyl terminus of a G-protein-coupled receptor kinase attenuates Gβγ-mediated signaling. *J. Biol. Chem.*, **269**, 6193–7

26. Pitcher, J. A., Inglese, J., Higgins, J. B., Arriza, J. L., Casey, P. J., Kim, C., Benovic, J. L., Kwatra, M. W., Caron, M. G. and Lefkowitz, R. J. (1992). Role of βγ subunits of G-proteins in targeting the β-adrenergic receptor kinase to membrane-bound receptors. *Science*, **257**, 1264–7

27. Boyer, J. L., Graber, S. G., Waldo, G. L., Harden, T. K. and Garrison, J. C. (1994). Selective activation of phospholipase C by recombinant G-protein α- and βγ- subunits. *J. Biol. Chem.*, **269**, 2814–9

28. Reuveny, E., Slesinger, P. A., Inglese, J., Morales, J. M., Inlguez-Lluhi, J. A., Lefkowitz, R. J., Bourne, H. R., Jan, Y. N. and Jan, L. Y. (1994). Activation of the cloned muscarinic potassium channel by G-protein βγ subunits. *Nature*, **370**, 143–6

29. Jelsema, C. L. and Axelrod, J. (1987). Stimulation of phospholipase A2 activity in bovine rod outer segments by the βγ subunits of tranducin and its inhibition by the α subunit. *Proc. Natl. Acad. Sci. USA*, **84**, 3623–7

30. Inglese, J., Freedman, N. J., Koch, W. J. and Lefkowitz, R. J. (1993). Structure and mechanism of the G-protein-coupled receptor kinase. *J. Biol. Chem.*, **268**, 23735–8

31. Spiegel, A. M., Backlund, P. S. Jr., Butrynski, J. E., Jones, T. L. Z. and Simonds, W. F. (1991). The G-protein connection: molecular basis of membrane association. *Trends Biochem. Sci.*, **16**, 338–41

32. Tang, W. J. and Gilman, A. G. (1992). Adenylyl cyclase. *Cell*, **70**, 869–72

33. Rhee, S. G. and Choi, K. D. (1992). Regulation of inositol phospholipid-specific phospholipase C isozymes. *J. Biol Chem.*, **267**, 12393–6

34. Wu, D., Lee, C. H., Rhee, S. G. and Simon, M. I. (1992). Activation of phospholipase C by the α subunits of the G_q and G_{11} proteins in transfected cos-7 cells. *J. Biol. Chem.*, **267**, 1811–7

35. Ben-Menahem, D., Shraga, Z., Lewy, H., Limor, R., Hammel, I., Stein, R., and Naor, Z. (1992). Dissociation between release and gene expression of gonadotropin α-subunit in gonadotropin-releasing hormone-stimulated αT3-1 cell line. *Biochemistry*, **31**, 12893–8

GnRH antagonists: design, synthesis and side effects   2

*J. E. Rivier, G.-C. Jiang, S. C. Koerber, S. L. Lahrichi, J. Porter, J. Rizo, L. Gierasch,
A. Hagler, W. Vale, M. Karten and C. L. Rivier*

INTRODUCTION

One of the main interests in the authors[1] laboratories over the past 20 years has been to understand the mechanisms by which gonadotropin releasing hormone (GnRH) modulates the hypothalamic–pituitary–gonadal axis. These mechanisms were investigated with agonists: analogs that, with time, desensitize the pituitary, and with antagonists that compete for pituitary receptor occupancy and, as such, have an immediate action that lasts as long as they are present in sufficient concentration. Until recently, most studies carried out with antagonists used Nal-Glu $\{[Ac\text{-}DNal^1, DCpa^2, DPal^3, Arg^5, 4\text{-}(p\text{-methoxybenzoyl})\text{-}D\text{-}2\text{-}Abu^6, DAla^{10}]\text{-}GnRH\}$ which, although very potent in inhibiting gonadotropin secretion, also stimulates the release of histamine and is relatively short-acting[1]. These preliminary studies, however, suggested that a GnRH antagonist may ultimately be used for male contraception, the management or treatment of endometriosis, infertility, ovulation induction in women with chronic anovulation (i.e. polycystic ovarian syndrome), precocious puberty, uterine myoma, ovarian hyperandrogenism and hirsutism, premenstrual syndrome (PMS), controlled induction of ovulation in *in vitro* fertilization programs, and may also be a promising lead in the treatment of breast and gynecological cancers[2–15]. Most of these disorders were found originally to respond to long-acting preparations of the superagonists which desensitize the gonadotropes after approximately 2 weeks of treatment[16]. An antagonist will probably displace the agonists in the clinic because it avoids the initial up-regulation of the gonadotropin–gonadal axis, leads to rapid and predictable recovery, permits flexibility in the degree of gonadal suppression, and can be used as a diagnostic test of gonadotropin-dependent gonadal dysfunction. However, if preparations of GnRH antagonists are to be used successfully in humans, they need to be long-acting to avoid daily administration and exhibit negligible side effects such as stimulating histamine release. Indeed, when compared to the superagonist, GnRH antagonists suffer from the fact that they need to be present in the bloodstream at all times to effectively prevent the action of endogenous GnRH.

In the last several years, the authors and others have developed antagonists with reduced histamine releasing activity (antide[17] and azaline B[18]) while a number of other analogs (RS-26306, Org 30850, SB-75, Ganirelix, A-75998 and Antarelix) may be somewhat less selective[18]. Because potent antagonists with essentially no histamine releasing activity are available and because they may have to be administered at greater doses than the superagonists, it would appear reasonable to consider only the most innocuous for extended clinical investigations or prolonged therapeutic use. A recent report comparing the anaphylactoid activities of antide and azaline B suggests that of the two, azaline B has the least, if any, anaphylactoid activity in animal models[19]. One possible limitation of azaline B resides in its propensity to form gels in aqueous media at concentrations above 3 mg/ml. This is a general property of most GnRH antagonists, and significant efforts have been expanded in trying to find analogs with increased solubility. Such systematic study is illustrated in Table 1, where the biological properties of a series of azalines are described. Azaline $\{[Ac\text{-}DNal^1, DCpa^2, DPal^3, Lys^5(atz),$

DLys[6](atz),ILys[8],DAla[10]] GnRH}, (number 1 in Table 1) and azaline B {[Ac-DNal[1],DCpa[2], DPal[3],Aph[5](atz),DAph[6](atz),ILys[8],DAla[10]]-GnRH}, (number 3 in Table 1) are two closely related antagonists of GnRH with high potency in an anti-ovulatory assay, in an *in vitro* pituitary cell culture assay (not shown) and in the castrated male rat assay[18]. Both analogs have low histamine releasing activities, thus making members of this family particularly attractive for clinical investigation. For poorly understood reasons which may derive from the introduction of an aromatic side chain at positions 5 and 6 (compared to the aliphatic side chain of the two lysine residues at positions 5 and 6 in azaline). Azaline B is considerably longer-acting than azaline, especially after intravenous administration[18]. Although azaline B is among the most potent GnRH antagonists, there is still a need for a more potent analog which would meet rigorous criteria such as ease of formulation for acute or slow release and economical synthesis; two properties that may be best fulfilled by closely related analogs.

This chapter describes two independent approaches to understanding the structural basis for biological action of GnRH analogs. In the first approach, two series of azaline B precursor derivatives {Ac-DNal-DCpa-DPal-Ser-Aph(X)-DAph(Y)-Leu-ILys-Pro-DAla-NH$_2$} had the ω-amino functions of the 4-aminophenylalanine at positions 5 and 6 (X, Y) acylated with different carboxylic acids and amino acids, and N-methylation of residue 5 were used to reduce propensity of the analog to form β-sheets (Table 1). In the second approach, two means of constraining conformation were investigated which involved: (1) introducing side chain-to-side chain constraints to limit the number of backbone conformations; and (2) using betidamino acids to investigate the topography of the side chains of acyline in its bioactive conformation.

THE AZALINE B SUB-FAMILY

A series of antagonists of GnRH homologous to azaline B were synthesized, characterized and tested in a rat anti-ovulatory assay (AOA). Selected analogs were also tested in an *in vitro* histamine-release assay[20]. The duration of action of some of the most potent and safest analogs in those assays was also determined in the castrated male rat in order to measure the extent (efficacy and duration of action) of inhibition of luteinizing hormone (LH) release[21]. The authors will now summarize the salient results from that study. Structurally, this series of analogs (Table 1) has novel substitutions (X and Y) in the structure of the azaline B precursor: [Ac-DNal[1],DCpa[2],DPal[3], Aph[5](X),DAph[6](Y),ILys[8],DAla[10]]-GnRH. These substitutions were designed to confer increased hydrophilicity as compared to that of Azaline B or to make them more easily accessible synthetically.

Of all the analogs reported here, number 2 in Table 2 is the simplest (i.e. the most readily accessible because all starting materials are commercially available) and was made for comparison studies. The fact that it is only one-half to one-third as potent as number 1 in Table 1 in the AOA is particularly telling and suggested to us that the Atz (5'-3'-amino-1*H*-1',2',4'-triazolyl) function, although conferring unique properties to this family of analogs, was not necessarily unique as demonstrated later in the Aph (4-amino-phenylalanine) – containing series (see analogs number 3 and 6 in Table 1). Also unexpected was the observation that unsubstituted Aph, as in analog number 4 in Table 1, resulted in a peptide that was both potent and long-acting, although not quite to the extent of azaline B or acyline despite a positive charge at positions 5, 6 and 8. Although this analog was not tested for histamine-releasing activity, it is believed from past examples that the presence of two charges at positions 5 and 6, in addition to that at position 8, would result in a significant increase in histamine-releasing activity as seen for peptides such as Nal-Glu and Nal-Arg[28]. Because of the high potency of numbers 3 and 4 in Table 1, it was suspected that any small acylating agent would not dramatically influence the potency of the analogs; this was confirmed with the results obtained from formylation (number 5 in Table 1), and acetylation (number 6 and 7 in Table 1) of the 4-amino function of phenylalanine at positions 5 and 6. Less predictable was the observation that acylation with Ac-Gly (number 8 in Table 1) or Atz-Gly (number 9 in Table 1) would result in dramatic shortening of the duration of action which was restored upon lengthening of

Table 1 Anti-ovulatory activity of selected GnRH analogs with R = Ac-DNal[1]-DCpa[2]-DPal[3]-

| | | AOA* | | |
| | | Dosage (μg/rat) | Rats ovulating/ total no. of rats | Duration of action[†] |
ID no.	Compounds			
1	[R,Lys[5](Atz),DLys[6](Atz),ILys[8],DAla[10]]-GnRH (**Azaline**)	2.0	1/10	short acting
2	[R,Lys[5](Ac),DLys[6](Ac),ILys[8],DAla[10]]-GnRH	2.5	3/3	v. short acting
		5.0	2/7	
3	[R,Aph[5](Atz),DAph[6](Atz),ILys[8],DAla[10]]-GnRH (**Azaline B**)	1.0	0/7	long acting
4	[R,Aph[5],DAph[6],ILys[8],DAla[10]]-GnRH	1.0	7/8	long acting
		2.0	0/7	
5	[R,Aph[5](For),DAph[6](For),ILys[8],DAla[10]]-GnRH	1.0	3/9	long acting
		2.5	0/8	
6	[R,Aph[5](Ac),DAph[6](Ac),ILys[8],DAla[10]]-GnRH (**Acyline**)	1.0	5/13	long acting
		2.5	0/7	
7	[R,Aph[5](Atz),DAph[6](Ac),ILys[8],DAla[10]]-GnRH	1.0	7/14	long acting
		2.5	0/8	
8	[R,Aph[5](Ac-Gly),DAph[6](Ac-Gly),ILys[8],DAla[10]]-GnRH	0.5	3/4	short acting
		1.0	5/8	
9	[R,Aph[5](Atz-Gly),DAph[6](Atz-Gly),ILys[8],DAla[10]]-GnRH	0.5	3/4	intermediate
		1.0	5/8	
10	[R,Aph[5](Atz-βAla),DAph[6](Atz-βAla),ILys[8],DAla[10]]-GnRH	1.0	9/18	long acting
		2.5	0/6	
11	[R,Aph[5](Atz-Gab),DAph[6](Atz-Gab),ILys[8],DAla[10]]-GnRH	0.5	10/14	long acting
		1.0	1/8	
12	[R,Aph[5](Atz-Ahx),DAph[6](Atz-Ahx),ILys[8],DAla[10]]-GnRH	0.5	6/6	intermediate
		1.0	2/10	
13	[R,Aph[5](Atz-DAla),DAph[6](Atz-DAla),ILys[8],DAla[10]]-GnRH	1.0	2/8	short acting
14	[R,Aph[5](Ac-DSer),DAph[6](Ac-DSer),ILys[8],DAla[10]]-GnRH	1.0	2/7	short acting
15	[R,Aph[5](Atz-Ser),DAph[6](Atz-Ser),ILys[8],DAla[10]]-GnRH	1.0	8/12	short acting
16	[R,N$^{\alpha}$MeAph[5](Atz),DAph[6](Atz),ILys[8],DAla[10]]-GnRH (**Azaline C**)	1.0	2/9	short acting
		2.5	0/8	

*The anti-ovulatory assay (AOA) was carried out as described by Corbin and Beattie[22] using an aqueous (1–2% dimethyl sulfoxide [DMSO]) vehicle: dosage in μg (rats ovulating/total). Results are expressed in terms of the dosage in μg/rat (rats ovulating/total number of treated rats). [†]Castrated male rat assay measurement of circulating luteinizing hormone (LH) levels in castrated rats treated subcutaneously with the peptides was carried out over a period extending up to 120 hours as reported earlier[18,23–25]. Long duration of action, fully active after 72 hours; intermediate, fully active at 48 hours but not at 72 hours; short acting, fully active at 24 hours but not at 48 hours; very short acting, inactive at 24 hours. *In vitro*, the peptides were tested for their ability to release histamine by rat mast cells (see data in text)[26,27]

Table 2 Potent and constrained GnRH antagonists

| | | AOA* | |
| | | Dosage (μg/rat) | Rats ovulating/ total no. of rats |
ID no.	Compounds		
17	Cyclo(1-10)-[Δ^3-Pro^1,DCpa^2,DTrp^3,DTrp^6,N$_{Me}$Leu^7, βAla^{10}]-GnRH	1500	9/10
18	Cyclo(4-10)-[Ac-Δ^3-Pro^1,DFpa^2-,Trp^3,Asp^4,DNal^6,Dpr^{10}]-GnRH	10	2/10
19	Bicyclo(4-10,5-8)-[Ac-DNal^1,DCpa^2,DTrp^3,Asp^4,Glu^5,DArg^6, Dpr^{10}]-GnRH	5	2/10
20	Bicyclo(4-10/5,5'-8)[Ac-DNal^1,DCpa^2,DPal^3,Asp^4,Glu^5(Gly), DArg^6,Dbu^8,DDpr^{10}]-GnRH	10 25	4/6 0/5
21	Bicyclo(1,1'-5/4-10)[Ac-Glu^1(Gly),DCpa^2,DTrp^3,Asp^4,Dbu^5, DNal^6,Dpr^{10}]-GnRH	2.5 5.0	2/8 1/7

*Anti-ovulatory assay (AOA) in *circa* 1% DMSO

the side chain [At-βAla (number 10 in Table 1) and Atz-Gaba (number 11 in Table 1)] and lost again with the substitution by Atz-Ahx (number 12 in Table 1).

Similarly, acylation by Atz-DAla (number 13), Ac-DSer (number 14) and Atz-Ser (number 15 in Table 1) led to shortened duration of action. These examples and others suggest that minor modifications of structure yield dramatic changes in biological efficacy; the possible result of subtle differences in bioavailability and affinity for both the receptor and other yet to be defined sites, including blood proteins.

The results obtained for histamine release, were more predictable and show the following order: concentration of peptide which triggers half maximal response (EC$_{50}$): 3 = 6 = 10 > GnRH = 1 > 2 = 16 > 5. Based on the limited number of compounds tested, the authors can suggest that most members of the azaline and azaline B family, but not of the azaline C family (characterized by an NαMe substitution at position 5) will have EC$_{50}$ equal to or greater than that of GnRH, and that the introduction of a polar side chain such as formyl (compound number 5 in Table 1) but not 4-(N-5'-(3'-amino-1H-1',2',4'-triazolyl) (number 3) or acetyl (number 6 in Table 1) may be somewhat deleterious.

In order to refine our understanding of the role of the aminotriazolyl moiety at positions 5 and 6 of azaline B, the authors synthesized number 7 in Table 1 (which is as efficacious as azaline B in the castrated male rat assay) with Aph(Atz) (i.e. 4-(N-5'-3'-amino-1H-1',2',4'-triazolyl)phenylalanine in position 5 and DAph(Ac) (i.e. acetyl-4-amino-D-phenylalanine) in position 6. Although this observation helped them to further define the structural requirements for long duration of action, it is not clear whether substitutions at the 5 position of the kind shown here [Aph(Atz), Aph(Ac), Aph(Atz-βAla)] are indeed solely responsible for such property.

THE AZALINE C FAMILY

Less desirable were analogs belonging to the series where we introduced α-methyl substitutions at position 5. The introduction of this substitution was prompted by the observation[29] that the introduction of a methyl group on the backbone nitrogen of residue 5 resulted in an analog that is significantly more soluble in aqueous buffers. We confirmed this observation[30] by introducing that modification in compound number 16 (azaline C) in Table 1. It is generally accepted that the solubility of a compound in a particular solvent (g/l) is a constant. In the case of peptides, this notion can be challenged. Indeed, a peptide may be very easily soluble in an aqueous buffer and may remain in solution for an indefinite period of time. However, it is not unusual (as is the case for many of the GnRH antagonists developed so far) that, with time, the peptide, which first assumed a random conformation in solution, slowly rearranges itself to yield a significant and critical concentration of an ordered and less soluble conformer which then gels. In the case of GnRH, it was suggested that the stabilized form consisted of beta sheets which aggregate and are less soluble[29]. The introduction of a backbone methyl group at position 5 would prevent formation of such beta sheets. Because of the presence of acetonitrile in our high performance liquid chromotography (HPLC) systems (a denaturing solvent) it is not surprising that this increased solubility in aqueous media is not reflected by a shortening in retention times in the HPLC system. It is unfortunate that this favorable modification, which increases solubility, also results in the loss of some potency in the AOA, in the loss of long duration of action and in significantly greater histamine releasing property[21].

CYCLIC GnRH ANALOGS

The fact that neither agonists nor antagonists of GnRH are orally active is a disadvantage. The authors and others have hypothesized that the bioactive conformation of GnRH or of one of its analogs could help in the design of a non-peptide mimetic that would be orally active. While there are reports that non-peptide antagonists of some peptide hormones have been developed that are orally active, evidence exists that these peptidomimetics do not interact with their respective receptors at loci identical to that at which peptide antagonists act (substance P is a good example[31]). This suggests that these antagonists will not necessarily have the 'identical and only' and (as in the case of GnRH) desired pharmacological properties of their peptidic counterparts.

Like many peptide hormones, GnRH is a highly flexible molecule that exists in solution as an equilibrium mixture of multiple conformers[32-34]. Nonetheless, working models of its preferred conformation that may coincide with its receptor-

bound conformation have been proposed. For example, a feature common to many models is a β-turn at Gly[6]-Leu[7] originally suggested by empirical conformational energy calculations[35,36]. Support for the presence of this turn has been provided by D-amino acid substitution studies[37, 38], an analog incorporating N-methyl Leu[7, 38, 39] and a lactam bridged analog that forced the ψ angle of Gly[6] and the ϕ angle of Leu[7] to values characteristic of a β-turn[38].

Chronologically, the development of potent cyclic GnRH antagonists and the study of their secondary structure is as follows: the most potent analog in the family representing head-to-tail cyclization, compound number 17 in Table 2, was found to exhibit a type II' β-turn involving residues 6–7 and a type II β-turn involving residues 1–2, connected by extended anti-parallel β-like strands[40-43]. Detailed theoretical and experimental analysis of the conformation of compound number 17 in Table 2 revealed a close proximity of residues 4–10 which served as a design lead for compound number 18 in Table 2.

Extensive nuclear magnetic resonance (NMR) and theoretical analysis of the conformation of compound number 18 in Table 2 revealed a type II' β-turn involving residues 6–7, a γ-turn at D-Trp[3], and a likely type II β-turn around residues 1–2[44-46]. In order to further constrain this lead compound and based upon available the structural activity relationship (SAR), a lactam bridge was incorporated between residues 5–8 to give the bicyclic compound number 19 in Table 2. The high resolution NMR and theoretical analysis of compound number 19 in Table 2 suggested a solution conformation very similar to that of compound number 18. SAR conducted on the family of bicyclic GnRH antagonists represented by 19 suggested that optimization of the 5–8 bridge could lead to more potent compounds. Thus compound number 20 in Table 2 was designed and synthesized to incorporate an intervening glycine in the Glu[5]-(Gly)-Dbu[8] bridge. To the authors' knowledge, the dicyclic compound number 20 is the first highly potent, constrained GnRH antagonist that has been observed to form a type I' β-turn, rather than a type II' β-turn, around residues 6–7. Although it could be that compound number 20 changes conformation upon binding to the GnRH receptor to form a type II' β-turn, it is also possible that the presence of a 6–7 turn, rather than the turn type, is important for biological activity. In fact, different types of turn may bring about two ends of a molecule in a similar fashion, so that analogous surfaces are offered for binding to the receptor. Yet another possibility is that the conformation observed for compound number 20 in Table 2 is biologically relevant and all other compounds that the authors have studied previously adopt such conformation upon receptor binding. From the point of view of the design of GnRH antagonists, more puzzling than the different type of turn around residues 6–7 is the radically different orientation of the tail formed by residue 1–3 with respect to the rest of the molecule observed in compounds number 19 and 20 in Table 2.

These results indicated that a type II' β-turn may not be required for GnRH antagonist activity and stressed the need to further constrain the N-terminal. This could be achieved with a Glu[1]-(Gly)-Dbu[5] cycle in addition to the optimized 4–10 cycle in compound number 21 in Table 2. The NMR and conformational analysis of this compound suggests a common conformation with that of compounds 18 and 19 which includes a type II' β-turn at residues 6–7 (Rizo *et al.*, in prep.).

Additionally, other investigators have developed computer approaches to determine the conformation of small bioactive peptides in general and GnRH in particular[47–49]. While the favored GnRH structure reported by Gupta *et al.*[47] appears to have little resemblance to any structure found by NMR[50–53] Nikiforovich's models[48,49] accommodate, at least in the case of a highly constrained (4–10/5–8) antagonist, those structural features determined from NMR studies[46].

BETIDES, AN APPROACH TO SIDE CHAIN CONSTRAINTS

The authors have approached the design of conformationally constrained bioactive peptides by investigating ways to constrain backbone (see above) as well as side chain conformations while maintaining high affinity for the receptors. This was achieved by us and others using methylation of the backbone. Further constraints, however,

can be achieved by methylation of the side chain at the β-position as shown by Kazmierski *et al.*[54] and us in the case of GnRH (Jiang *et al.*, in prep.). More recently, we described a novel approach to side chain stabilization using a new class of amino acids, the betidamino acids (betide is a contraction of '**bet**a' position and 'am**ide**'), which are N'-monoacylated aminoglycine (Agl) derivatives where each N'-acyl group may mimic amino acid side chains or introduce novel function.

With the report of the synthesis of racemic α-Fmoc, α'Boc-aminoglycine [Fmoc-Agl(Boc)] by Qasmi *et al.*[55] we recognized that the introduction of an acyl moiety resembling an amino acid side chain on one of the two amino functions would leave the other free to form the peptide backbone thus generating betidamino acids.

Betidamino acids offer several advantages over other amino acids in SAR studies.

(1) Side chain diversity in betidamino acids is virtually unlimited due to the availability of numerous acylating agents.

(2) The side chain nitrogen can be acylated as well as alkylated and acylated. The structural constraints introduced by the presence of a betidamino acid were of particular interest to the authors in the identification of bioactive conformations of peptide hormones and for the design of receptor selective analogs[56, 57].

(3) The authors have shown that betides are more hydrophilic than the corresponding peptides or β-methyl amino acid containing peptides; a property of particular appeal in the design of GnRH antagonists. Nevertheless, it is premature to conclude that such betidamino acid-containing analogs would be less prone to gelling.

To investigate biocompatibility of the betide scaffold, the authors prepared Agl(acyl)-substituted analogs of the GnRH antagonist acyline [Ac-D2Nal-D4Cpa-D3Pal-Ser-4Aph(Ac)-D4Aph(Ac)-Leu-ILys-Pro-DAla-NH$_2$] (compound number 6 in Table 3)[56,57]. Acyline is fully active in an anti-ovulatory assay at 2.5 μg/rat and is long acting; replacement of D-2Nal with L-2Nal (compound number 22 in Table 3) decreases the potency by a factor greater than 5 (full inhibition

Table 3 Betidamino acid-containing GnRH antagonists

		AOA*	
ID no.	Compounds	Dosage (μg/rat)	Rats ovulating/ total no. of rats
6	[Ac-DNal^1,DCpa^2,DPal^3,Aph^5(Ac),DAph^6(Ac),ILys^8, DAla^{10}]-GnRH (**Acyline**)	2.5 1.0	0/7 5/13
22	[Ac-L-Nal^1,DCpa^2,DPal^3,Aph(Ac)^5,DAph(Ac)^6,ILys^8,DAla^{10}]-GnRH	25 10	0/3 2/6
23	[Ac-L- or D-Agl(2-naphthoyl)^1,DCpa^2,DPal^3,Aph^5(Ac),DAph^6(Ac), ILys^8,DAla^{10}]-GnRH	2.5 1.0	0/8 2/4
24	[Ac-D- or L-Agl(2-naphthoyl)^1,DCpa^2,DPal^3,Aph^5(Ac),DAph^6(Ac),ILys^8, DAla^{10}]-GnRH	5.0 2.5	0/8 5/5
25	[Ac-DNal^1,DCpa^2,L- or D-Agl(nicotinoyl)^3,Aph^5(Ac),DAph^6(Ac),ILys^8, DAla^{10}]-GnRH	2.5 1.0	0/7 3/3
26	[Ac-DNal^1,DCpa^2,D- or L-Agl(nicotinoyl)^3,Aph^5(Ac),DAph^6(Ac), ILys^8,DAla^{10}]-GnRH	2.5 1.0	0/5 6/14

*Anti-ovulatory assay (AOA) dosage

at 25 μg/rat). Using the corresponding achiral betidamino derivative D/LAgl(2-naphthoyl) (bDNal), one diastereomer was obtained (compound number 23 in Table 3) that was equipotent to acyline ([Ac-L- or D-b2Nal^1]acyline) and one (compound number 24 in Table 3) that was less potent by only a factor of two ([Ac-D- or L-b2Nal^1]acyline). Replacing the D3Pal at position 3 with D or L-Agl(3-nicotinoyl)(bDPal) gave two diasteromeric peptides (compounds 25 and 26 in Table 3) that are equipotent to the parent acyline. These results (along with others) have led to the conclusion that acylated Agl substitutions are compatible with biological systems and that D- and L-betidamino acid containing peptides (most of the time) only differ in potency by a factor of 1 to 5 (versus 5–100-fold difference for the corresponding D- and L-amino acid substitutions in most peptides), suggesting that peptides with D- and L-betidamino acid substitutions may assume similar conformations; more specifically, present the amino acid side chains ??? defined and overlapping sites. A preliminary explanation is suggested by the fact that the volume spanned by a betidamino acid side chain is greater than that for the corresponding amino acids because of the difference in length of the bearing arm (betidamino acids have an amide bond replacing the methylene group found in conventional amino acids).

CONCLUSION

While the clinical significance of GnRH agonists is well recognized, the therapeutic use of GnRH antagonists in humans has awaited the availability of potent analogs with no untoward side effects. Several families of linear antagonists with high potency in inhibiting ovulation in the rat have been identified; some members of these families release histamine while others do not and have no anaphylactoid activity. Because none have physicochemical properties (solubility characteristics) similar to that of the superagonists for which long-term delivery systems are available, further structure activity relationship studies are warranted unless delivery systems can be adapted. Oddly, within the azaline B family, the authors have identified, using a castrated male rat model, analogs exhibiting short (<12 hours), intermediate (>12<72 hours) and long (>72 hours) duration of action after subcutaneous injection of 50 µg of the analog per rat. They concluded that the basis for such vulnerability/resistance to degradation and elimination must be specific. From this series, two long-acting and safe analogs stand out: azaline B (Ac-D2Nal-DCpa-D3Pal-Ser-Aph(Atz)-DAph(Atz)-Leu-ILys-Pro-DAla-NH$_2$) (where Aph is 4-amino phenylalanine and Atz is aminotriazolyl) and acyline (Ac-D2Nal-DCpa-D3Pal-Ser-Aph(Ac)-DAph(Ac)-Leu-ILys-Pro-DAla-NH$_2$). Both are relatively soluble in aqueous buffers and, for comparison purposes, are significantly more synthetically accessible than the Nal-Glu antagonist.

The authors' academic interest is in understanding the mechanism by which GnRH agonists and antagonists interact with the GnRH receptor to elicit or prevent gonadotropin secretion. This can be achieved in several ways, all of which are dependent on the structural analysis of the ligand, its receptor and their interaction. In the authors[1] efforts to more clearly define the bioactive conformation of GnRH antagonists, they have demonstrated the usefulness of several strategies in drug development. These include optimization of the chirality of the backbone, optimization of the functionality of the side chains, the use of betidamino acids to limit side chain rotational freedom and the introduction of side chain-to-side chain constraints. Although all GnRH analogs that are currently in the clinic are linear analogs, it is expected that the stuctural knowledge, derived from the discovery of highly constrained and potent analogs, will lead to the discovery of constrained peptidomimetics with oral activity.

ACKNOWLEDGEMENTS

This work was supported by National Institutes of Health (NIH) under contracts NO1-HD-9-2903 and NO1-HD-0-2906 and in part by NIH grant HD 13527 and the Hearst Foundation. The authors thank Dr J. Reel for the histamine release data as well as for some of the antiovulatory data obtained at Bioqual Inc. under contract NO1-HD-1-3130 with the Contraceptive Development Branch, Center for Population Research, National Institute for Child Health and Development. They are also grateful to C. Miller, R. Kaiser, D. Pantoja, S. Johnson and Y. Haas for their outstanding technical contributions, and D. Johns the manuscript preparation.

References

1. Rivier, J., Porter, J., Rivier, C., Perrin, M., Corrigan, A., Hook, W. A., Siraganian, R.P. and Vale, W.W. (1986). New effective gonadotropin releasing hormone antagonists with minimal potency for histamine release *in vitro. J. Med. Chem.*, **29**, 1846–51

2. Lunenfeld, B. and Insler, V. (1993). *GnRH Analogues. The State of the Art 1993.* (Carnforth, UK: Parthenon Publishing Group)

3. Hall, J. E., Bhatta, N., Adams, J. M., Rivier, J. Vale, W. W. and Crowley, W.F. (1990). Variable tolerance of the developing follicle and corpus luteum to GnRH antagonist-induced gonadotropin withdrawal in the human. *J. Clin. Endocrinol. Metab.*, **72**, 993–1000

4. Pavlou, S. N., Veldhuis, J., Lindner, J., Souza, K.H., Urban, R.J., Rivier, J. E., Vale, W. W. and Stallard, D. J. (1990). Persistence of concordant luteinizing hormone (LH), testosterone and α-subunit pulses following LH-releasing hormone antagonists administration in normal men. *J. Clin. Endocrinol. Metab.*, **70**, 1472–78

5. Urban, R.J., Pavlou, S. N., Rivier, J. E., Vale, W. W., Dufau, M. L. and Veldhuis, J. D. (1990). Suppressive actions of a gonadotropin-releasing hormone (GnRH) antagonist on LH, FSH, and prolactin release in estrogen-deficient post-menopausal women. *Am. J. Obstet. Gynecol.*, **162**, 1255–60

6. Daneshdoost, L., Pavlou, S. N., Molich, M. E., Gennarelli, T. A., Savino, P. J., Sergott, R.C., Bosley, T. M., Rivier, J., Vale, W. W. and Snyder, P. J. (1990). Inhibition of follicle-stimulating hormone secretion from gonadotroph adenomas by repetitive administration of a GnRH antagonist. *J. Clin. Endocrinol. Metab.*, **71**, 92–7

7. Pavlou, S. N., Rivier, J., Vale, W. and Kamilaris, T. (1990). Clinical pharmacology of LHRH antagonists. In Vickery, B. H. and Lunenfeld, B.

(eds.) *Precocious Puberty, Contraception and Safety Issues,* pp. 127–31. (Dordrecht: Kluwer Academic Publishers)

8. McGrath, G. A., Goncalvez, R., Udupa, J., Grossman, R. I., Pavlou, S. N., Molitch, M. E., Rivier, J., Vale, W. W. and Snyder, P. J. (1992). New technique for quantitation of pituitary adenoma size: use in evaluating treatment of gonadotroph adenomas with a GnRH antagonist. *J. Clin. Endocrinol. Metab.,* **76**, 1363–8

9. Kolp, L. A., Pavlou, S. N., Urban, R. J., Rivier, J. E., Vale, W. W. and Veldhuis, J. D. (1992). Abrogation by a potent gonadotropin-releasing hormone antagonist of the estrogen progesterone-stimulated surge-like release of luteinizing hormone and follicle-stimulating hormone in postmenopausal women. *J. Clin. Endocrinol. Metab.,* **75**, 993–7

10. Bagatell, C. J., Matsumoto, A. M., Christensen, R. B., Rivier, J. E. and Bremner, W. J. (1993). Comparison of a gonadotropin releasing-hormone antagonist plus testosterone (T) versus T alone as potential male contraceptive regimens. *J. Clin. Endocrinol. Metab.,* **77**, 427–32

11. Soules, M. R., Bremner, W. J., Dahl, K. D., Rivier, J. E., Vale, W. W. and Clifton, D. K. (1990). The induction of premature luteolysis in normal women–follicular LH secretion and corpus luteum function in the subsequent cycle. *Am. J. Obstet. Gynecol.,* **164**, 989–96

12. Tenover, J. S., Dahl, K. D., Vale, W. W., Rivier, J. E. and Bremner, W. J. (1990). Hormonal responses to a potent gonadotropin hormone-releasing antagonist in normal elderly men. *J. Clin. Endocrinol. Metab.,* **71**, 881–8

13. Roseff, S. J., Kettel, L. M., Rivier, J., Burger, H. G., Baulieu, E. and Yen, S. S. C. (1990). Accelerated dissolution of luteal–endometrial integrity by the administration of antagonists of GnRH and prosterone to late luteal phase women. *Fertil. Steril.,* **54**, 805–10

14. Ditkoff, E. C., Cassidenti, D. L., Paulson, R. J., Sauer, M. v., Wellington, L. P., Rivier, J., Yen, S. S. C. and Lobo, R. A. (1992). The gonadotropin-releasing hormone antagonist (Nal-Glu) acutely blocks the luteinizing hormone surge but allows for resumption of folliculogenesis in normal women. *Am. J. Obstet. Gynecol.,* **165**, 1811–17

15. Kettel, L. M., Murphy, A. A., Morales, A. J., Rivier, J., Vale, W. and Yen, S. S. C. (1993). Rapid regression of uterine leiomyoma in response to long-term daily administration of GnRH antagonist. *Fertil. Steril.,* **60**, 642–6

16. Bergqvist, I. A. (1995). Hormonal regulation of endometriosis and the rationales and effects of gonadotrophin-releasing hormone agonist treatment: a review. *Hum. Reprod.,* **10**, 446–52

17. Ljungqvist, A., Feng, D.-M., Bowers, C., Hook, W. and Folkers, K. (1990). Antagonists of LHRH superior to antide: effective sequence/activity relationships. *Tetrahedron,* **46**, 3297–304

18. Rivier, J., Porter, J., Hoeger, C., Theobald, P., Craig, A. G., Dykert, J., Corrigan, A., Perrin, M., Hook, W. A., Siraganian, R. P., Vale, W. and Rivier, C. (1992). Gonadotropin releasing hormone antagonists with Nω-triazolyl-ornithine, -lysine or -para-aminophenyl-alanine residues at positions 5 and 6. *J. Med. Chem.,* **35**, 4270–8

19. Campen, C. A., Lai, M.-T., Kraft, P., Kirchner, T., Phillips, A., Hahn, D. W. and Rivier, J. (1995). Potent pituitary-gonadal axis suppression and extremely low anaphylactoid activity of a new gonadotropin releasing hormone (GnRH) receptor antagonist 'azaline B'. *Biochem. Pharmacol.,* **49**, 1313–21

20. Karten, M. J., Hoeger, C. A., Hook, W. A., Lindbert, M. C. and Naqvi, R. H. (1990). The development of safer GnRH antagonists: strategy and status. In Bouchard, P., Haour, F., Franchimont, P. and Schatz, B. (eds.) *Recent Progress on GnRH and Gonadal Peptides,* pp. 147–158. (Paris Elsevier)

21. Rivier, J. E., Jiang, G., Porter, J., Hoeger, C., Craig, A. G., Corrigan, A., Vale, W. and Rivier, C. L. (1995). GnRH antagonists: novel members of the azaline B family. *J. Med. Chem.,* **38**, 2649–62

22. Corbin, A. and Beattie, C. W. (1975). Inhibition of the pre-ovulatory proestrous gonadotropin surge, ovulation and pregnancy with a peptide analogue of luteinizing hormone releasing hormone. *Endocr. Res. Commun.,* **2**, 1–23

23. Rivier, C., Rivier, J., Perrin, M. and Vale, W. (1983). Comparison of the effect of several GnRH antagonists on LH secretion, receptor binding and ovulation. *Biol. Reprod.,* **29**, 374–8

24. Rivier, C., Rivier, J. and Vale, W. (1986). Stress-induced inhibition of reproductive functions: role of endogenous corticotropin-releasing factor. *Science,* **231**, 607–9

25. Rivier, C. and Vale, W. (1989). In the rat, interleukin-1α acts at the level of the brain and the gonads to interfere with gonadotropin and sex steroid secretion. *Endocrinology,* **124**, 2105–9

26. Karten, M. J., Hook, W. A., Siraganian, R. P., Coy, D. H., Folkers, K., Rivier, J. E. and Roeske, R. W. (1987). *In vitro* histamine release with LHRH analogs. In Vickery, B. H. and Nestor, J. (eds.) *LHRH and Its Analogs, Contraceptive and Therapeutic*

Applications, part 2, pp. 179–190. (Lancaster, Boston, The Hague: MTP Press, Ltd)

27. Hook, W. A., Karten, M. and Siraganian, R. P. (1985). Histamine release by structural analogs of LHRH. *Fed. Proc.,* **44**, 1323

28. Karten, M. J. (1992). An overview of GnRH antagonists development: two decades of progress. In Crowley, W. F. Jr and Conn, P. M. (eds.) *Modes of Action of GnRH and GnRH Analogs,* pp. 277–97. (New York: Springer-Verlag)

29. Haviv, F., Fitzpatrick, T. D., Nichols, C. J., Swenson, R. E., Mort, N. A., Bush, E. N., Diaz, G., Nguyen, A. T., Holst, M. R., Cybulski, V. A., Leal, J. A., Bammert, G., Rhutasel, N. S., Dodge, P. W., Johnson, E. S., Cannon, J. B., Knittle, J. and Greer, J. (1993). The effect of NMeTyr⁵ substitution in luteinizing hormone-releasing hormone antagonists. *J. Med. Chem.,* **36**, 928–33

30. Rivier, J. (1993). Novel antagonists of GnRH: a compendium of their physicochemical properties, activities, relative potencies and efficacy in humans. In *GnRH Analogues. The State of the Art 1993,* pp. 13–26. (Carnforth, UK: Parthenon Publishing Group)

31. Lowe, J. A. III, Drozda, S. E., Snider, R. M., Longo, K. P., Zorn, S. H., Morrone, J., Jackson, E. R., McLean, S., Bryce, D. K., Bordner, J., Nagahisa, A., Kanai, Y., Suga, O. and Tsuchiya, M. (1992). The discovery of (2S,3S)-*cis*-2-(Diphenylmethyl)-N-[(2-methoxyphenyl)-methyl]-1-azabicyclo[2.2.2]-octan-3-amine as a novel, nonpeptide substance P antagonist. *J. Med. Chem.,* **35**, 2591–600

32. Sprecher, R. F. and Momany, F.A. (1979). On the conformation of luteinizing hormone-releasing hormone, nuclear overhauser observations. *Biochem. Biophys. Res. Commun.,* **87**, 72–7

33. Kopple, K. D. (1983). Peptide backbone folding in LHRH and analogs. In *Peptides: Synthesis–Structure–Function,* pp. 295–8. (Rockford, IL: Pierce Chemical Co.)

34. Kopple, K. D. (1983). Nitroxyl-induced T₁ relaxation rates as a probe of conformation in peptide hormones. *Int. J. Pept. Protein Res.,* **21**, 43–8

35. Momany, F. A. (1976). Conformational energy analysis of the molecule, luteinizing hormone-releasing hormone. 1. Native decapeptide. *J. Am. Chem. Soc.,* **98**, 2990–6

36. Momany, F. A. (1976). Conformational energy analysis of the molecule, luteinizing hormone-releasing hormone. 2. Tetrapeptide and decapeptide analogues. *J. Am. Chem. Soc.,* **98**, 2996–3000

37. Chandrasekaren, R., Lakshminarayanan, A. V., Pandya, U. V. and Ramachandran, G. N. (1973). Conformation of the LL and LD hairpin bends with internal hydrogen bonds in proteins and peptides. *Biochim. Biophys. Acta,* **303**, 14–27

38. Monahan, M., Amoss, M., Anderson, H. and Vale, W. (1973). Synthetic analogs of the hypothalamic luteinizing hormone releasing factor with increased agonist or antagonist properties. *Biochemistry,* **12**, 4616–20

39. Tonelli, A.E. (1976). The effects of isolated *N*-methylated residues on the conformational characteristics of polypeptides. *Biopolymers,* **15**, 1615–22

40. Rivier, J., Koerber, S., Struthers, S., Tanaka, G., Rivier, C., Perrin, M., Porter, J., Corrigan, A., Vale, W. and Hagler, A. (1988). Design of active multicyclic gonadotropin releasing hormone antagonists. In *Proceedings of the Banbury Ctr. Conference on Therapeutic Peptides and Proteins: Formulation, Delivery and Targeting,* pp. 85–91. (Cold Spring Harbor, New York: Cold Spring Harbor Press)

41. Rivier, J., Koerber, S., Rivier, C., Porter, J. and Hagler, A. (1990). Design, computer derived structure and biological activity of three bicyclic gonadotropin releasing hormone (GnRH) antagonists. In *Current Research in Protein Chemistry,* pp. 273–81. (Academic Press)

42. Rivier, J., Kupryszewski, G., Theobald, P., Hoeger, C., Porter, J., Perrin, M., Corrigan, A., Struthers, S., Koerber, S., Hagler, A., Vale, W. and Rivier, C. (1991). Two distinct approaches for the design of potent GnRH antagonists. In *Proceedings of the 2nd International Symposium on GnRH Analogues in Cancer and Human Reproduction,* Vol. 2, pp. 123–35. (Carnforth, UK: Parthenon Publishing)

43. Rivier, J., Kupryszewski, G., Varga, J., Porter, J., Rivier, C., Perrin, M., Hagler, A., Struthers, S., Corrigan, A. and Vale, W. (1988). Design of potent cyclic gonadotropin releasing hormone (GnRH) antagonists. *J. Med. Chem.,* **31**, 677–82

44. Rizo, J., Koerber, S. C., Bienstock, R. J., Rivier, J., Hagler, A. T. and Gierasch, L. M. (1992). Conformational analysis of a highly potent, constrained gonadotropin-releasing hormone antagonist. 1. Nuclear magnetic resonance. *J. Am. Chem. Soc.,* **114**, 2852–9

45. Rizo, J., Koerber, S. C., Bienstock, R. J., Rivier, J., Gierasch, L. M. and Hagler, A. T. (1992). Conformational analysis of a highly potent, constrained gonadotropin-releasing hormone antagonist. 2. Molecular dynamics simulations. *J. Am. Chem. Soc.,* **114**, 2860–71

46. Bienstock, R. J., Rizo, J., Koerber, S. C., Rivier, J. E., Hagler, A. T. and Gierasch, L. M. (1993).

Conformational analysis of a highly potent dicyclic gonadotropin-releasing hormone antagonist by nuclear magnetic resonance and molecular dynamics. *J. Med. Chem.*, **36**, 3265–73

47. Gupta, H. M., Talwar, G. P. and Salunke, D. M. (1993). A novel computer modeling approach to the structures of small bioactive peptides: the structure of gonadotropin releasing hormone. *Proteins,* **16**, 48–56

48. Nikiforovich, G. V. and Marshall, G. R. (1993). Conformation–function relationships in LHRH analogs. I. Conformation of LHRH peptide backbone. *Int. J. Pept. Protein Res.*, **42**, 171–80

49. Nikiforovich, G. V. and Marshall, G. R. (1993). Conformation–function relationships in LHRH analogs. II. Conformations of LHRH peptide agonists and antagonists. *Int. J. Pept. Protein Res.*, **42**, 181–93

50. Kawaguchi, K., Maruyama, T., Terasawa, I., Kohda, D., Shimada, I. and Inagaki, F. (1989). Structure of luteinizing hormone-releasing hormone bound to perdeuterated dodecylphosphocholine micelles as studies by 2D-NMR. *Pept. Chem.*, 337–40

51. Wessels, P. L., Feeney, J., Gergory, H. and Gormley, J. J. (1973). High resolution nuclear magnetic resonance studies of the con-formation of the luteinizing hormone-releasing hormone (LH-RH) and its component peptides. *J. Chem. Sci. Perkin*, II, 1691–8

52. Deslauriers, R., Levy, G. C., McGregor, W. H., Sarantakis, D. and Smith, I.C.P. (1975). Conformational flexibility of luteinizing hormone-releasing hormone in aqueous solution. A carbon-13 spin-lattice relaxation time study. *Biochemistry,* **14**, 4335–43

53. Chary, V. R., Srivastava, S., Hosur, R. V., Roy, K. B. and Govil, G. (1986). Molecular conformation of gonadoliberin using two-dimensional NMR spectroscopy. *Eur. J. Biochem.*, **158**, 323–32

54. Kazmierski, W.M., Urbanczyk-Lipkowska, Z. and Hruby, V.J. (1994). New amino acids for the topographical control of peptide conformation: synthesis of all the isomers of α,β-Dimethyl-phenylalanine and α,β-dimethyl-1,2,3,4-tetrahydroisoquinoline-3-carboxylic acid of high optical purity. *J. Org. Chem.*, **59**, 1789–95

55. Qasmi, D., René, L. and Badet, B. (1993). An α-aminoglycine derivative suitable for solid phase peptide synthesis using Fmoc strategy. *Tetrahedron Lett.*, **34**, 3861–2

56. Rivier, J. E., Jiang, G.-C., Simon, L., Koerber, S. C., Porter, J., Craig, A. G. and Hoeger, C. A. (1995). Betidamino acids: versatile and constrained scaffolds for drug discovery. In Kaumaya, P. T. P. and Hodges, R. S. (eds.) *Peptides: Chemistry, Structure and Biology.* (Mayflower Scientific Ltd)

57. Hoeger, C. A., Jiang, G.-C., Koerber, S. C., Reisine, T., Liapakis, G. and Rivier, J. E. (1995). Betide based strategy for the design of selective somatostatin analogs. In Kaumaya, P. T. P. and Hodges, R. S. (eds.) *Peptides: Chemistry, Structure and Biology.* (Mayflower Scientific Ltd)

Extrapituitary sites of action of LHRH agonists

M. Motta, D. Dondi, P. Limonta, R. Maggi, M. Montagnani, R. M. Moretti and F. Pimpinelli

INTRODUCTION

Many experimental and clinical studies indicate that luteinizing hormone releasing hormone (LHRH) agonists represent useful therapeutic agents for the treatment of sex steroid-dependent tumors, such as advanced carcinoma of the prostate and of the breast[1]. The anti-tumoral effect of LHRH agonists was believed, until recently, to be mediated exclusively by down-regulation of the pituitary–gonadal axis. LHRH agonists, given continuously and in pharmacological doses inhibit LH secretion and decrease serum sex hormone levels by down-regulating LHRH receptors at the pituitary level[1–3]. Subsequent studies have demonstrated that LHRH and its agonists may also exhibit direct inhibitory effects on the gonads, where they may interfere with the steroidogenic process[4]. This occurs because, in a similar manner to the pituitary, the gonads have been shown to contain specific LHRH receptors[5]. Moreover, receptors for LHRH analogs have been reported to be present in specimens of both human prostatic and mammary tumoral tissues[6,7], as well as in rat prostate and breast[6,8,9]. These observations suggest that LHRH agonists might affect the growth of sex hormone-dependent cancers also acting directly at the level of the tumor.

Growth factors mainly endowed with stimulatory activity such as epidermal growth factor (EGF), transforming growth factor-alpha (TGF-α), bovine fibroblast growth factor (bFGF), insulin-like growth factors (IGFs), etc., appear to be involved in the control of the growth of prostate and breast cancers (for references see[1,10–12]). The presence of locally produced growth factors in the tumoral cell lines[11,13–16], the existence of growth factor receptors in the same cell line[6,12,17,18], and the demonstration that binding to the receptors is followed by the activation of intracellular signals[12] suggest that the proliferation of human prostate and breast cancer cell lines are regulated locally by functional growth stimulatory loops; the EGF/TGFα system is particularly well documented[11,12,19–21].

This chapter will summarize some recent studies on the effects of LHRH agonists on prostatic tumors carried out in the authors' laboratory. The objectives of these investigations were:

(1) To explore the possibility that LHRH agonists might possess a direct inhibitory effect on prostatic tumoral tissue;

(2) To study, in more detail, the mechanisms involved in these potential direct anti-tumoral effects; in particular, it was deemed of interest to analyze whether the possible inhibition of the growth of human prostatic cancer cells induced by LHRH agonists might involve the inhibition of the activity of the locally expressed EGF/TGFα system;

(3) To study the expression of LHRH messenger ribonucleic acid (mRNA);

(4) To analyze whether a LHRH degrading activity (LHRH-DA) could be present at the level of the prostatic tumor.

As models of human prostatic cancer *in vitro*, the androgen-dependent LNCaP (lymph node carcinoma of the prostate) cells , derived from a metastatic human prostatic carcinoma, and the androgen-independent DU145 cells, originated from a brain metastasis of a human prostatic carcinoma, have been used. These human prostatic cancer cell lines represent useful experimental tools, since they maintain the peculiar characteristics of the original tumors: the LNCaP cells retain the androgen-responsiveness, the expression of androgen receptors[22,23], the production of acid phosphatases, etc., while the DU145 cells maintain the androgen independence of the original tumors[24] and do not express androgen receptors[25].

INHIBITORY EFFECT OF LHRH AGONISTS ON THE PROLIFERATION OF LNCaP AND DU145 CELLS

Research

The hypothesis of a direct anti-tumoral effect of LHRH agonists at the level of the prostatic tumor has been tested by studying the effects of two potent LHRH agonists (Zoladex and buserelin) on the proliferation of LNCaP and DU145 cells. The cells, cultured in a medium containing fetal calf serum (FCS), were treated with different doses of the LHRH agonists (10^{-12}–10^{-6} M); at the end of the period of treatment (9 and 4 days for LNCaP and DU145, respectively), cells were harvested and counted by hemocytometer[26,27]. Both LHRH analogs significantly inhibited LNCaP and DU145 cell proliferation at doses ranging from 10^{-10} to 10^{-6} M; lower concentrations of both drugs proved inactive. To verify the specificity of the anti-proliferation action of LHRH agonists on both cell lines, the authors investigated whether their inhibitory action on LNCaP and DU145 cell proliferation could be counteracted by simultaneous treatment of the cells with a potent LHRH antagonist (ANT, Nal-Arg-LHRH kindly provided by Dr W. Vale, Salk Institute, La Jolla, CA, USA). ANT, when given alone at the dose of 10^{-8} M, had no effect on cell proliferation in the presence of FCS, while the same dose of this peptide was able to reverse totally the anti-proliferation action exhibited by the two LHRH agonists. This last observation has prompted the authors to investigate the possible involvement of specific LHRH receptors. This hypothesis has been verified by means of a receptor binding assay[26,27.] It has been shown that receptors for the LHRH agonists are expressed on LNCaP and DU145 cell membranes only when the cells are grown, respectively, with FCS deprived of steroids and in a chemical medium devoid of possible growth factors. Computer analysis of binding data revealed the presence of a single class of low affinity (dissociation constant $[K_d]$ = 100 nM and 10 mM for LNCaP and DU145 cells, respectively) high capacity (maximum binding capacity $[B_{max}]$ = 629 fmol/mg protein and 425–668 pmol/mg protein for LNCaP and DU145 cells, respectively) binding sites. The analysis of the binding parameters for LHRH receptors on rat pituitaries, tested in the present experiments as tissue of reference, showed K_d and B_{max} values of 0.14 nM and 107 fmol/mg protein, respectively, confirming the data reported previously[28].

Conclusions

These results suggest that LHRH agonists exert a direct anti-proliferative action on human prostatic tumor cells by acting through specific receptors. This effect appears to be specific, since it is counteracted by the simultaneous addition to the culture medium of a LHRH antagonist, and it is linked to the presence of specific receptors. It is interesting to note that LHRH receptors seem to be expressed on LNCaP cells only when the cells have been grown in a medium deprived of steroids. This observation seems to suggest that the expression of LHRH receptors on prostatic tumor may be negatively regulated by circulating levels of testicular androgens, since the androgen dependence of the prostatic tissue has been widely reported[1,29].

Taken together, these data seem to indicate that LHRH agonists, when utilized for the treatment of prostatic carcinoma, could inhibit tumor growth not only by suppressing the activity of the pituitary–testicular axis, but also by exerting a direct and specific anti-proliferative action at the level of the tumor. Finally, the observation that LHRH agonists are also inhibitory on the growth of DU145 cells (derived from androgen-independent human prostatic carcinoma) suggests that these agents could be of therapeutic significance, particularly in those conditions in which the original or metastatic tumor is no longer androgen-dependent. Obviously, these observations, although encouraging, need to be verified in clinical situations before any definite conclusion might be drawn.

INTERACTION BETWEEN LHRH AGONISTS AND GROWTH STIMULATORY FACTORS IN LNCaP AND DU145 CELLS

Research

The following experiments have been performed to clarify whether, in LNCaP as well as in DU145 cells, LHRH agonists could inhibit cell proliferation by interfering with the activity of locally produced growth stimulatory factors. Precisely, the effects of a LHRH agonist (Zoladex) on the proliferative action of EGF and on the concentration of EGF/TGFα receptors have been analyzed in LNCaP as well as in DU145 cells. To study the effects of a LHRH agonist on the EGF-induced proliferation of LNCaP and DU145 cells, they have been treated with EGF (5 ng/ml) either in the absence or in the presence of different doses of the LHRH agonists (10^{-10}–10^{-6} M). After 7 days of treatment, cells were harvested and counted by hemocytometer. As expected, EGF significantly stimulated both LNCaP and DU145 cell proliferation; this effect was completely counteracted by the simultaneous treatment of the cells with the highest dose of the LHRH agonist (10^{-6} M). Furthermore, to verify whether the LHRH agonist could modify the binding characteristics of the EGF/TGFα receptor, LNCaP and DU145 cells have been treated with the LHRH agonist (10^{-6} M) for 1.5 and 3 hours. The binding parameters of the EGF/TGFα receptor (B_{max} and K_d) have been evaluated by a receptor binding assay, using ^{125}I-EGF as the specific ligand[12]. The treatment resulted in a significant decrease of the concentration of EGF binding sites in both cell lines and at both time intervals considered, while the K_d values of the receptors for their ligand were not affected by the treatment.

Conclusions

These results suggest that, in prostatic tumor cells, LHRH agonists could act by counteracting the mitogenic action of the EGF/TGFα system. The inhibitory effect of LHRH agonists on the EGF-induced growth of LNCaP cells is probably explained by the observed decrease in the concentration of EGF/TGFα receptors; this, in turn, might be followed by the inhibition of its signal transduction mechanisms. This issue is currently investigated in the authors' laboratory by measuring the levels of phosphorylation of tyrosine residues of the EGF/TGFα receptor.

EXPRESSION OF LHRH mRNA IN LNCaP AND DU145 CELLS: EVIDENCE FOR AN AUTOCRINE INHIBITORY LHRH LOOP

Research

The significance of the presence of specific binding sites for LHRH on prostatic tumor cells (data reported here and[30]) as well as on fragments of human and rat prostatic tumoral tissue[6,9] is open to speculation. Since hypothalamic LHRH is rapidly degraded at the pituitary level[31] the possibility that the decapeptide could reach the prostate through the general circulation seems to be extremely unlikely. In the authors' opinion, it appears more logical to postulate that these receptors respond to some locally produced LHRH-like peptides, which may participate in the mechanisms controlling tumor growth by acting as an autocrine and/or paracrine factor. To test this hypothesis, the expression of LHRH mRNA in both LNCaP and DU145 cells has been analyzed by using the reverse transcription–polymerase chain reaction (RT–PCR) technique[32]. Briefly, the ribonucleic acid (RNA) extracted from both tumoral cell lines, from rat hypothalamus (positive control) and from rat pituitary (negative control) was reverse transcribed, and then amplified by PCR using two pairs of primers, one specific for human (LNCaP and DU145 cells) and the other specific for rat (hypothalamus and pituitary) LHRH complementary (c) DNAs[33]. In these conditions, a PCR product of 228 base pairs was expected. After the PCR reaction, the amplified cDNAs were electrophoresed on a 1.5% agarose gel containing ethidium bromide. The predicted 228-base pair fragment was obtained in LNCaP and DU145 cells as well as in the rat hypothalamus. After Southern blot[34], this fragment hybridized with a synthetic ^{32}P-labeled LHRH oligonucleotide- probe. The 228 base pair RT–PCR product from LNCaP and DU145 cells was further subcloned in *Escherichia coli*; the sequence of this product, which shows a complete match with the human placental LHRH cDNA sequence[33], unequivocally demonstrates that a mRNA for LHRH is expressed in human prostatic cancer cells.

The presence of LHRH mRNA in LNCaP and DU145 cells seems to be in line with the hypothesis that LHRH or a LHRH-like peptide could be produced by prostatic tumor cells and act as an autocrine/paracrine factor in the local control of tumor proliferation. To verify the role of the locally produced LHRH, the effects of a treatment with a LHRH antagonist (ANT, 10^{-8}M) on LNCaP and DU145 cell proliferation have been studied. LNCaP and DU145 cells were cultured with FCS deprived of steroids and in serum-free conditions, respectively, since both LHRH receptors[26,27,30] and LHRH-immunoreactivity[30,35] have been found previously in cells grown in these specific culture conditions. The results show that treatment with ANT resulted in a significant stimulation of prostatic tumor cell proliferation. It is interesting to note that, as mentioned previously, a similar treatment with the same compound did not affect proliferation of LNCaP cells grown with FCS (i.e. in the presence of steroids).

Conclusions

The present data indicate that both LNCaP and DU145 cells express a specific LHRH mRNA which is translated into a peptide which may act as a local inhibitory growth factor on tumor cell proliferation; this is suggested by the observation that the LHRH antagonist was able to stimulate the growth of both cell lines. This LHRH system seems to be negatively regulated by different factors: for example, testicular androgens in the case of LNCaP cells, and growth factors present in the serum in the case of DU145 cells. Moreover, the observation that LHRH antagonists may exert, in given experimental conditions, proliferative effects on LNCaP and DU145 cells may suggest a word of caution in their clinical utilization. We do not wish to over emphasize our results, which could be due solely to the use of cell cultures grown in particular conditions; however, the present data suggest that the relationship between LHRH antagonistic analogs and normal and pathological

cell proliferation should be given particular attention in the future, especially in connection with prostatic pathology.

PRESENCE OF LHRH DEGRADING ACTIVITY IN LNCaP CELLS

Research

It is known that LHRH is actively hydrolyzed in its most relevant target tissue, the pituitary, by membrane-bound and soluble peptidases[31]; the activity of these peptidases may locally influence the biological effects of LHRH and its analogs (e.g. by modifying their duration of action at the receptor level)[36,37].

Since, as mentioned in the preceding sections, LNCaP cells express a LHRH-like system (e.g. mRNA, receptors and peptide)[32], it was deemed of interest to investigate whether a LHRH-degrading activity (LHRH-DA) could be present in human prostatic cancer cells, an extrapituitary target for LHRH and its analogs. To this end, soluble fractions of LNCaP cell homogenates were utilized. Using high pressure liquid chroma-tography it has been shown that the degradation pattern of LHRH is characterized by two major initial products identified as the LHRH 1-5 and LHRH 1-6 fragments[38]. These results indicate that a LHRH-DA is present in the soluble fraction of LNCaP cells. The involvement of the Tyr^5–Gly^6 bond in the initial degradation of LHRH was also observed, when the soluble fraction of the rat ventral prostate or the whole homogenates or fractions of brain, pituitary, liver, lung, ovary and testis tissues were tested for the presence of LHRH-DA[36,37]. In subsequent experiments, the LHRH-DA present in LNCaP cells was monitored by the cation-exchanger batchwise method described by Berger et al.[39,40]. For this assay [pGlu-^{3}H]-LHRH was used as a substrate for the LHRH-DA and its degradation was evaluated as the remaining radioactivity in the incubation cocktail after treatment at alkaline pH with the Dowex 50W-X2 resin, which strongly binds the positively charged intact labeled peptide, but only very weakly binds the negatively charged labeled degradation products. The results obtained by the radio-chemical method show that the crude soluble fraction of the LNCaP cell homogenate induced a time-dependent (from 0 to 60 min at 30°C) degradation of [pGlu-^{3}H]-LHRH described by first-order kinetics (rate constant=0.0073 min^{-1}). This LHRH-DA showed apparent K_m and V_{max} values of 31.6 μM and 4.5 pmol/min/μg protein, respectively. Co-incubation of [pGlu-^{3}H]-LHRH with unlabeled LHRH resulted in a dose-dependent inhibition (IC$_{50}$=7.9 μM) of tracer degradation by the LNCaP LHRH-DA, indicating a specific competition. LHRH agonists were also able to inhibit the degradation of [pGlu-^{3}H]-LHRH with different kinetics and potencies; the LHRH agonist [DSer-(tBu)^6,Gly^{10}-Aza]-LHRH resulted to be the most potent blocker of LHRH-DA present in LNCaP cells. It is interesting to underline that somatostatin is also able to inhibit the degradation of LHRH by the LNCaP soluble fraction. This effect is of particular interest, since the hormone and its analogs are currently studied as a potential tool for the treatment of the carcinoma of the prostate[1]. It is not surprising that the LHRH-DA present in the soluble fraction of LNCaP cells is not fully specific for LHRH; it must also be underlined that the endopeptidase, which degrades LHRH at the pituitary level, does not appear absolutely specific for LHRH (it also hydrolyzes enkephalin precursors, bradykinin, neurotensin, etc.)[41].

Conclusions

These results suggest the presence in LNCaP cells of a soluble peptidase able to degrade LHRH. This finding reinforces the concept that the prostate is a target for the action of LHRH and of its analogs. This observation should be taken into consideration when LHRH agonists are used for the treatment of prostatic carcinoma, especially when they have reached the stage of androgen-independence. The utilization of LHRH analogs, which are resistant to the degradation by the prostatic LHRH-DA and which reduce the degradation of the endogenous inhibiting LHRH-like peptide, will certainly improve the treatment of carcinoma of the prostate.

GENERAL CONCLUSIONS

Collectively, the present studies indicate, first, that LHRH agonists can inhibit the growth of prostatic cancer by acting not only through the inhibition of gonadotropin secretion, but also directly on cellular growth and replication. Secondly, these studies suggest that LNCaP and DU145 cells express a LHRH (or LHRH-like) loop possibly endowed with inhibitory activity on tumor cell proliferation. Finally, the present studies, which are aimed at investigating the mechanisms through which LHRH agonists exert their action at the level of prostatic tumors, suggest an intimate interplay among the inhibitory actions of these agents and the stimulatory role exerted by growth factors. In particular these data support the hypothesis that LHRH agonists may interfere with the proliferation promoting effects exerted on human prostatic tumor growth by the locally expressed EGF/TGFα loop.

ACKNOWLEDGEMENTS

The experiments performed in the authors' laboratory and reported here have been supported by AIRC, by CNR through the Special Projects ACRO (contract number 94.01162.PF 39), FATMA (contract number 95.00868.PF 41), Aging (contract number 94.00470.PF 40) and by MURST.

References

1. Motta, M. and Serio, M. (eds.) (1994). *Sex hormones and antihormones in endocrine dependent pathology: basic and clinical aspects.* (Netherlands: Elsevier)

2. Belchetz, P. E. (1983). Gonadotropin regulation and clinical applications of GnRH. *Clin. Endocrinol. Metab.*, **12**, 619–40

3. Clayton, R. N. (1987). Gonadotropin releasing hormone: from physiology to pharmacology. *Clin. Endocrinol.*, **26**, 361–8

4. Hsueh, A. J. W. and Jones, P. B. C. (1981). Extrapituitary actions of GnRH. *Endocrinol. Rev.*, **2**, 437–61

5. Clayton, R. N. and Catt, K. J. (1981). Gonadotropin-releasing hormone receptors: characterization, physiological regulation, and relationship to reproductive function. *Endocr. Rev.*, **2**, 186–209

6. Fekete, M., Redding, T. W., Comaru-Schally, A. M., Pontes, J. E., Connelly, R. W., Srkalovic, G. and Schally, A. V. (1989). Receptors for luteinizing hormone-releasing hormone, somatostatin, prolactin, and epidermal growth factor in rat and human prostate cancers and in benign prostate hyperplasia. *Prostate*, **14**, 191–208

7. Baumann, H. H., Kiesel, L. Kaufman, M., Bastert, G. and Runnebaum, B. (1993). Characterization of binding sites for a GnRH-agonist (buserelin) in human breast cancer biopsies and their distribution in relation to tumor parameters. *Breast Cancer Res. Treat.*, **25**, 37–46

8. Milanovic, S. R., Monje, E., Szepeshazi, K., Radulovic, S. and Schally, A. (1993). Effect of treatment with LHRH analogs containing cytotoxic radicals on the binding characteristics of receptors for luteinizing-hormone-releasing hormone in MXT mouse mammary carcinoma. *J. Cancer Res. Clin. Oncol.*, **119**, 273–8

9. Srkalovic, G., Bokser, L., Radulovic, S., Korkut, E. and Schally, A. V. (1990). Receptors for luteinizing hormone-releasing hormone (LHRH) in Dunning R3327 prostate cancers and rat anterior pituitaries after treatment with a sustained delivery system of LHRH antagonist SB-75 *Endocrinology*, **127**, 3052–60

10. Voigt, K. D. and Knabbe, C. (eds.) 1991. *Endocrine-dependent Tumors.* (New York: Raven Press)

11. Dickson, R. B. and Lippman, M. E. (1987). Estrogenic regulation of growth and polypeptide growth factor secretion in human breast carcinoma. *Endocr. Rev.*, **8**, 29–43

12. Limonta, P., Moretti, R. M., Dondi, D., Montagnani Marelli, M. and Motta, M. (1994). The EGF/TGFα system as an autocrine growth stimulatory loop in LNCaP cells. *Endocr. Rel. Cancer*, **5**, 5–13

13. Osborne, C. K., Coronado, E. B., Kitten, L. J. Arteaga, C. I., Fuqua, S. A. W., Ramasharma, K., Marshall, M. and Li, C. H. (1989). Insulin-like growth factor-II (IGF-II): a potential autocrine/ paracrine growth factor for human breast cancer acting via the IGF-I receptor. *Mol. Endocrinol.*, **3**, 1701–9

14. Connolly, J. M. and Rose, D. P. (1990). Production of epidermal growth factor and transforming growth factor-α by the androgen-responsive LNCaP human cancer cell line. *Prostate*, **16**, 209–18

15. Schuurmans, A. L. G., Bolt, J., Veldscholte, J. and Mulder, E. (1991). Regulation of growth of LNCaP human prostate tumor cells by growth factors and steroid hormones. *J. Steroid Biochem. Mol. Biol.*, **40**, 193–7

16. MacDonald, A. and Habib, F. K. (1992). Divergent responses to epidermal growth factor in hormone sensitive and insensitive human prostate cancer cell lines. *Br. J. Cancer*, **65**, 177–82

17. Furlanetto, R. W. and DiCarlo, J. N. (1984). Somatomedin-C receptors and growth effects in human breast cells maintained in long-term tissue culture. *Cancer Res.*, **44**, 2122–8

18. Huff, K. K., Kaufman, D., Gabbay, K. H., Spencer, E. M., Lippman, M. E. and Dickson, R. B. (1986). Human breast cancer cells secrete an insulin-like growth factor-I-related polypeptide. *Cancer Res.*, **46**, 4613

19. Connolly, J. M. and Rose, D. P. (1991). Autocrine regulation of DU145 human prostate cancer cell growth by epidermal growth factor-related polypeptides. *Prostate*, **19**, 173–80

20. Hofer, D. R., Sherwood, E. R., Bromberg, W. D., Mendelsohn, J., Lee, C. and Kozlowski, J. M. (1991). Autonomous growth of androgen-independent human prostatic carcinoma cells: role of transforming growth factor α. *Cancer Res.*, **51**, 2780–5

21. Tillotson, J. K. and Rose, D. P. (1991). Endogenous secretion of epidermal growth factor peptides stimulates growth of DU145 prostate cancer cells. *Cancer Lett.*, **60**, 109–12

22. Horoszewicz, J. S., Leong, S. S., Kawinski, E., Karr, J. P., Rosenthal, H., Ming Chu, T., Mirand, E. A. and Murphy, G. P. (1983). LNCaP model of human prostatic carcinoma. *Cancer Res.*, **43**, 1809–18

23. Veldscholte, J., Ris-Stalper, C., Kuiper, G. G. J. M., Jenster, G., Berrevoets, C., Claassen, E., van Rooij, H. C. J., Trapman, J. Brinkmann, A. O. and Mulder, E. (1990). A mutation in the ligand binding domain of the androgen receptor of human LNCaP cells affects steroid binding characteristics and response to anti-androgens. *Biochem. Biophys. Res. Commun.*, **17** (3), 534–40

24. Stone, K. R., Mickey, D. D., Wunderli, H., Mickey,

G. H. and Paulson, D. F. (1978). Isolation of a human prostate carcinoma cell line (DU145). *Int. J. Cancer*, **21** (3), 274–81

25. Culig, Z., Klocker, H., Eberle, J., Kaspar, F., Hobisch, A., Cronauer, M. V. and Bartsch, G. (1993). DNA sequence of the androgen receptor in prostatic tumor cell lines and tissue specimens assessed by means of the polymerase-chain reaction. *Prostate*, **22**, 11–22

26. Limonta, P., Dondi, D., Moretti, R. M., Maggi, R. and Motta, M. (1992). Antiproliferative effects of luteinizing hormone-releasing hormone agonists on the human prostatic cancer cell line LNCaP. *J. Clin. Endocrinol. Metab.*, **75**, 207–12

27. Dondi, D., Limonta, P., Moretti, R. M., Montagnani Marelli, M., Garattini, E. and Motta, M. (1994). Antiproliferative effects of luteinizing hormone-releasing hormone (LHRH) agonists on human androgen-independent prostate cancer cell line DU145: evidence for an autocrine-inhibitory LHRH loop. *Cancer Res.*, **54**, 4091–5

28. Limonta, P., Dondi, D., Maggi, R., Martini, L. and Piva, F. (1987). Effects of aging on pituitary and testicular luteinizing hormone-releasing hormone receptors in the rat. *Life Sci.*, **42**, 335–42

29. Eaton, C. L., Davies, P., Harper, M., France, T., Rushmere, N. and Griffiths, K. (1991). Steroids and the prostate. *J. Steroid Biochem. Mol. Biol.*, **40**, 175–83

30. Qayum, A., Gullick, W., Clayton, R. C., Sikora, K. and Waxman, J. (1990). The effects of gonadotropin releasing hormone analogues in prostate cancer are mediated through specific tumor receptors. *Br. J. Cancer*, **62**, 96–9

31. Horsthemke, B., Knisatschek, H., Rivier, J., Sandow, J. and Bauer, K. (1981). Degradation of luteinizing hormone-releasing hormone and analogues by adenohypophyseal peptidases. *Biochem. Biophys. Res. Commun.*, **100**, 753–9

32. Limonta, P., Dondi, D., Moretti, R. M., Fermo, D., Garattini, E. and Motta, M. (1993). Expression of luteinizing hormone-releasing hormone mRNA in the human prostatic cancer cell line LNCaP. *J. Clin Endocrinol. Metab.*, **76**, 797–800

33. Adelman, J. P., Mason, A. J., Hayflyck, J. S. and Seeburg, P. H. (1986). Isolation of the gene and hypothalamic cDNA for the common precursor of gonadotropin-releasing hormone and prolactin release-inhibiting factor in human and rat. *Proc. Natl Acad. Sci. USA*, **83**, 179–83

34. Wood, W. I., Gitschier, J., Lasky, L. A. and Lawn, R. M. (1985). Base composition-independent hybridization in tetramethyl-ammonium chloride: a method for oligonucleotide screening of highly complex gene libraries. *Proc. Natl. Acad. Sci. USA*, **82**, 1585–8

35. Qayum, A., Gullick, W. J., Mellon, K., Krausz, T., Neal, D., Sikora, K. and Waxman, J. (1990). The partial purification and characterization of GnRH-like activity from prostatic biopsy specimens and prostatic cancer cell lines. *J. Steroid Biochem. Mol. Biol.*, **37**, 899–902

36. Lasdun, A., Reznik, S., Molineaux, C. J. and Orlowski, M. (1989). Inhibition of endopeptidase 24.15 slows the *in vivo* degradation of LHRH. *J. Pharm. Exp. Ther.*, **251**, 439–47

37. Molineaux, C. J., Lasdun, A., Michaud, C. and Orlowski, M. (1988). Endopeptidase-24.15 is the primary enzyme that degrades LHRH both *in vitro* and *in vivo*. *J. Neurochem.*, **51**, 624–33

38. Maggi, R., Moretti, R. M., Montagnani Marelli, M., Pimpinelli, F. and Motta, M. (1995). Human prostatic carcinoma cell line LNCaP degrades luteinizing hormone-releasing hormone. *Int. J. Oncol.*, **6**, 1231–6

39. Berger, H., Schafer, H. Klauschenz, E., Albrecht, E. and Mehlis, B. (1982). Rapid assay for *in vitro* degradation of luteinizing hormone releasing hormone. *Anal. Biochem.*, **127**, 418–25

40. Berger, H., Pliet, R., Mann, L. and Mehlis, B. (1988). Proteolytic inactivation of luteinizing hormone-releasing hormone (LHRH) by the whole rat ovary *in vitro*. *Peptides*, **9**, 7–12

41. Carone, F. A., Stetler-Stevenson, M. A., May, V., LaBarbera, A. and Flouret, G. (1987). Differences between *in vitro* and *in vivo* degradation of LHRH by rat brain and other organs. *Am. J. Physiol.*, **253**, E317–21

LHRH analogs with cytotoxic radicals 4

A. V. Schally, A. Nagy, K. Szepeshazi, J. Pinski, G. Halmos, P. Armatis, M. Miyazaki, A. M. Comaru-Schally, T. Yano and G. Emons

INTRODUCTION AND BACKGROUND

Two classes of luteinizing hormone releasing hormone (LHRH) analogs consisting of agonists and antagonists have been developed so far for oncological and gynecological uses[1,2]. LHRH agonists provide the preferred primary treatment for advanced prostate carcinoma[2,3]. The use of LHRH agonists is an established therapy for estrogen-dependent premenopausal breast cancer[1,2]. LHRH agonists have been also used for the treatment of advanced epithelial ovarian cancer[1,4] and more recently endometrial cancer[1,5].

The efficacy of modern LHRH antagonists such as Cetrorelix (SB-75) have already been demonstrated in patients with prostate cancer[6,7] and benign prostate hyperplasia[6]. LHRH antagonists offer therapeutic advantages over the agonists because of rapidity of action and avoidance of flare-up in the disease[2,7,8]. Better responses to Cetrorelix than to LHRH agonists have been obtained in experimental models of breast and ovarian cancer[1,2,8–11]. Thus, LHRH antagonists such as Cetrorelix could also be of potential clinical value for the treatment of breast, ovarian and endometrial cancer[1,2].

Theoretical considerations for the targeting approach

The mechanism of action of LHRH analogs in oncology is based mainly on the inhibition of the pituitary–gonadal axis, but direct effects on various tumors may also play a role[1,2,8,12–14]. In patients with advanced breast or prostate cancer, the suppression of sex steroid secretion (medical castration) produced by administration of LHRH analogs accounts for most benefits derived from the treatment[1,2,12–14]. However, there is also evidence that LHRH agonists and antagonists can have direct effects on tumor cells[1,2]. In epithelial ovarian cancer, LHRH analogs might exert anti-tumor activity through the suppression of gonadotropin secretion (selective medical hypophysectomy)[1,2,10] but, in addition, direct anti-proliferative effects of LHRH analogs on ovarian cancer cells have been shown *in vitro*[1,2,10,15]. In endometrial cancer, experimental studies have similarly demonstrated direct anti-proliferative activity of LHRH analogs[1,2,16]. Estrogen deprivation induced by LHRH analogs, combined with these direct effects, might be used for treatment of some cases of endometrial cancer. The concept of direct action of LHRH analogs on cancers is based on evidence provided by clinical results, the effects on tumor cell lines in cultures and the detection of high-affinity binding sites for LHRH in various cancers[1,2,12–16].

Medical castration would not benefit postmenopausal women with breast cancer or patients with estrogen receptor (ER)-negative tumors, and responses to LHRH agonists in a small percentage of these cases are tentatively explained by direct effects of LHRH analogs on tumors[1,2,17–20].

Observations on growth inhibition of cultured tumor cells by LHRH analogs strongly support the concept of their direct effects. Significant inhibition *in vitro* of human breast and prostatic cancer cells by LHRH agonists is now well documented[21–27]. New LHRH antagonists such as Cetrorelix similarly cause a marked inhibition of proliferation of mammary, ovarian and endometrial cancer cell lines *in vitro*[1,10,27]. The presence of LHRH immunoreactivity and messenger ribonucleic acid (mRNA) for LHRH in human mammary cancer cells also suggests that LHRH may play a role in the growth of mammary tumors[21]. Similarly, the evidence for production of an LHRH-like peptide and/or expression of mRNA for LHRH was obtained in human prostate cancer and human ovarian and endometrial cancer lines[28–30]. Thus, LHRH-like peptides may function as local regulators of tumor growth.

Direct effects of LHRH analogs could be mediated by receptors found on tumor cells. Specific membrane receptors for LHRH have been found in specimens of human prostate cancers[13,31] and LNCaP and DU145 human prostate cancer lines[23,26]. Various investigators found LHRH receptors in several human mammary carcinoma cell lines[25,32,33]. Two classes of [D-Trp[6]]-LHRH binding sites were also detected in 260 of 500 samples of human breast cancers (52%), one class showing high affinity[34]. Both high-affinity and low-affinity LHRH receptors were found in human ovarian epithelial cancers and in EFO-21 and EFO-27 human ovarian cancer lines[1,15]. In human endometrial carcinomas and in HFC-1A and Ishikawa endometrial cancer lines, the presence of high-affinity membrane receptors for [D-Trp[6]]-LHRH was established[1,16]. LHRH receptors were also found in human pancreatic cancers[2,8,14]. The expression of the LHRH receptor gene in human breast and ovarian cancer cell lines was also demonstrated[1,21,28]. Nucleotide sequence of the LHRH receptor mRNA in human ovarian tumors and in the breast tumor MCF-7 cell line is identical with the human pituitary LHRH receptor mRNA[35]. These findings provide a rationale for devising therapeutic approaches based on the presence of LHRH receptors in malignancies in which these receptors are found.

This chapter discusses the development of a new class of anti-tumor agents based on LHRH agonists or antagonists linked to various cytotoxic radicals. After the agonists and antagonists, this could be the third class of LHRH analogs with anti-tumor activity.

Conventional versus targeted chemotherapy

Chemotherapy has been, for many decades, one of the main modalities for the systemic treatment of malignant neoplasms[36–41]. Chemotherapy can also be used as an adjuvant therapy to surgery, radiotherapy or hormone treatment[4,37–41]. In spite of the development of modern, more specific cytotoxic drugs, their non-selective toxic action on cells other than cancerous cells remains a major problem[36–44]. In addition, conventional chemotherapy is associated with a varying degree of response in the prostate, breast, ovarian and endometrial cancer[1,2,4,5,8,13,14,36–44].

In patients with advanced prostatic carcinoma, all palliative hormone therapies aimed at androgen deprivation, including LHRH analogs, can provide a clinical response in 70–80% of cases, but the duration of remission is limited and most patients will relapse in 18–36 months[2,3,13,40,43,45]. The relapse of prostate cancer is due to proliferation of androgen-independent cancer cells[40,45] and therapeutic options are limited for these patients. Conventional chemotherapy shows low response rates and high toxicity[2,40]. Targeted chemotherapy may be more effective and would greatly reduce the peripheral toxicity of cytotoxic agents.

Combination chemotherapy can be of substantial benefit to women with advanced, aggressive breast cancer who cannot be treated with endocrine therapy, but high doses which have to be employed produce toxic side effects[37–39,41,46]. Although chemotherapy is used in advanced epithelial ovarian cancer and in disseminated endometrial cancer, it is associated with significant side effects[1,2,4]. Frequently, in all these malignancies, the required doses of antineoplastic agents may not be applied or cannot be tolerated by patients[40].

Local delivery of therapeutic molecules to tumor cells would solve these complications. A new approach which is being developed to overcome the problem of non-selective toxic effects on normal cells is the targeting of tumor cells, which is based upon the selectivity of carrier molecules for specific binding sites in tumor tissues[1,2,8,12–16,36,47]. Chemotherapeutic compounds and toxins can be covalently attached to various carriers, including hormones, for which receptors are present on cancer cells or to antibodies that preferentially recognize tumor cells[2,36,47]. Such conjugates are designed to deliver cytotoxic agents more selectively to cancer cells. Ideally, tumor cells that bind these conjugates would be killed, while normal cells that do not have the receptors would be spared[2,8,47]. The cytotoxic conjugate could exert its effect after internalization or simply by binding to the cell surface, without entering the cell[48–51].

Since specific high-affinity binding sites for LHRH are present in about 50% of breast cancer specimens[34], including estrogen-receptor (ER)-negative samples[34], as well as about 80% of ovarian cancers[1,15], 77% of endometrial carcinomas[1,16] and a very high percentage of prostate cancers[31], targeted chemotherapy based on cytotoxic LHRH analogs could be more efficacious and less toxic than conventional regimens of antineoplastic agents[2,12–14].

On the basis of the presence of specific LHRH receptors on human tumor cells and reports on the direct action of LHRH analogs, a new class of anti-tumor drugs has been developed in our institute by linking cytotoxic radicals to LHRH agonists and antagonists[2,8,12–14,46,52–60]. Such cytotoxic hybrids could be tried, not only for treatment of prostate and breast cancers, but also ovarian and endometrial cancer[1,2]. Cytotoxic compounds linked to hormonal peptides such as LHRH, that might be targeted to certain cancers having receptors for those peptides, and that would more selectively kill cancer cells, could be of major therapeutic importance[2]. This approach might extend the applications of analogs of LHRH from the current palliation toward an eventual cure[2].

DESIGN AND SYNTHESIS OF CYTOTOXIC LHRH ANALOGS

The first targeted chemotherapeutic agents developed for the treatment of prostate cancer and breast cancer used estrogenic steroid molecules as carriers for various alkylating agents[44]. Nitrogen mustard compounds were chemically coupled to carrier estrogens for enhancing selectivity and cytotoxicity on ER-positive cells[42–44]. These cytotoxic estrogens, such as estracyte (estramustine), accumulate in the rat prostate due to the presence in the ventral lobe of the prostate of a protein that binds estramustine with high affinity and high capacity. However, estramustine has low affinity for the 'conventional' ERs[42,43]. Estracyte has been used clinically in

patients with hormone refractory prostate cancer[43] and in women with advanced carcinoma of the breast[61], but objective response rates are low. The use of other hormonal carriers that could increase the efficacy of chemotherapeutic agents appeared to be worthy of extensive exploration[2].

In order to take advantage of the presence of LHRH receptors on various tumors we designed, synthesized and developed a novel class of anti-tumor peptides based on LHRH agonists and antagonists linked to various cytotoxic radicals[36,52–54,60]. Our early compounds contained nitrogen mustard or metal complexes. Thus, metal complexes related to cisplatin [*cis*-diammine-dichloroplatinum] were incorporated into LHRH analogs containing D-lysine at position 6. Some of the metallopeptides thus obtained proved to be highly active LHRH agonists or antagonists. For instance, SB-40, a $PtCl_2$-containing metallopeptide in which platinum is incorporated into an N^ε-(D,L-2,3-diaminopropionyl)-D-lysine residue [D-Lys(D,L-A_2pr)] at position 6, showed 50 times higher LH releasing potency than the native hormone. Most metallopeptide analogs of LHRH showed high-binding affinities for the membrane receptors of rat pituitary and human breast cancer cells[53]. Some of these cytotoxic compounds had endocrine and/or tumoricidal activity *in vivo*[53].

The alkylating-nitrogen mustard derivatives of phenylalanine (Melphalan, Mel) (Figure 1) have been also linked to LHRH analogs. To obtain highly potent alkylating analogs of LHRH, the D enantiomer of Mel was incorporated into position 6 of the native hormone and some of its antagonistic analogs[52]. [D-Mel[6]]-LHRH (SB-05) and [Ac-D-Nal(2)[1], D-Phe(4Cl)[2], D-Pal(3)[3], Arg[5], D-Mel[6], D-Ala[10]]-LHRH (SB-86) possessed the expected high agonistic and antagonistic activities, respectively, and also showed high affinities for the membrane receptors of rat pituitary cells and rat Dunning R-3327 prostate tumor cells[52]. These two analogs exerted cytotoxic effects on human and rat mammary cancer cells *in vitro*, as shown by inhibition of [³H]thymidine incorporation into DNA. Thus, these two alkylating D-Mel[6] analogs of LHRH seemed to be suitable for interfering with intracellular events in certain cancer cells[52]. Nitrogen mustard compounds (chlorambucil, cyclophosphamide, Melphalan) are among the

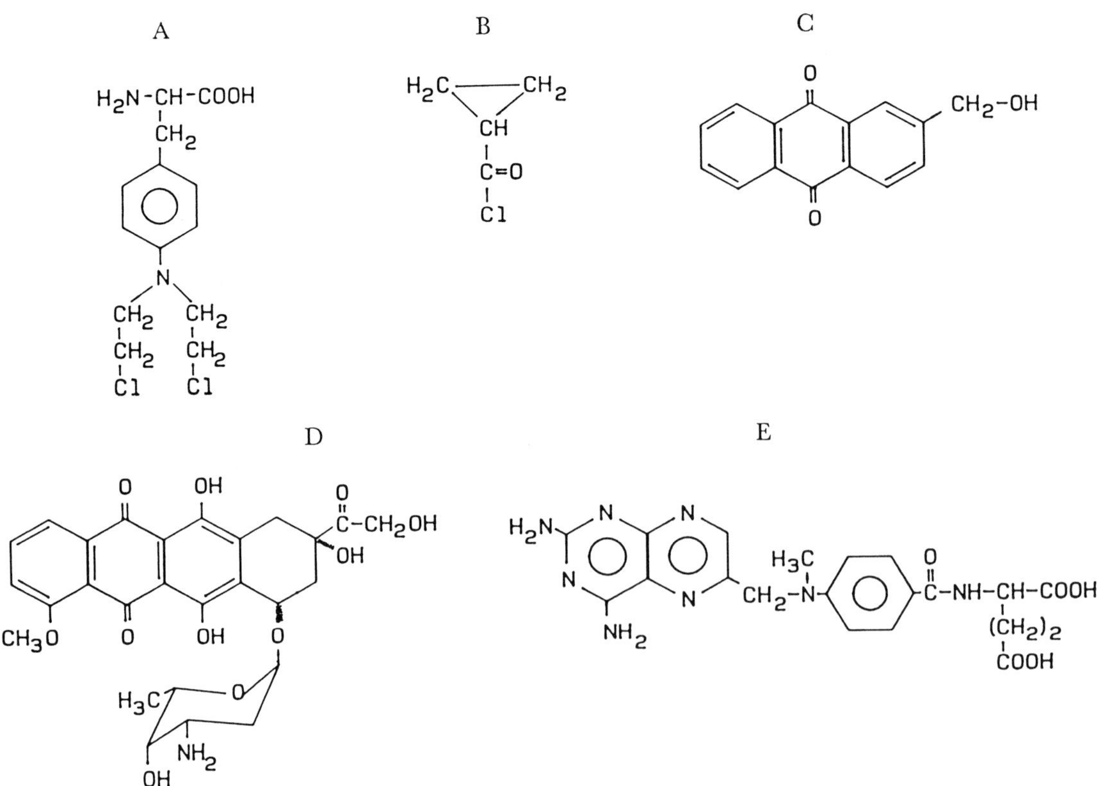

Figure 1 Structures of some cytotoxic compounds that can be incorporated into peptide analogs: (A) Melphalan (Mel); (B) cyclopropanecarbonyl (CPC) chloride; (C) (2-hydroxymethyl)anthraquinone (HMAQ); (D) Doxorubicin (DOX); and (E) methotrexate (MTX). Modified from Janáky, T., Juhász, A., Rékási, Z. *et al.* (1992) Short-chain analogs of luteinizing hormone-releasing hormone containing cytotoxic moieties. *Proc. Natl. Acad. Sci. USA*, **89**, 10203–7[54]. Reproduced with permission of the National Academy of Sciences

oldest anti-cancer drugs in clinical use. Alkylating agents used in the treatment of cancer exert cytotoxic effects through transfer of their alkyl groups to various cell components. Alkylation of DNA within the nucleus probably represents the main interaction that leads to cell death.

In an effort to produce better cytotoxic analogs, chemotherapeutic–antineoplastic radicals, including reactive cyclopropane, an alkylating agent, anthraquinone derivatives (2-hydroxymethyl)anthraquinone (HMAQ) and anti-cancer antibiotic adriamycin (Doxorubicin) and antimetabolite, methotrexate (MTX) (Figure 1), were linked to suitably modified agonists and antagonists of LHRH which function as carriers[2,8,36].

Anthraquinone derivatives, including the anthracycline antibiotic adriamycin, daunomycin, and Novantrone (mitoxantrone dihydrochloride), an anthracenedione with some structural similarities to adriamycin, are also widely used as bioreductive intercalating antineoplastic agents[36,41,48–51,57]. These compounds bind to DNA through intercalation between specific bases, inhibit RNA and DNA synthesis, cause DNA strand scission and interfere with cell replication. Although derivatives of 2-(hydroxymethyl) anthraquinone (HMAQ) show less cytotoxic activity than Adriamycin or Novantrone, they are stable and suitable for coupling to peptides[36,57]. In order to attach this anthraquinone derivative to a free amino group in the peptide, glutaric acid was used as a spacer in G-HMAQ[36].

MTX was used as the cytotoxic radical, because of its efficacy as an anti-cancer agent in clinical use, its chemical stability and suitability for coupling to amino acids. MTX is a folic acid antagonist that inhibits dihydrofolic acid reductase and interferes with DNA, RNA and protein synthesis and cellular replication[36,41,57,60]. These cytotoxic compounds were linked to agonistic analogs with D-lysine[6] or antagonist such as [Ac-D-Nal(2)[1], D-Phe(4Cl)[2], D-Trp[3], Arg[5], D-Lys[6], D-Ala[10]]-LHRH[36]. Two cytotoxic molecules could be conjugated to one carrier through (2,3-diaminopropionyl)-substituents on the N^ε of D-lysine[36]. The enhanced biological activities produced by the incorporation of D amino acids into position 6 of the agonistic analogs were further increased by the attachment of hydrophobic cytotoxic groups, resulting in compounds with much higher hormonal activity than LHRH. Most of the hybrid agonistic analogs showed high binding affinities for the membrane receptors of human breast cancer cells[36]. The hybrid antagonist inhibited ovulation in rats and suppressed LH release *in vitro*. The binding affinity of cytotoxic antagonists to receptors on human breast cancer membranes was decreased compared to the precursor peptides, although analogs with 2-(hydroxymethyl)anthraquinone hemiglutarate have high affinity[36]. All the cytotoxic analogs tested inhibited [³H]thymidine incorporation into DNA in cultures of various human breast cancer lines such as MCF-7 and MDA-MB-231 and prostate cancer cell lines, PC-3- and LNCaP[36]. Some cytotoxic analogs also significantly suppressed the growth of mammary and prostate cancers *in vivo* in animal models (see below)[40,46,57]. Preliminary testing in the ovarian cancer cell lines EFO-21 and EFO-27 showed that their *in vitro* proliferation was inhibited by cytotoxic antagonist T-144 containing two residues of G-HMAQ and agonistic analog AJ-04 with methotrexate. This inhibition was significantly greater than that exerted by the respective carrier peptides. Similarly, in the endometrial cancer cell lines Ishikawa and HEC-1, another cytotoxic antagonist T-121/B as well as T-144 had strong anti-proliferative activity, which was markedly higher than that of the respective carrier peptides. A systemic evaluation in ovarian and endometrial cancer lines is in progress (Emons *et al.*, in prep.).

Short-chain hexapeptide and heptapeptide analogs of LHRH were also synthesized for use as carriers for cytotoxic compounds[54]. Short cytotoxic analogs would be easier to test because their short carriers based on LHRH sequences[3–9] were expected to have no biological and therefore no oncological activity *in vivo*, in contrast to long-decapeptide carriers. Melphalan, Doxorubicin, methotrexate and cisplatin-like platinum complex were linked to these peptides in position 6. The hybrid molecules showed no LHRH agonistic activity or characteristic antagonistic activity *in vitro* and *in vivo*. Several of these analogs showed high receptor-binding affinities to rat pituitaries, human breast cancer and rat Dunning prostate cancer, and exerted some cytotoxic effects on MCF-7 breast cancer cell line[54]. However, no conclusive oncological activity could be demonstrated *in vivo* in Dunning prostate cancer in rats or MXT-breast cancer models in mice.

ONCOLOGICAL TESTS *IN VIVO*

Inhibition of growth of Dunning R-3327H prostate cancer in rats

The effects of hybrid cytotoxic LHRH analogs produced by linking anthraquinone or methotrexate to carrier agonist [D-Lys[6]]-LHRH were evaluated[40] in rats bearing Dunning R-3327H prostate adenocarcinoma. The two cytotoxic analogs T-98 [(D-Lys[6])-LHRH coupled to glutaryl-2-(hydroxymethyl)anthraquinone (G-HMAQ)], and AJ-04 [(D-Lys[6])-LHRH linked to methotrexate (MTX)], carrier [D-Lys[6]]-LHRH, or the free cytotoxic compounds MTX and G-HMAQ were administered from osmotic minipumps for 7–8 weeks. The cytotoxic LHRH analogs caused somewhat greater tumor growth inhibition than the carrier peptide, while anthraquinone or methotrexate alone, given in equimolar doses, were ineffective. Histological evaluation showed that the inhibition of mitosis and the frequency of apoptosis were higher in tumors treated with AJ-04, T-98, [D-Lys[6]]-LHRH than in control tumors. Serum LH and testosterone levels were lowered by both carrier peptide and cytotoxic analogs. Since suppression of androgen sensitive organs (testes, ventral prostates and seminal vesicles) was similar with both carrier and cytotoxic analogs, a somewhat greater inhibition of tumor growth after treatment with T-98 and AJ-04, compared with [D-Lys[6]]-LHRH, implies more than a simple endocrine action in inhibition of tumor growth. T-98 administration at a therapeutically effective dose does not cause any myelosuppression in rats. No signs of suppression or damage to the hematopoietic system such as lymphopenia, erythropenia or neutropenia were observed. The total and differential blood count was not significantly different in animals treated with T-98 as compared to controls[40]. These results indicate that LHRH analogs containing cytotoxic radicals anthraquinone or methotrexate retain their hormonal activity after administration *in vivo* and can effectively inhibit prostate cancer growth[40].

Inhibition of growth of estrogen-independent MXT mouse mammary carcinoma *in vivo*

Three cytotoxic LHRH analogs were tested in mice bearing MXT estrogen-independent mammary tumors[57]. Cytotoxic LHRH analogs AJ-04, (agonist [D-Lys[6]]-LHRH linked to methotrexate [MTX]), T-98 ([D-Lys[6]]-LHRH coupled to glutaryl-2-(hydroxymethyl)anthraquinone (G-HMAQ) and T-121/B (antagonist T-147, Ac-D-Nal(2)-D-Phe(4Cl)-D-Trp-Ser-Arg-D-Lys[A$_2$pr]-Leu-Arg-Pro-D-Ala-NH$_2$ containing two residues of G-HMAQ) were administered from osmotic minipumps for 3 weeks to female BDF$_1$ mice bearing MXT ((3.2)/Ovex) estrogen-independent mammary tumors. All three cytotoxic LHRH analogs produced a significant inhibition of tumor growth. The effects of T-98 and T121/B were superior to those obtained by treatment with equimolar doses of cytotoxic moiety anthraquinone or with LHRH carriers. MTX alone also had an anti-tumor effect, which can be explained by a strong inhibitory action of this cytotoxic agent on fast growing tumors. In contrast, G-HMAQ alone had no significant effect on tumor growth and was toxic. Treatment with the carrier agonist [D-Lys[6]]-LHRH resulted in a slight inhibition of tumor growth, but the cytotoxic analogs based on this agonist linked to cytotoxic radical MTX or G-HMAQ were more effective than the carrier in both experiments. The carrier antagonist T-147 had little effect on tumor growth[57]. It appeared that cytotoxic LHRH analogs inhibit tumor growth through a combined hormonal and cytotoxic effect and that linking to the carrier reduces toxicity after administration *in vivo*[57].

Chronic *in vivo* treatment of mice bearing MXT cancers with cytotoxic LHRH analogs AJ-04 and T-121/B, but not with T-98, produced a significant down-regulation of membrane receptors for LHRH on mammary tumors[58]. Administration of cytotoxic LHRH analogs, AJ-04, T-98 and especially T-121/B also reduced maximal binding capacity of epidermal growth factor (EGF) receptors[58]. This interference with EGF receptors might be useful in the treatment of breast and other cancers[58].

Studies in estrogen-dependent MXT mouse breast cancers

In a subsequent study, the authors investigated the accumulation of analog in tumors and correlation between growth characteristics and epidermal growth factor (EGF) receptor content of estrogen-dependent MXT mouse mammary cancers during treatment with cytotoxic LHRH analog T-98[46]. Female BDF mice bearing estrogen-dependent MXT mouse mammary cancers were treated for 4 weeks with T-98 (agonist [D-Lys[6]]-LHRH linked to glutaryl-2(hydroxy-methyl)anthraquinone) or equimolar amounts of the cytotoxic moiety G-HMAQ and carrier [D-Lys[6]]-LHRH[46]. Both T-98 and [D-Lys[6]]-LHRH significantly inhibited the growth of MXT cancers, but G-HMAQ had only a minor effect. Cytotoxic analog T-98 and the carrier [D-Lys[6]]-LHRH inhibited ovarian and uterine weights and serum estradiol to a similar extent, but T-98 caused a greater reduction in tumor volume and mitotic activity in tumor cells than the carrier[46]. Tumor inhibition by T-98 was linked to a significant decrease in binding capacity of EGF receptors in tumor cell membranes. The concentration of EGF receptors remained high in tumors that continued to enlarge in spite of treatment and in all control untreated tumors, even small ones[46]. Thus, the reduction in EGF receptors is probably due to the therapy with T-98. Three hours after the injection of radiolabeled T-98, a higher radioactivity was accumulated in tumors as compared to other organs. The pituitaries showed higher radio-activities at later periods. This indicates that specific targeting and local delivery of T-98 might play a role in the anti-tumor effect exerted by this cytotoxic analog[46].

Growth inhibition of MCF-7 MIII human breast cancer xenografts in nude mice by treatment with cytotoxic LHRH analog AJ-04 containing methotrexate

In nude mice bearing MCF-7 MIII human breast cancer, cytotoxic analog AJ-04 also inhibited tumor growth (Yano *et al.*, in prep.). The reduction in tumor volume and tumor weight produced by administration of 16.7 μg (8.7 nmol)/day of AJ-04 was highly significant in comparison to controls and greater than that caused by the daily injection of equimolar amounts of methotrexate or carrier [D-Lys^6]-LHRH. There were no changes in body weights between various groups. AJ-04 also reduced percentage increase in tumor volume, tumor burden and increased tumor doubling time (Yano *et al.*, in prep.).

MECHANISM-MODE OF ACTION OF CYTOTOXIC ANALOGS OF LHRH

The authors' work shows that LHRH analogs might serve as carriers for chemotherapeutic agents. The conjugates would deliver cytotoxic agents more selectively to target cells by binding to receptors on cell membranes of tumors. The conjugate must preserve the binding affinity of the carrier to the specific binding sites. Binding kinetics and analyses of displacement curves of [^{125}I][D-Trp^6]-LHRH and [^{125}I]T-98 in membranes of human breast cancer and estrogen-independent MXT mouse mammary cancer suggest that binding of the cytotoxic analog T-98 to the LHRH receptor proceeds reversibly, like that of its congeners without cytotoxic radicals[59]. The

cytotoxic conjugate may exert its effect after internalization[62] or simply by binding to the cell surface, without entering the cell[48–51]. The release of the cytotoxic radical is likely to occur following endocytosis of the hybrid molecules if the carrier or the chemical bond of conjugation is sensitive to enzymatic cleavage within the cell. This could be followed by a chain of events that might result in interference with the replication of neoplastic cells, or even their destruction. The binding and internalization of the cytotoxic analog T-98 (agonist [D-Lys^6]-LHRH linked to glutaryl-2-(hydroxymethyl)anthraquinone), by rat anterior pituitary cells was investigated[56]. Analog T-98 was bound to pituitary membrane binding sites for LHRH with a high affinity (K_d = 1.2 nM) and was 17 times more potent in releasing luteinizing hormone (LH) than LHRH. The labeling of this cytotoxic LHRH analog with radioactive [^{125}I] did not significantly affect its binding affinity, but greatly decreased its LH-releasing activity. In cultured pituitary cells, binding and internalization of [^{125}I]T-98 were observed, which were time and temperature-dependent. Binding resistant to 0.2 M acetic acid assumed to be due to the internalized analogue was small at 6 min, but increased continuously in time and exceeded the surface binding at about 45 min. At 2 hours, about 70% of total cell-associated radioactivity was found to be acid resistant[36]. The authors' results indicate that T-98 is internalized by pituitary gonadotropes through receptor-mediated endocytosis[56]. Their findings also suggest that this cytotoxic LHRH agonist may also be internalized by LHRH receptors present in breast, prostate, ovarian and endometrial cancers[56]. However, the internalization or the release of the cytotoxic moieties from the carrier hormone by the splitting of the bond between the drug and the peptide may not be an essential requirement, since cytotoxic drugs linked to peptides by non-hydrolyzable covalent bonds can produce active drug carrier conjugates, as shown by Varga[48,49] and others[50,51]. When daunomycin was coupled to peptide melanocyte stimulating hormone (MSH), the conjugate proved to be more toxic to murine melanoma cells than the free drug[48].

The damage caused by cytotoxic analogs to pituitary LH- and follicle stimulating hormone

(FSH)-secreting cells would not be detrimental to the cancer patient, since hypophysectomy has been used for treatment of some sex hormone-dependent cancers. A possible damage to other cells (e.g. corticotropes, thyrotropes) could be also alleviated by appropriate replacement therapy[2]. The authors' work indicates that in the pituitary cell superfusion system, cytotoxic LHRH analogs selectively affected LH cells, but not growth hormone (GH) and prolactin (PRL) cells[55]. Thus, four cytotoxic LHRH analogs were tested in a long-term superfusion system in order to determine their effects on different types of rat pituitary cells[55]. The compounds investigated included two cytotoxic agonists, T-98 ([D-Lys^6]-LHRH coupled to glutaryl-2-(hydroxy-methyl)anthraquinone [G-HMAQ]) and T-107 ([DLys^6]-LHRH linked to Doxorubicin through glutaric acid spacer), and two cytotoxic antagonists T-121 and T-144, both containing two residues of G-HMAQ. The analogs were infused for 24 hours at pharmacological concentrations. The secretions of LH, GH and PRL after the treatment were compared to those before the analog infusion. All four cytotoxic LHRH analogs selectively decreased the stimulated LH response, while the release of GH and PRL was not influenced. The inhibitory effects of cytotoxic LHRH agonists and antagonists on LHRH-induced LH release were significantly greater than those of their parent peptides. Cytotoxic LHRH agonists and their carriers caused depletion of LH pools, while cytotoxic LHRH antagonists or their parent peptides decreased the available binding sites for LHRH. Equimolar concentrations of cytotoxic radicals alone (Doxorubicin or G-HMAQ), however, caused functional damage to all types of cells tested. The inhibitory effect of Doxorubicin on stimulated secretion of LH, GH and PRL in the authors' system could be due to an action on cell membranes. The authors' work indicated that, in the pituitary cell superfusion system, targeted cytotoxic LHRH analogs selectively affect LH cells, in contrast to unconjugated cytotoxic radicals, which also damage GH and PRL cells. Based on our results in the course of clinical applications of these analogs, the damage to gonadotrope cells can be expected as the only side effect on the pituitary.

CONCLUSION

In conclusion, various cytotoxic LHRH analogs have been synthesized and tested in diverse *in vitro* and *in vivo* systems. Because the anti-tumor action of such analogs may be exerted to a greater degree at selective sites that have the cell membrane receptors, the peripheral toxicity on normal cells that do not bind cytotoxic analogs would be reduced[2]. Improved cytotoxic compounds containing Doxorubicin derivatives linked to LHRH analogs have now been synthesized. An advantage of using Doxorubicin as a radical for linking to peptide analogs is that anthracyclin antibiotics may be cytotoxic without entering the cells[48–51]. Such analogs containing Doxorubicin may kill cancer cells by membrane action on the cell surface[48–51]. These new cytotoxic LHRH analogs are undergoing complex mass spectra and nuclear magnetic resonance (NMR) analyses aimed at the structural confirmation (Nagy *et al.*, in prep.). In parallel *in vivo* studies, oncological responses and toxicity are being investigated in animal tumor models and in human breast, ovarian, prostate and pancreatic cancer cell lines xenografted into nude mice. Preliminary results indicate that the activity of these new cytotoxic LHRH analogs may be one or two orders of magnitude higher than that of previous cytotoxic hybrids (Nagy *et al.*, in prep.). The ongoing development of LHRH analogs as carriers for targeted cytotoxic radicals, such as Doxorubicin derivatives, could result in therapeutic agents endowed with both a hormonal action and a local tumoricidal effect[2]. This approach, which still remains to be tested clinically, may improve considerably present methods of treatment and convert the current palliative therapy produced by LHRH analogs into an eventual cure.

ACKNOWLEDGEMENTS

Some experimental work described in this paper was supported by USPHS Grants CA 40003 and 40004 and by the Medical Research Service of the Veterans Affairs Department. The authors are grateful to Professor Juergen Engel, Dr M. Bernd Asta Medica, Frankfurt/M and Dr E. Busker, Degussa, Hanau-Wolfgang, Germany, for valuable advice and extensive help with mass spectra and NMR analyses.

References

1. Emons, G. and Schally, A. V. (1994). The use of luteinizing hormone releasing hormone agonists and antagonists in gynaecological cancers. *Hum. Reprod.*, **9**, 1364–79

2. Schally, A. V., Comaru-Schally, A. M. and Hollander, V. (1993). Hypothalamic and other peptide hormones. In Holland J. F., Frei, E., Bast, R. C., Kufe, D. W., Morton, D. L. and Weichselbaum, R. R. (eds.) *Cancer Medicine*, 3rd ed., pp. 827–40. (Philadelphia, PA: Lea & Febiger)

3. Crawford, D .E. (1990). Hormonal therapy of prostatic carcinoma. Defining the challenge. *Oncology*, **66**, 1035–8

4. Parmar, H., Phillips, R. H., Rustin, G., Lightman, S. L. and Schally, A. V. (1988). Therapy of advanced ovarian cancer with D-Trp^6-LHRH (decapeptyl) microcapsules. *Biomed. Pharmacother.*, **42**, 531–8

5. Gallagher, C. J., Oliver, R. T. D., Oram, D. H., Fowler, C. G., Blake, P. R., Mantell, B. S., Slevin, M.L. and Hope-Stone, H.F. (1991). A new treatment for endometrial cancer with gonadotrophin-releasing hormone analogue. *Br. J. Obstet. Gynaecol.*, **98**, 1037–41

6. Gonzalez-Barcena, D., Vadillo-Buenfil, M., Gomez Orta, F., Fuentes-Garcia, M., Cardenas-Cornejo, I., Graef-Sanchez, A., Comaru-Schally, A. M. and Schally, A. V.(1994). Responses to the antagonistic analog of LH-RH (SB-75) (Cetrorelix) in patients with benign prostatic hyperplasia and prostatic cancer. *Prostate*, **24**, 84–92

7. Gonzalez-Barcena, B., Vadillo-Buenfil, M., Cortez-Morales, A., Fuentes-Garcia, M., Cardenas-Cornejo, I., Comaru-Schally, A. M. and Schally, A. V. (1995). LHRH antagonist SB-75 (Cetrorelix) as primary single therapy in patients with advanced prostatic cancer and paraplegia due to metastatic invasion of spinal cord. *Urology*, **45**, 275–81

8. Schally, A. V. (1994). Hypothalamic hormones: from neuroendocrinology to cancer therapy. *Anticancer Drugs*, **5**, 115–30

9. Szende, B., Srkalovic, G., Groot, K., Lapis, K. and Schally, A. V. (1990). Growth inhibition of mouse MXT mammary tumor by the luteinizing hormone-releasing hormone antagonist SB-75. *J. Natl. Cancer Inst.*, **82**, 513–17

10. Yano, T., Pinski, J., Halmos, G., Szepeshazi, K., Groot, K. and Schally, A. V. (1994). Inhibition of growth of OV-1063 human epithelial ovarian cancer xenografts in nude mice by treatment with luteinizing hormone-releasing hormone antagonist SB-75. *Proc. Natl. Acad. Sci. USA*, **91**, 7090–4

11. Yano, T., Pinski, J., Szepeshazi, K., Halmos, G., Radulovic, S., Groot, K., and Schally, A. V. (1994). Inhibitory effect of bombesin/gastrin releasing peptide antagonist RC-3095 and luteinizing hormone-releasing hormone antagonist SB-75 on the growth of MCF-7 MIII human breast cancer xenografts in athymic nude mice. *Cancer*, **73**, 1229–38

12. Schally, A. V., Bajusz, S., Redding, T. W., Zalatnai, A. and Comaru-Schally, A. M. (1989). Analogs of LHRH: the present and the future. In Vickery, B.H. and Lunenfeld, V. (eds.) *GnRH Analogues in Cancer and in Human Reproduction, Basic Aspects*, Vol. 1, pp. 5–31. (Dordrecht/Boston/London: Kluwer Academic Publishers)

13. Schally, A. V., Comaru-Schally, A. M. and Gonzalez-Barcena, D. (1992). Present status of agonistic and antagonistic analogs of LHRH in the treatment of advanced prostate cancer. *Biomed. Pharmacother.*, **46**, 465–47

14. Schally, A. V., Radulovic, S., and Comaru-Schally, A. M. (1993). Experimental and clinical studies in hormone dependent cancers. In Mazzaferri, E. and Samaan, N. (eds.) *Endocrine Tumors*, pp. 49–73. (Boston: Blackwell Scientific Publications Inc.)

15. Emons, G., Ortmann, O., Becker, M., Irmer, G., Springer, B., Laun, R., Hölzel, F., Schulz, K.-D. and Schally, A. V. (1993). High affinity binding and direct antiproliferative effects of LHRH analogues in human ovarian cancer cell lines. *Cancer Res.*, **53**, 5439–46

16. Emons, G., Schröder, B., Ortmann, O., Westphalen, S., Schulz, K.-D. and Schally, A.V. (1993). High affinity binding and direct antiproliferative effects of LHRH analogues in human endometrial cancer cell lines. *J. Clin. Endocrinol. Metab.*, **77**, 1458–64

17. Harris, A. L., Carmichael, J., Cantwell, B. M. J. and Dowsett, M. (1989). Zoladex: endocrine and therapeutic effects in post-menopausal breast cancer. *Br. J. Cancer*, **59**, 97–9

18. Saphner, T., Troxel, A. B., Tormey, D. C., Neuberg, D., Robert, N. J., Pandya, K. J., Edmonson, J. H., Rosenbluth, R. J. and Abeloff, M. D. (1993). Phase II study of goserelin for patients

with postmenopausal metastatic breast cancer. *J. Clin. Oncology*, **11**, 1529–35

19. Plowman, P. N., Nicholson, R. I. and Walker, K. J. (1986). Remission of postmenopausal breast cancer during treatment with the luteinizing hormone releasing hormone agonist ICI 118630. *Br. J. Cancer*, **54**, 903–9

20. Kaufmann, M., Jonat, W., Kleeburg, U., Eirmann, W., Janicke, F., Hilfrich, J., Kreienberg, R., Albrecht, M., Weitzel, H. K., Schmid, H., Strunz, P., Schachner-Wunschmann, E., Bastert, G. and Maass, H. (1989). The German zoladex trial group: goserelin, a depot gonadotropin releasing hormone agonist in the treatment of premenopausal patients with metastatic breast cancer. *J. Clin. Oncol.*, **7**, 1113–19

21. Harris, N. S., Dutlow, C., Eidne, K., Dong, K.-W., Roberts, J. and Millar, R. P. (1991). Gonadotropin-releasing hormone gene expression in MDA-MB-231 and ZR-75-1 breast carcinoma cell lines. *Cancer Res.*, **51**, 2577–81

22. Klijn, J. G. M., de Jong F. H., Lamberts F. W. and Blankenstein M. A. (1985). LHRH agonist treatment in clinical and experimental human breast cancer. *J. Steroid Biochem.*, **23**, 867–73

23. Limonta, P., Dondi, D., Moretti, R. M., Maggi, R. and Motta, M. (1992). Antiproliferative effects of luteinizing hormone-releasing hormone agonists on the human prostatic cancer cell line LNCaP. *J. Clin. Endocrinol. Metab.*, **75**, 207–12

24. Loop, S. M., Gorder, C. A., Lewis, S. M., Drivdahl, R. H. and Ostenson, R. C. (1995). Growth inhibition of human prostate tumor cells by an agonist of gonadotrophin-releasing hormone. *Prostate*, **26**, 179–88

25. Miller, W. R., Scott W. N., Morris, R., Fraser, H. M. and Sharpe, R. M. (1985). Growth of human breast cancer cells inhibited by a luteinizing hormone-releasing hormone agonist. *Nature*, **313**, 231–3

26. Qayum, A., Gullick, W., Clayton, R. C., Sikora K. and Waxman, J. (1990). The effects of gonadotrophin releasing hormone analogues in prostate cancer are mediated through specific tumor receptors. *Br. J. Cancer*, **62**, 96–9

27. Sharoni, Y., Bosin, E., Miinster, A., Levy, J., and Schally, A. V. (1989). Inhibition of growth of human mammary tumor cells by potent antagonists of luteinizing hormone-releasing hormone. *Proc. Natl. Acad. Sci. USA*, **86**, 1648–51

28. Irmer, G., Bürger, C., Müller, R., Ortmann, O., Peter, U., Kakar, S. S., Neill, J. D., Schulz, K.-D. and Emons, G. (1995). Expression of the messenger ribonucleic acids for luteinizing hormone-releasing hormone and its receptor in human ovarian epithelial carcinoma. *Cancer Res.*, **55**, 817–22

29. Limonta, P., Dondi, D., Moretti, R. M., Fermo, D., Garattini, E. and Motta, M. (1993). Expression of luteinizing hormone-releasing hormone mRNA in the human prostatic cancer cell line LNCaP. *J. Clin. Endocrinol. Metab.*, **76**, 797–800

30. Irmer, G., Bürger, C., Ortmann, O., Schulz, K.-D., and Emons, G. (1994). Expression of luteinizing hormone releasing hormone and its mRNA in human endometrial cancer cell lines. *J. Clin. Endocrinol. Metab.*, **79**, 916–19

31. Fekete, M., Redding, T. W., Comaru-Schally, A. M., Pontes, A. E., Connelly, R. W., Srkalovic ,G., and Schally, A. V. (1989). Receptors for luteinizing hormone-releasing hormone, somatostatin, prolactin and epidermal growth factor in rat and human prostate cancers and in benign prostatic hyperplasia. *Prostate*, **14**, 191–208

32. Eidne, K. A., Flanagan, C. A., Harris, N. S. and Millar, R. P. (1987). Gonadotropin-releasing hormone (GnRH)-binding sites in human breast cancer cell lines and inhibitory effects of GnRH antagonists. *J. Clin. Endocrinol. Metab.*, **64**, 425–32

33. Yano, T., Korkut, E., Pinski, J., Szepeshazi, K., Milovanovic, S., Groot, K., Clarke, R., Comaru-Schally, A. M., and Schally, A. V. (1992). Inhibition of growth of MCF-7 MIII human breast carcinoma in nude mice by treatment with agonists or antagonists of LH-RH. *Breast Cancer Res. Treat.*, **21**, 35–45

34. Fekete, M., Wittliff, J. L. and Schally, A. V. (1989). Characteristics and distribution of receptors for [D-Trp6]-luteinizing hormone-releasing hormone, somatostatin, epidermal growth factor, and sex steroids in 500 biopsy samples of human breast cancer. *J. Clin. Lab. Anal.*, **3**, 137–47

35. Kakar, S. S., Grizzle, W. E. and Neill, J. D. (1994). The nucleotide sequences of human GnRH receptors in breast and ovarian tumors are identical with that found in pituitary. *Mol. Cell Endocrinol.*, **106**, 145–9

36. Janáky, T., Juhász, A., Bajusz, S., Csernus, V., Srkalovic, G., Bokser, L., Milovanovic, S. R., Redding, T. W., Rékási, Z., Nagy, A. and Schally, A. V. (1992). Analogues of luteinizing hormone-releasing hormone containing cytotoxic groups. *Proc. Natl. Acad. Sci. USA*, **89**, 972–6

37. Carbone, P. P., Nixon, D. W., Fennelly, J., Greenberg, E., Henderson, I. C., Hortobagyi, G.,

Kennedy, B. J., Trainin, N. and Scanlon, E. F. (1990). Adjuvant systemic therapy. *Cancer*, **65**, 2108–9

38. Tormey, D. C., Gray, R., Gilchrist, K., Grage, T., Carbone, P. P., Wolter, J., Woll, J. E. and Cummings, F.J. (1990). Adjuvant chemohormonal therapy with cyclophosphamide, methotrexate, 5-fluorouracil, and prednisone (CMFP) or CMFP plus tamoxifen compared with CMF for premenopausal breast cancer patients. *Cancer*, **65**, 200–6

39. Bonadonna, G. (1993) From adjuvant to neo-adjuvant chemotherapy in high-risk breast cancer: the experience of the Milan Cancer Institute. Steiner Award Lecture 1992. *Int. J. Cancer*, **55**, 1–4

40. Pinski, J., Schally, A. V., Yano, T., Szepeshazi, K., Halmos, G., Groot, K., Comaru-Schally, A. M., Radulovic, S. and Nagy, A. (1993). Inhibition of growth of experimental prostate cancer in rats by LHRH analogs linked to cytotoxic radicals. *Prostate*, **23**, 165–78

41. Chabner, B. (1990). *Cancer Chemotherapy. Principles and Practice*. (Philadelphia: J.B. Lippincott)

42. Konyves, I. (1989). Estramustine phosphate (Estracyt) in the treatment of prostate carcinoma. *Int. Urol. Nephrol.*, 21, 393–7

43. Konyves, I., Muntzing, J. and Rozencweig, M. (1984). Chemotherapy principles in the treatment of prostatic cancer. *Prostate*, **5**, 55–62

44. Konyves, I. and Liljekvist, J. (1975). The steroid molecule as a carrier of cytotoxic groups. In *Biological Characterization of Human Tumors. Excerpta Medica International Congress Series 375*, pp. 98–105. (Amsterdam/Oxford: Elsevier)

45. Isaacs, J. T. (1984). The timing of androgen ablation therapy and/or chemotherapy in the treatment of prostatic cancer. *Prostate*, **5**, 1–17

46. Szepeshazi, K., Schally, A. V., Halmos, G., Szoke, B., Groot, K. and Nagy, A. (1996). Effect of a cytotoxic analog of LH-RH (T-98) on the growth of estrogen-dependent MXT mouse mammary cancers: correlations between growth characteristics and EGF receptor content of tumors. *Breast Cancer Res. Treat.*, in press

47. FitzGerald, D. and Pastan, I. (1989). Targeted toxin therapy for the treatment of cancer. *J. Natl. Cancer Inst.*, **81**, 1455–63

48. Varga, J. M. (1985). Hormone-drug conjugates. *Methods Enzymol.*, **112**, 259–69

49. Varga, J. M., Asato, N., Lande, S. and Lerner, A. B. (1977). Melanotropin–daunomycin conjugates shows receptor-mediated cytotoxicity in cultured murine melanoma cells. *Nature*, **267**, 56–8

50. Tritton, T. R. and Yee, G. (1982). The anticancer agent adriamycin can be actively cytotoxic without entering cells. *Science*, **217**, 248–50

51. Tritton, T.R. (1991). Cell surface actions of adriamycin. *Pharmacol. Ther.*, **49**, 293–309

52. Bajusz, S., Janáky, T., Csernus, V. J., Bokser, L., Fekete, M., Srkalovic, G., Redding, T. W. and Schally, A. V. (1989). Highly potent analogues of luteinizing hormone-releasing hormone containing D-phenylalanine nitrogen mustard in position 6. *Proc. Natl. Acad. Sci. USA*, **86**, 6318–22

53. Bajusz, S., Janáky, T., Csernus, V. J., Bokser, L., Fekete, M., Srkalovic, G., Redding, T. W. and Schally. A. V. (1992). Highly potent metallopeptide analogues of luteinizing hormone-releasing hormone. *Proc. Natl. Acad. Sci. USA*, **86**, 6313–17

54. Janáky, T., Juhász, A., Rékási, Z., Serfözö, P., Pinski, J., Bokser, L., Srkalovic, G., Milovanovic, S., Redding, T. W., Halmos, G., Nagy, A. and Schally, A.V. (1992). Short-chain analogs of luteinizing hormone-releasing hormone containing cytotoxic moieties. *Proc. Natl. Acad. Sci. USA*, **89**, 10203–7

55. Rékási, Z., Szöke, B., Nagy, A., Groot, K., Rékási E. S. and Schally, A. V.(1993). Effect of luteinizing hormone-releasing hormone analogs containing cytotoxic radicals on the function of rat pituitary cells: tests in a long term superfusion system. *Endocrinology*, **132**, 1991–2000

56. Szöke, B., Horvath, J., Halmos, G., Rékási, Z., Groot, K., Nagy, A., Schally, A. V. (1994). LH-RH analogue carrying a cytotoxic radical is internalized by rat pituitary cells *in vitro*. *Peptides*, **15**, 359–66

57. Szepeshazi, K., Schally, A. V., Juhász, A., Nagy, A. and Janáky, T. (1992). Effect of LH-RH analogs containing cytotoxic radicals on growth of estrogen independent MXT mouse mammary carcinoma *in vivo*. *Anticancer Drugs*, **3**, 109–16

58. Milovanovic, S. R., Monje, E., Szepeshazi, K., Radulovic, S. and Schally, A. (1993). Effect of treatment with LHRH analogs containing cytotoxic radicals on the binding characteristics of receptors for luteinizing hormone-releasing hormone in MXT mouse mammary carcinoma. *J. Cancer Res. Clin. Oncol.*, **119**, 273–8

59. Milovanovic, S. R., Radulovic, R. and Schally, A. V. (1992). Evaluation of binding of cytotoxic analogs of luteinizing hormone-releasing hormone to human breast cancer and mouse MXT mammary tumor. *Breast Cancer Res. Treat.*, **24**, 147–58

60. Nagy, A., Szöke, B., and Schally, A. V. (1993). Selective coupling of methotrexate to peptide hormone carriers through a γ-carboxamide linkage of its glutamic acid moiety: benzotriazol-1-yloxytris(dimethylamino)phosphonium hexafluorophosphate activation in salt coupling. *Proc. Natl. Acad. Sci. USA*, **90**, 6373–6

61. Dawes, P. J. D. K. (1982). A pilot study of Estracyt in advanced breast cancer. *Cancer. Treat. Rep.*, **66**, 581–2

62. Wynn, P. C., Suarez-Quian, D. A., Childs, G. V. and Catt, K. J. (1986). Pituitary binding and internalization of radioiodinated gonadotropin-releasing hormone agonists and antagonist ligands *in vitro* and *in vivo*. *Endocrinology*, **119**, 1852–63

Section 2

Delivery systems

Small-size microcapsules for long-term GnRH agonist administration

Y. Ogawa

INTRODUCTION

Repeated injections of a high potency gonadotropin releasing hormone (GnRH) agonist induce reversible hyposteroidogenesis as a result of down-regulation of the pituitary–gonadal axis, and a reduction in GnRH receptor numbers[1,2]. Since repeated injections have several disadvantages, a new dosage form was designed to overcome them. To obtain efficient down-regulation the maintenance of a certain critical serum drug level is required. In an attempt to achieve this several prolonged-release dosage forms have been investigated and developed, including a rod-shaped depot implant and microcapsule depot forms[3–5]. These depot formulations undergo bioerosion as the drug is released to avoid empty form remaining at the injection site. Co-polymers composed of lactic and glycolic acids (PLGA) are most suitable for use as the biodegradable or bioerodible polymer in these formulations, because PLGA has been used safely in surgical sutures and has physicochemical properties which allow easy depot manufacture. As the erosion rate of PLGA depends on the co-polymer ratio between lactic and glycolic acid and the average molecular weight, the optimal co-polymer ratio and molecular weight must be selected according to the intended dose period[6,7]. The purpose of this study was to obtain a microcapsule depot form, prepared with PLGA, which could constantly release a high-potency GnRH analog, leuprorelin, for 1 month after a single injection. The microcapsules are small enough to be able to pass easily through a conventional needle for subcutaneous injection.

MATERIALS AND METHODS

Preparation of the microcapsules

Copoly (lactic/glycolic) acid (PLGA) with a free carboxyl group on one side (Figure 1) was synthesized using a polycondensation process without a catalyst. A PLGA with a lactic/glycolic

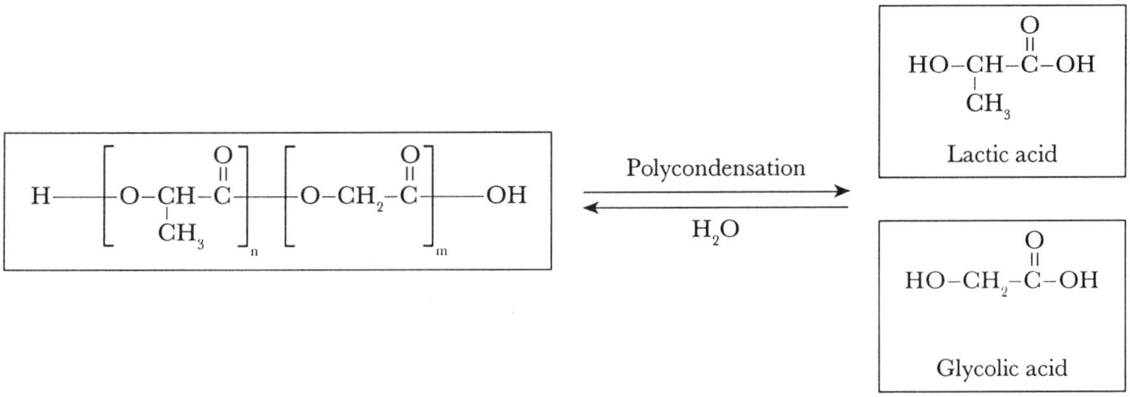

Figure 1 Structure and biodegradation products of copolyl(lactic/glycolic) acid

"

co-polymer ration of 75/25 and an average molecular weight of about 10 000 met the requirements for the monthly release of leuprorelin most effectively[7].

Microcapsules containing 10% leuprorelin were prepared by an in-water drying procedure, a novel production procedure designed to obtain monolithic microcapsules, as described previously[8]. The procedure was briefly as follows: an aqueous drug solution and a dichloromethane PLGA solution were mixed with stirring to make a water/oil emulsion, then the mixture was poured into an aqeuous polyvinyl alcohol solution to make a dual water/oil/water emulsion. The dichloromethane was evaporated to harden the PLGA microparticles containing the aqueous drug solution. The hardened microparticles were lyophilized to remove the water and leave the microcapsules in powder form. Selection of an optimal processing temperature and optimal viscosities of the aqueous drug solution and the water/oil emulsion were essential to allow well-shaped microcapsules to be obtained and to entrap the water-soluble drug efficiently.

Animal experiments

The microcapsules were injected subcutaneously or intramuscularly into the nape or thigh of Sprague–Dawley (SD) rats (3 mg/kg as the drug) using a dispersing vehicle and a conventional subcutaneous syringe with a 23-gauge needle. Microcapsules remaining at the injection site were excised periodically to allow determination of the amount of leuprorelin released by high performance liquid chromatography (HPLC).

Endometriosis in rats was surgically induced by a previously reported method[9,10]. In brief, female rats underwent abdominal incision and a 5 ¥ 5 mm endometrial section of the right uterine horn was sutured to the body wall of the peritoneal cavity. The growth of the explant was determined 3 weeks after transplantation, then treatment with the subcutaneous microcapsule depot injection was begun. The rats were killed 3 weeks after beginning treatment, and endometriosis was graded according to the following four categories: I, explant disappeared; II, explant present but no fluid; III, some fluid in explant; and IV, growth approximates that before treatment.

Determination of remaining leuprorelin and serum leuprorelin and testosterone levels

The methods employed have been described previously[11]. Briefly, the amount of drug remaining at the injection site was assayed by an HPLC procedure with ultraviolet detection after extraction from the microcapsules into a buffer (pH 6.0). This indicated the likelihood of *in vivo* release. The serum drug level was determined by a double antibody radioimmunoassay method. Serum testosterone was assayed after extraction with diethyl ether by a radioimmunoassay method, using a commercially available kit (Testosterone-H-3; Green Cross Co., Osaka, Japan).

Determination of particle size distribution

The particle size distribution of the microcapsules was determined by Coulter Counter TA-II (Coulter Electronics Inc., Hialeah, FL, USA) with an aperture of 280 μm.

In vitro release of leuprorelin and gel permeation chromatography of PLGA

The *in vitro* release of the drug and the average molecular weight of the PLGA in a pH 7.0 solution was determined by a previously reported method[7,12]. Sealed glass vials containing 10 ml of buffer solution and 50 mg microcapsules were incubated with horizontal oscillation at 37°C. For further analysis of leuprorelin and PLGA, the microcapsules were collected by filtering periodically. The leuprorelin content was assayed by the HPLC procedure described above. After dissolving the collected microcapsules in tetrahydrofuran, the average molecular weight of the PLGA was assayed by gel permeation chromatography (GPC) using the refractive index. The molecular weight was calculated by microcomputer software developed by Shimadzu (Kyoto, Japan).

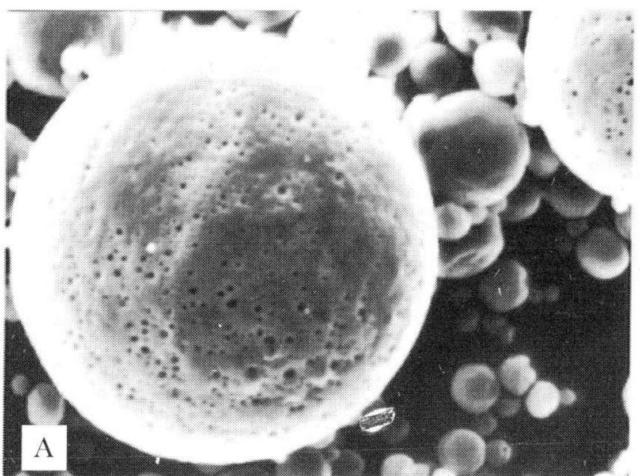
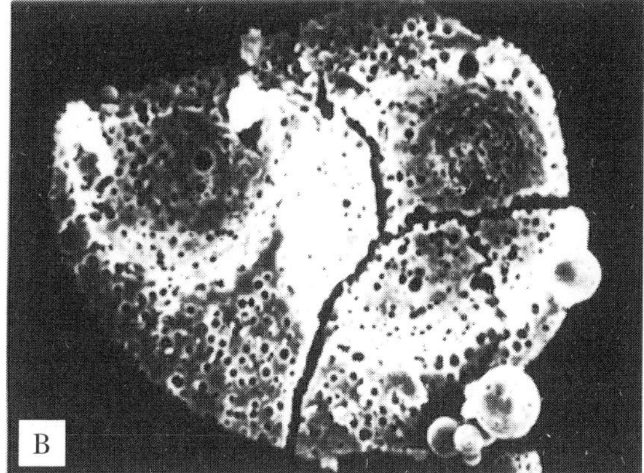

Figure 2   Scanning electron photomicrographs of the microcapsules: (A) surface; (B) cross-section. Figure 2A has been reproduced with permission of the Copyright Council of Academic Society from *Chemical and Pharmaceutical Bulletin 1980*, **36**, 1502

RESULTS AND DISCUSSION

Appearance of the microcapsules and particle size distribution

A scanning electron photomicrograph of the microcapsules is shown in Figure 2. The microcapsules were fairly spherical with numerous micropores or microvesicles on the surface. The right-hand picture shows a cross-section of the microcapsules, showing numerous micropores dotted on the inside and indicating that the micropores on the surface do not penetrate deeply inside.

Particle sizes ranged between 8 and 70 μm and their distribution conformed to the log-normal. The mean diameter was 20 μm. The particles were small enough to pass through a 23-gauge needle.

Remaining leuprorelin and serum leuprorelin and testosterone level profiles after administration of the microcapsules

The microcapsules remaining at the injection site were excised periodically to determine the *in vivo* release. Leuprorelin was released somewhat rapidly during the first day but then linearly for 4 weeks. There were almost no microcapsules remaining at the injection site on day 28.

Figure 3 shows the mean serum level profiles for leuprorelin (as leuprorelin acetate) after a single

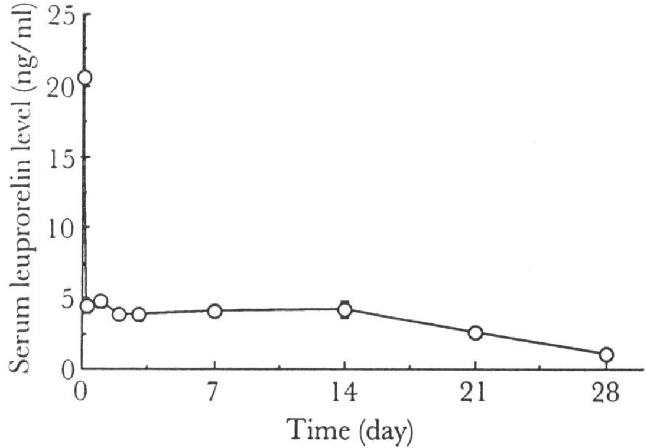

Figure 3   Serum leuprorelin levels in rats after a single intramuscular injection of the microcapsules at a dose of 3 mg/kg (as leuprorelin acetate). Each point represents the mean for five rats with standard error

subcutaneous or intramuscular injection of the microcapsules in five rats. Initial release of the drug produced a sharp increase in the serum level, but following this the levels were sustained at a reasonably steady level for 4 weeks.

Serum testosterone levels in the rats increased during the early stages due to the stimulative effects of the drug, but then decreased to below normal due to the paradoxical effect and remained at the suppressed level. Figure 4 shows the mean serum testosterone levels after repeated administration of the microcapsules to rats once

Table 1 Effect of treatment with the microcapsules on experimental endometriosis in rats

Treatment	Dose (μg/kg/day)	No. of rats	Grade of response*			
			I	II	III	IV
None		5	0	0	1	4
Ovariectomy		5	3	2	0	0
Microcapsule	100	13	7	5	0	1
	10	5	1	1	2	1
	1	5	0	1	0	4
Daily aqueous solution	100	4	0	4	0	0
Daily nasal**	100	4	1	1	2	0

*: I, explant disappeared; II, explant present but no fluid; III, some fluid in explant; IV, growth approximates that before treatment; **: with 5% α-cyclodextrin

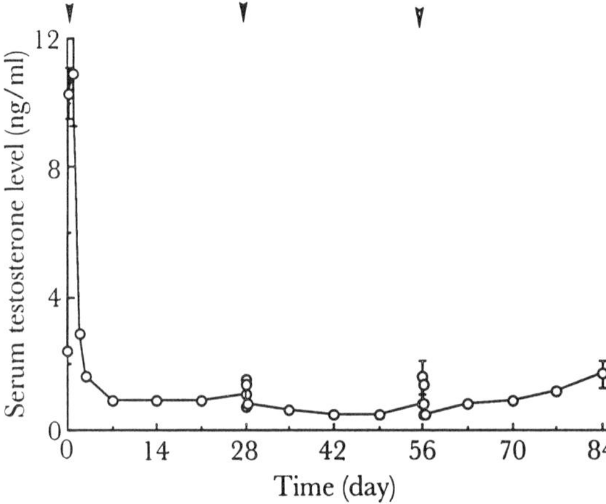

Figure 4 Serum testosterone levels in rats after repeated subcutaneous administration of the microcapsules every 4 weeks at a dose of 3 mg/kg (as leuprorelin acetate). Each point represents the mean of the results for five rats with standard error. Arrows show an injection of the microcapsules

every 4 weeks. No elevation of the serum testosterone level was observed after the second and third administration, indicating that no acute-on-chronic effect occurred due to the continuous presence of the drug in the blood.

Effects of the microcapsules on experimental endometriosis in rats

The pharmacological effects on experimental endometriosis produced by ovariectomy, daily subcutaneous and nasal administration of 3 mg/kg of leuprorelin acetate, and a single subcutaneous injection of the microcapsules are summarized in Table 1. All explants in the non-treated controls had grown by the third week after treatment. In contrast, all explants in the ovariectomy group had obviously regressed. Treatment with the microcapsules which provided a leuprorelin dose of 3 mg/kg (100 μg/kg/day in Table 1) produced the same level of regression as ovariectomy. Treatment with the microcapsules providing 0.3 mg/kg resulted in slightly lower efficacy. Daily injection of a saline drug solution produced regressive effects in all four rats, but did not reduce the severity to grade I. Treatment by nasal administration with 5% a-cyclodextrin, an excellent absorption promoter, led to the same level of regression as that produced by a dose equivalent to one-tenth that found in full-strength microcapsules.

Degradation of the PLGA and drug release

As reported previously, leuprorelin was released rapidly when the microcapsules were prepared with a PLGA which degraded rapidly, but was released slowly when the microcapsules were prepared with a PLGA which degraded slowly[7]. The drug remaining and the molecular weight of the polymer were determined simultaneously in an *in vitro* release test. After rapid release over the first day, the amount of leuprorelin remaining

● Leuprorelin remaining (as leuprorelin acetate)
○ The areas under the curve of the co-polymer by gel permeation chromatography

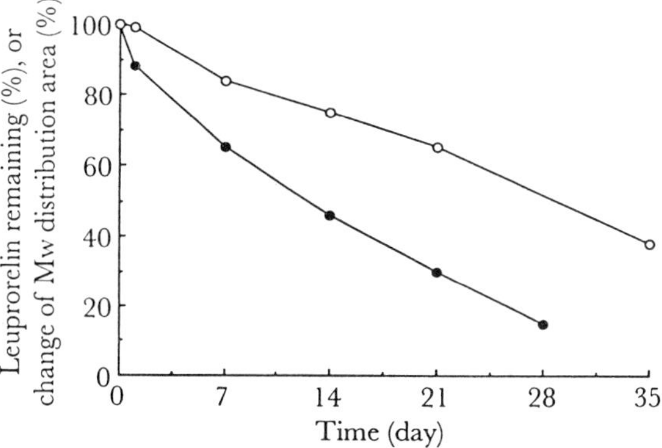

Figure 5 Relationship between remaining leuprorelin and degradation of the co-polymer in *in vitro* release test

Advantages and disadvantages of small-size microcapsules

was almost proportional to the decrease in the molecular weight of the PLGA, as shown in Figure 5. This means that the drug was released in parallel with the erosion of the PLGA after an initial rapid release, and that the initial rapid release over the first day was not related to the polymer erosion. As also reported previously, leuprorelin is involved in an interaction with PLGA within the microcapsules[7]. The initial rapid release occurs because the matrices of the microcapsules are swollen by the infiltration of water and the free drug, which has no or only a weak interaction with PLGA, is diffused through water channels at the initial stages.

As described above, microcapsules containing 10% leuprorelin as acetate salt were prepared using a new PLGA containing a free carboxyl group by a new technique. The mean diameter of the microcapsules was about 20 μm, which is relatively small. These microcapsules have the following advantages: a small amount of dichloromethane was used as a solvent for the PLGA in the new production procedure, so hardly any residual solvent was detected in the microcapsules (less than 30 p.p.m. [w/w]). The microcapsules could be produced easily on a large scale, because their preparation requires only a small amount of organic solvent. No metal was used as a catalyst in the new PLGA due to synthesis by polycondensation without a catalyst. The microcapsules could be injected easily using a conventional 23-gauge needle for subcutaneous injection.

However, there is a disadvantage. A certain amount of the drug in the microcapsules was released initially within 24 hours after injection. The amount of the dose released initially depends on the particle size and the water solubility of the drug contained. Leuprorelin, which dissolves easily in water, exhibited initial release of up to 15% of the dose from 20 μm microcapsules. We, however, adopted the use of the small-size microcapsules because of their many merits, in spite of the disadvantage of initial release, because leuprorelin has few adverse effects.

References

1. Heber, D., Dodson, R., Stoskopf, C., Peterson, M. and Swerdloff, R. S. (1982). Pituitary desensitization and the regulation of pituitary gonadotropin-releasing hormone (GnRH) receptors following chronic administration of a superactive GnRH analog and testosterone. *Life Sci.*, **30**, 2301–8

2. Mann, D. R., Gould, K. G. and Collins, D. C. (1984). Influence of continuous gonadotropin-releasing hormone (GnRH) agonist treatment on luteinizing hormone and testosterone secretion, the response to GnRH, and the testicular response to human chorionic gonadotropin in male rhesus monkeys. *J. Clin. Endocrinol. Metab.*, **58**, 262–7

3. Ogawa, Y. (1992). Monthly microcapsule-depot form of LHRH agonist leuprorelin acetate (Enantone depot): formulation and pharmacokinetics in animals. *Eur. J. Hosp. Pharm.*, **2**, 120–7

4. Redding, T. W., Schally, A. V., Tice, T. R. and Meyers, W. E. (1984). Long-acting delivery

systems for peptide: inhibition of rat prostate tumors by controlled release of [D-Trp6] luteinizing hormone releasing hormone from injectable microcapsules. *Proc. Natl Acad. Sci. USA*, **81**, 5845–8

5. Huchinson, F. G. and Furr, B. J. A. (1986). Biodegradable polymers for sustained release of polypeptides. In Davis, S. S., Illum, L. and Tomlinson, E. (eds) *Delivery System for Peptide Drugs*, pp. 115–23. (New York: Plenum Press)

6. Ogawa, Y., Okada, H., Yamamoto, M. and Shimamoto, T. (1988). *In vivo* release profiles of leuprolide acetate from microcapsules prepared with polylactic acids or copoly(lactic/glycolic) acids and *in vivo* degradation of these polymers. *Chem. Pharm. Bull.*, **36**, 2576–81

7. Ogawa, Y., Yamamoto, M., Takada, S., Okada, H. and Shimamoto, T. (1988). Controlled-release of leuprolide acetate from polylactic acid or copoly(lactic/glycolic) acid microcapsules: influence of molecular weight and copolymer ratio of polymer. *Chem. Pharm. Bull.*, **36**, 1502–7

8. Ogawa, Y., Yamamoto, M., Okada, H., Yashiki, T. and Shimamoto, T. (1988). A new technique to efficiently entrap leuprolide acetate into microcapsules of polylactic acid or copoly(lactic/glycolic) acid. *Chem. Pharm. Bull.*, **36**, 1095–103

9. Okada, H., Heya, T., Ogawa, Y. and Shimamoto, T. (1988). One-month release injectable microcapsules of a luteinizing hormone-releasing hormone agonist (leuprolide acetate) for treating experimental endometriosis in rats. *J. Pharmacol. Exp. Ther.*, **244**, 744–50

10. Jones, R. C. (1984). The effect of a luteininzing hormone releasing hormone (LRH) agonist (Wy-40,972), levonorgestrel, danazol and ovariectomy on experimental endometriosis in the rat. *Acta Endcrinol.*, **106**, 282–8

11. Ogawa, Y., Okada, H., Heya, T. and Shimamoto, T. (1989). Controlled release of LHRH agonist, leuprolide acetate, from microcapsules: serum drug level profiles and pharmacological effects in animals. *J. Pharm. Pharmacol.*, **41**, 439–44

12. Kamei, S., Iinuma, Y., Yuasa, Y., Saikawa, A., Igari, Y. and Ogawa, Y. (1995). LHRH agonist depot formulations: comparative studies of Decapeptyl with Enantone. *Eur. Hosp. Pharm*, **1**, 113–20

Implants and other controlled release systems for long-term LHRH agonist administration

6

J. Sandow, G. Seidel, W. von Rechenberg, G. Jerabek-Sandow and B. Krauss

INTRODUCTION

Hormone therapy by substitution of a physiological secretion pattern has a long history. The pharmacotherapy by infusion of luteinizing hormone-releasing hormone (LHRH) and LHRH agonists leads to changes in the response of hormone secretory cells; for example, pituitary gland receptors are down-regulated. This regulatory principle has found wide application for control of the gonadotrope cells of the pituitary gland and gonadal steroid secretion in gynecology and oncology[1,2]. The observations that long-term subcutaneous infusion of buserelin in animals was highly effective in reducing the pituitary luteinizing hormone (LH) and follicle stimulating hormone (FSH) content[1] and in suppression of the estradiol secretion to the postmenopausal range in patients with endometriosis and leiomyoma was the starting point of our search for biodegradable implants[3,4] and other injectable dosage forms (e.g. microparticles with a steady release rate suitable for a dose interval of 1–4 months).

SELECTION OF POLYMER

The co-polymers of polylactide–glycolide (PLG) are widely used as biodegradable matrix material for the controlled release of drug substances[5,10]. Research in this area has been very active, using steroid hormones for contraceptive applications, and has been extended to the range of peptides by the goserelin implant[6-8]. An important advantage of LHRH agonists in this respect is their thermal stability during manufacture by melting of the implant material and subsequent extrusion. In our initial studies we compared release profiles of buserelin using fast degrading PLG 50:50 and slow degrading PLG 75:25[9].

One major advantage of implants is the high drug load of peptide that can be incorporated, in contrast to microparticles. In the range of 20–35% of drug load, it was possible to obtain suppression of gonadal steroids for up to 180 days in rats and dogs at a buserelin dose of 3.3 mg. The most consistent results were obtained with a drug load of 22.5%, in contrast with an average of 6–8% in microparticles. An extensive comparison was performed of PLG 50:50 and PLG 75:25 implant material of similar average molecular weight (intrinsic viscosity 0.6–0.8). Cumulative release of these implants in rats, dogs and monkeys showed an average amount of 5–10% remaining to be released on day 30 after injection of PLG 50:50 implants (residual buserelin content in the implants), and an average amount of 18% remaining to be released after day 60 PLG 75:25. This prolonged release period was considered a significant advantage. It was therefore decided to evaluate the slow degrading polymer in more detail in clinical studies.

Release profiles

The release rate in rats, dogs and monkeys was estimated from buserelin excretion using conversion factors determined experimentally for each species. In rats, quantitative urine collection is possible and a conversion factor of 3.84 was applied for a 26% dose excreted in the urine. In dogs and monkeys, quantitative urine collection was more difficult and the creatinine (CR) correction was therefore applied to estimate the daily urine volume, based on the average amount of CR excreted in these animal species within 24 hours. The conversion factor in male beagle dogs was 0.88, and the conversion factor in male rhesus monkeys was 1.26 based on the percentage of the drug (buserelin) excreted in urine and the average amount of CR found in urine within 24 hours. For clinical pharmacokinetics, a similar approach was developed to estimate release rates by a non-invasive procedure and to compare them with the therapeutic serum concentration achieved. The conversion factor in clinical studies from buserelin excretion (μg/g CR) to the release rate (μg/24 hours) was 4.95 based on 30% buserelin excretion and an average human CR excretion of 1.5 g/24 hours.

Effect of coating

The initial release from implants is determined by diffusion from the surface. This process can be delayed considerably by coating implants with a diffusion barrier (e.g. cyanoacrylate). Such implants provide a much longer suppression period: they reduce the initial release by 30–40% in favor of an extended release period[2] and longer dose interval. In dogs, the suppression of testosterone was extended from 120 to 142 days.

Animal studies

Two implant materials of buserelin implants were compared, a slow degrading polylactide–glycolide (PLG 75:25) and a fast degrading polylactide–glycolide (PLG 50:50). The biological tests were performed by subcutaneous implantation in male rats (Figure 1). Each rat received a dose of 3.3 mg buserelin for a dose interval (test period) of 28 days or 56 days. The parameters were the prostate and testes weight, urinary buserelin excretion (for calculation of the release rate) and residual drug content in implants at the end of the dose interval. Buserelin excretion is closely related to serum concentrations of buserelin, as established in animals and in humans by subcutaneous infusions at controlled rates similar to those found by release from implants[11–13]. The amount released during the dose interval was calculated from the initial content before implantation and residual content in implants recovered from rats on days 28 or 56. The percentage of the dose released during the

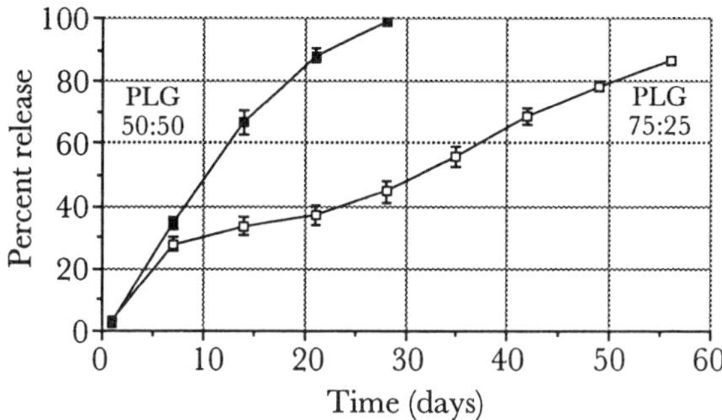

Figure 1 Selection of a suitable polymer for extended release periods in rats. Cumulative buserelin release from fast degrading PLG 50:50 (seven batches tested) and slow degrading PLG 75:25 (18 batches tested) in rats at a dose of 3.3 mg buserelin per implant. There is a considerable release reserve on day 30 using PLG 75:25

dose interval was calculated from the cumulative buserelin excretion with correction for residual drug content.

PLG 75:25 implants (slow release) suppressed testosterone secretion in rats for the 56-day dose interval. They released 82.2% of the drug content within 56 days and the average release rate R_{av} was 48.4 μg/day. The PLG 50:50 implants (rapid release) suppressed testosterone secretion in rats for 28 days, with release of 98.6% of the drug content within 28 days, and an R_{av} of 116.2 μg/day.

To confirm consistent release profiles, 18 batches of implants PLG 75:25 were tested in male rats by subcutaneous implantation for 56 days (dose 3.3 mg buserelin). The release rate was estimated from the buserelin excretion using a conversion factor of 3.84 (26% of the amount released per day are excreted in the urine of rats). The pharmacokinetics showed a maximum release (R_{max}) of 299 μg/24 hours (range 172–583) on day 1 and a minimum release (R_{min}) of 41.8 μg/24 hours (range 16.1–126) on day 56 of the dose interval. During the dose interval 86.3% of the dose was released (range 75.7–93.8), and the average rate R_{av} (days 1–56) was 50.9 μg/day (range 44.6– 55.3).

CLINICAL USE OF IMPLANTS

PLG 50:50 implants (28-day dose interval) were used in clinical trials in mammary carcinoma and benign mastopathia[14]. PLG 75:25 implants (56-day dose interval) were used in clinical trials in prostate carcinoma (multiple dose regimen)[4,5,16] and endometriosis (single dose regimen)[3,17–20]. Single dose biopharmaceutical studies were performed in normal male test controls[21], patients with benign prostate hyperplasia (BPH) and postmenopausal women.

The preclinical rat data were predictive for the release profile and release rates found in clinical studies. The release rate R_{min} in rats (day 56) was 24.3 µg/24 hours at a dose of 3.3 mg buserelin. When compared with the human pharmacokinetics of the PLG 75:25 implant to assess the relevance of the animal model for predicting the release rate in man, R_{min} on day 56 of the test period in normal test controls was 30–45 µg/24 hours at a dose of 6.6 mg[2,4,15,31]. The PLG 75:25 implant was fully effective in suppression of serum testosterone for a dose interval of 56 days in men with BPH and prostate carcinoma. With a dose increment to 10 mg buserelin, a dose interval of 3 months was covered[16]; this interval was also reported for goserelin implants[38].

For comparison of rat and human kinetics, all data were adjusted to a dose size of 3.3 mg and the percentage of dose released during the dose interval was calculated. In rats 82.2% of the buserelin dose was released within 56 days. In normal male test controls 82.0% and 83.5% of the dose were released until day 56 (two dose sizes tested). The release rate R_{min} on day 56 of the dose interval estimated by the rat model and the corresponding human release rate R_{min} were similar (Figure 2). The average release R_{av} during the dose interval (days 1–56) was 48.4 µg/day in the rat model, and 48.7 µg/day in human test controls.

R_{max} is the release rate on day 1 of the dose interval, R_{min} is the release rate on the last day of the dose interval. R_{av} is the average release rate during dose interval, and minimum therapeutic concentration (MTR) is the minimum therapeutic concentration at end of dose interval. The safety interval is the time period after the end of the dose interval from R_{min} until reaching the minimum therapeutic concentration.

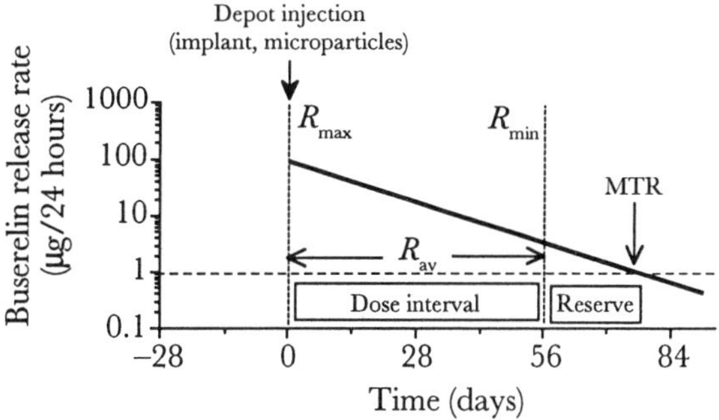

Figure 2 Pharmacokinetic parameters for the evaluation of buserelin release from implants and microparticles during the dose interval and until reaching the minimum therapeutic release rate MTR for suppression of estradiol and testosterone. R_{max}, initial release; R_{av}, average rate during dose interval (e.g. days 1–56); R_{min}, release at end of dose interval; MTR minimum therapeutic release rate before end of gonadal steroid suppression; reserve, amount remaining to be released after the end of the dose interval

In clinical studies with implants similar average release rates R_{av} during the dose interval were found, as in rats. The release rate R_{min} at the end of the dose interval of 28 days for a dose of 3.3 mg was similar to R_{min} after 56 days for a dose of 6.6 mg, R_{min} being 36.6 and 33.7 µg/24 hours, respectively (Table 1).

Biodegradation and tissue tolerance

Implants of PLG 50:50 and PLG 75:25 were tested by subcutaneous injection in male rats. Animals were sacrificed after 2–10 weeks, and implants were retrieved for analysis of residual content. The tissue capsule surrounding the implantation site was analyzed by histology, and in each group remaining implants were studied by scanning electron microscopy to characterize the process of physical disintegration[9]. The biodegradation of PLG 50:50 implants (from days 14–28) was much more rapid than that of PLG 75:25 implants. The terminal half-life of buserelin release from PLG 50:50 implants was 6 days, and the terminal half-life of release from PLG 75:25 (from days 42–56) was 20 days. This half-life reflects the different rates of biodegradation of the two polymer matrices.

Table 1 Therapeutic serum concentrations and release rates in patients with prostate carcinoma treated with buserelin implants dose size 3.3 mg and 6.6 mg. C_{max}, C_{min} are serum concentrations on first and last day of dose interval, R_{max} and R_{min} are release rates on the same days. Testosterone suppression is maintained by a release rate above 5 μg/24 hours

Buserelin implants dose size (mg)	Serum concentration (ng/ml)		Buserelin excretion (μg/g CR)		Dose interval (days)
	C_{max}	C_{min}	R_{max}	R_{min}	
3.3	4.96	0.47	685	36.6	28
6.6	8.24	0.41	1157	33.7	56

The buserelin release rate is calculated from buserelin excretion using a conversion factor of 4.95 from excretion (μg/g CR) to release rate (μg/24 hours). CR, creatinine

Histology of the PLG 50:50 implants showed degradation products in the surrounding tissue from the fifth week of implantation onwards (macrophage cells of the tissue capsule containing polylactide/glycolide plaques identified by double refraction). These implants (rapid release) caused an enhanced tissue reaction with appearance of degradation products on day 35 after implantation. Scanning electron microscopy indicated that disintegration began 14 days after implantation.

Degradation of the PLG 75:25 implants was markedly delayed. In the connective tissue capsule surrounding the PLG 75:25 implants, no degradation products were visible until week 10 after implantation. The tissue reaction to the PLG 75:25 slow degrading implant was extremely mild, consisting of a thin connective tissue capsule rich in collagen fibres with few cellular elements (mainly fibrocytes and macrophage cells). The physical disintegration process was monitored by weight changes of implants. Wet weight is related to the uptake of water by the implant material, and dry weight is related to the mass loss by the formation of water-soluble oligomers and monomers during disappearance of the implants from the injection site. The wet weight of PLG 50:50 implants increased until day 14 due to initial swelling caused by uptake of water, with subsequent rapid weight loss until day 42. The PLG 75:25 implants exhibited slow and prolonged swelling caused by uptake of water until day 56; accelerated weight loss by disintegration occurred between days 56 and 70 after implantation. The dry weight of the PLG 75:25 implants showed a slow and steady mass loss[9]. Scanning electron micrographs of the implant surface of the slow degrading polymer confirmed integrity of the structure up to 8 weeks after implantation and increasing dissolution after 10 weeks. It was concluded that the tissue tolerance of PLG 75:25 implant material (slow release) is excellent, with only a mild tissue reaction present. Such implants are degraded slowly, with an accelerated period of disintegration beginning on day 56 after implantation. The terminal half-life of buserelin release of 20 days in rats reflects the terminal phase of biodegradation.

STUDIES IN DOGS

Suppression of testosterone secretion

In adult male dogs, the duration of testosterone suppression and the minimum therapeutic release rate (MTR) were investigated. Implants of PLG 75:25 (slow release) of a dose size of 3.3 mg buserelin suppressed testosterone secretion in dogs for 170 days (range 164–176) and PLG 50:50 implants suppressed testosterone for 108 days (range 100–121). The minimum therapeutic release rate (MTR) required for testosterone suppression in dogs was 0.48–0.82 μg buserelin per day (range 10 animals) independent of the different duration of suppression achieved by the two implant materials.

MTR in dogs was calculated from the buserelin excretion (54% of the amount released per day), and the average amount in urine of dogs (0.48 g CR per day) using a conversion factor of 0.88 from buserelin excretion (μg/g CR) to release rate (μg/24 hours).

In the second study in dogs, testosterone suppression and MTR were confirmed. A single implant of PLG 75:25 suppressed testosterone for 148 days (range 126–168), whereas a single implant of PLG 50:50 was effective for 93 days (range 70–126). The MTR for testosterone suppression in this study was 0.26–0.93 μg buserelin/day (range nine dogs). The PLG 75:25 implants released 71.6% of the drug content within 56 days and the PLG 50:50 implants released 96.2 % of the drug content within 28 days (Figure 3).

The dogs described in this study were treated four times with buserelin implants separated by appropriate recovery periods (wash-out periods). Normal testosterone secretion was established after each treatment. At autopsy, after a total study period of 5.5 years the histology showed normal pituitary tissue and normal spermatogenesis.

Inhibition of sexual maturation

Buserelin implant treatment (12 months, seven consecutive implants of a dose of 3.3 mg, dose interval 56 days) suppressed testosterone secretion

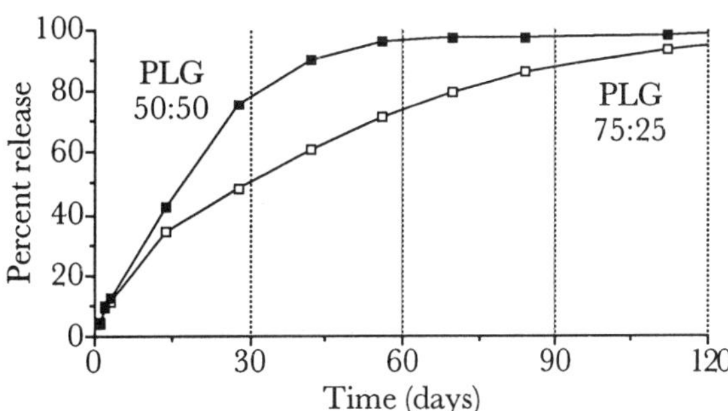

Figure 3 Cumulative release of buserelin from implants of different polymer composition in dogs. The slow degrading PLG 75:25 implants maintain a therapeutic release rate for a much longer period than the fast degrading polymer. At the end of a dose interval of 2 months, the release reserve is much higher with PLG 75:25 implants

and delayed sexual maturation for 15 months in male prepubertal dogs. Serum testosterone began to rise 20 weeks after the last implant (Figure 4). The adult range of serum testosterone was reached 22 weeks after treatment, and sexual maturation was completed in all animals within 1 year after treatment. Spermatogenesis was fully established in 8 of 10 dogs at this time, and testicular histology 2 years after treatment was normal. There were no changes in pituitary size or histology. This study in prepubertal dogs was performed to

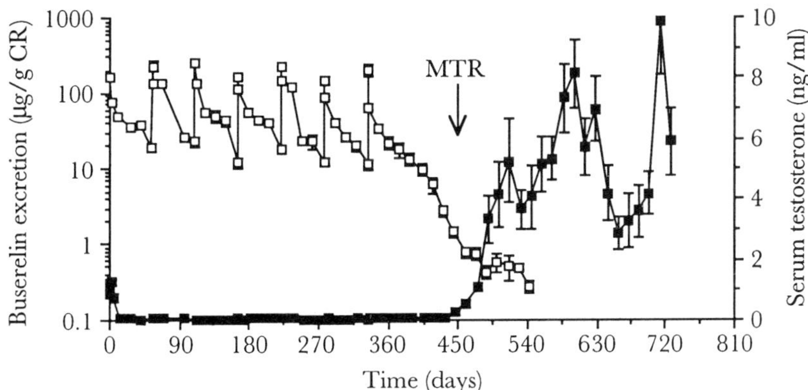

Figure 4 Relation of pharmacokinetics and pharmacodynamics in dogs treated for inhibition of sexual maturation, starting before puberty. Buserelin implants 3.3 mg at dose interval 56 days. Testosterone suppression is maintained until reaching the minimum therapeutic release rate (MTR) of 0.8 μg/24 hours. Normal sexual maturation started spontaneously; at the end of the study all dogs had normal testes volume and spermatogenesis. $\square$, excretion; $\blacksquare$, testosterone

investigate the effect of buserelin implants on sexual maturation and development of normal testosterone secretion and spermatogenesis after the end of implant treatment. During the treatment period, serum testosterone remained low in all dogs (prepubertal state of maturation). Serum testosterone began to rise 129 days (range 111–153) after the last implant in all animals. The buserelin release rate (MTR) at this time was 0.8 µg/24 hours (range 0.18–1.14). The pharmacokinetics of buserelin release were highly reproducible. The average release rate R_{av} was 47.1 µg (dose interval 56 days), the terminal half-life of release was 19–26 days, and 81% of the dose was released during each dose interval.

STUDIES IN MONKEYS

Suppression of ovarian function

Female monkeys *(Macaca arctoides)* were treated with single buserelin implants PLG 75:25 (dose size 2.6 mg). The pharmacokinetics of buserelin release were monitored by reference infusions from osmotic minipumps delivering a daily rate of 50 µg per monkey for 90 days[21]. During these infusions, serum estradiol remained suppressed as long as the infusion was continued at a rate of 50 µg/24 hours. The average buserelin excretion during infusions at steady state was 12.9 µg/g CR (26% of the dose infused). Estradiol suppression after one implant lasted 134 days (range 94–166), progesterone suppression lasted 149 days (range 105–182). Buserelin release showed a prolonged plateau phase from days 16–68. The terminal half-life of release was 25 days. After adjustment for a dose size of 3.3 mg for comparison with results in rats, dogs and monkeys, the average release R_{av} in female monkeys during the dose interval of 56 days was 36.4 µg/day. The release rate R_{min} on the last day of the dose interval (day 56) was 24.9 µg/day, and 81.1% of the drug contents were released until day 56.

Inhibition of sexual maturation

Buserelin implant treatment delayed sexual maturation for 20 months in male prepubertal rhesus monkeys[22]. Ten weeks after the last implant injection pubertal maturation began, and sexual maturation was completed in all animals within 1 year after treatment. At the end of the study the testicular volume and spermatogenesis of previously treated monkeys were similar to age-matched controls, indicating adult testicular function. This preclinical safety study with buserelin implants in juvenile rhesus monkeys was performed to assess the effect of delaying puberty for 20 months on development of the reproductive system. Eight prepubertal rhesus monkeys about 3 years of age were treated. Prepubertal status was confirmed by low serum testosterone and testicular volume. Buserelin implants were injected subcutaneously every 4 weeks. PLG 75:25 (slow release) was used for implants 1–8, and PLG 50:50 (rapid release) was used for implants 9–19 (dose size 3.3 mg, dose interval 28 days). Before and during treatment serum testosterone levels were low (0.25–0.5 ng/ml) in all monkeys; no ejaculates could be obtained at the end of the treatment period. There was no testosterone response in the LHRH test. Testicular volume remained prepubertal (about 2 ml) in all monkeys during the treatment period. Serum testosterone and testicular volume began to rise 10 weeks after the last implant. At this time the MTR was 3.46 µg buserelin per day. This estimate is similar to the MTR requirement in female monkeys for maintenance of estradiol suppression. Pubertal maturation proceeded normally and after 12 months testosterone remained in the adult range. Pituitary–testicular responsiveness was established in all monkeys within 17 weeks after the last implant (adequate rise of serum testosterone in the LHRH test). After 48 weeks, five out of seven monkeys had adult sperm counts. All animals had normal morphology and motility.

The histological examination at the end of the study period showed no abnormalities in any of the organ tissues examined; spermatogenesis was normal, and pituitary size and histology were normal. The pharmacokinetic analysis performed for the PLG 50:50 implants showed a release rate R_{min} at steady state (R_{ss}) of 11.6 µg/24 hours at the end of each dose interval (day 28). The PLG 50:50 implants had a terminal half-life of release of 14 days in contrast to the longer half-life of 25 days for release from PLG 75:25 implants in female monkeys[21].

Table 2 Ovarian suppression after buserelin implant at doses of 1.8–6.6 mg in women with endometriosis. Buserelin excretion, release rate and average duration of ovarian suppression is assessed by time until ovulation returns

Treatment implants dose size (mg)	Buserelin excretion (μg/g CR)	Buserelin release (μg/24 hours)	Return to ovulation (days)	
			Mean	*Range*
1.6	0.43	2.12	61	37–77
3.3	0.65	3.21	97	75–177
6.6	0.61	3.01	173	119–288

CR, creatinine

TREATMENT OF ENDOMETRIOSIS

It is generally accepted that serum estradiol suppression to the postmenopausal range is the critical end-point for indication of premenopausal mammary carcinoma, and testosterone suppression to the castrate range is the critical end-point for indication of prostate carcinoma. These surrogate end-points are considered to be closely related to clinical efficacy. For gynecological indications of endometriosis and leiomyoma the decrease in serum estradiol and a bleeding pattern consistent with secondary amenorrhea are the clinical parameters related to efficacy. Suppression aims at symptomatic relief and uterine myometrial–endometrical involution, achieved by profound estrogen deficiency. LHRH agonists have also found application in treatment of precocious puberty for temporary inhibition of sexual maturation. For this indication suppression of gonadal steroid secretion is also a critical end-point.

To estimate the therapeutic requirement for maintaining suppression of serum estradiol studies were performed (in women with intact ovaries) for indication of endometriosis and leiomyoma. Buserelin was initially administered by subcutaneous infusion[13,23], and later by implants and microparticles. The release rate R was calculated from buserelin excretion using the buserelin/CR ratio. From infusion studies in women, a conversion factor of 4.95 was established for the relation of buserelin excretion (μg/g CR) to the release rate (μg/24 hours)[12,28]. The MTR before the first estradiol rise found after repeated implant injections was 3–4 μg/24 hours. The duration of buserelin release after single injection of implants at a clinically effective rate was determined in women with endometriosis, measuring the serum estradiol concentrations, the urinary excretion of estrone glucuronide and the first progesterone rise after implantation indicating ovulation[12,18–20]. The first ovulation after a dose of 1.8–6.6 mg was found 61–173 days after treatment (Table 2), depending on the dose[28]. At the 6.6 mg dose, the range found in seven patients was extremely wide (199–288 days), whereas at a 1.8 mg dose the range was much more predictable (37–77 days). In a repeated dose study, the interval from the last implant injection to the rise in serum estradiol was 275 days (range 195–355 days)[3]. Such long suppression periods were considered suitable for treatment of the symptoms of endometriosis, with the intention of obtaining long-lasting regression of endometriotic lesions. The long interval until return of ovulation was, however, considered inappropriate for the treatment of endometriosis associated with infertility, where predictable return to ovulation is required.

In several biopharmaceutical studies the release profiles of the fast degrading PLG 50:50 implants[13] and the slow degrading PLG 75:25 implants[11] were determined, to establish the release rate at the end of a dose interval of R_{min} and the duration from R_{min} until reaching the MTR established for estradiol suppression in endometriosis (safety interval in case of delayed dose renewal). PLG 75:25 implants released 71.6–73.5% of drug content during the dose interval (days 1–56) with

Table 3 Biopharmaceutical studies with buserelin implants in normal test controls and patients. Percentage of dose released from implants during the dose interval. The remaining drug content is the release reserve in case of delayed dose interval

Treatment buserelin implants dose size	Dose released until day 180 (%)		Dose released until day 180 (%)	
	3.3 mg	6.6 mg	3.3 mg	6.6 mg
Adult males	81.9	83.5	99.6	99.5
Postmenopausal women	71.6	82.2	94.9	97.0
Women of reproductive age				
1, endometriosis, leiomyoma	82.2	80.9	99.8	98.1
2, endometriosis	79.5	72.7	100	93.1

1, 2: two study groups were evaluated for percentage release during test period

Table 4 Ovarian suppression by single subcutaneous injection of microparticles dose 1.8–7.2 mg buserelin. Average duration and range in days after microparticle injection in normal female test controls

Treatment microparticles dose size (mg)	Buserelin excretion (µg/g CR)	Buserelin release rate (µg/24 hours)	Return to ovulation (days)		Rate of response (amenorrhea)
			Mean	Range	
1.8	0.33	1.65	69	50–88	8/12
3.6	0.51	2.51	82	62–99	9/11
7.2	0.32	1.56	112	94–144	10/10

Rate of response: number of women suppressed for at least one menstrual cycle (amenorrhea) and number of women treated per dose. CR, creatinine

a considerable reserve amount remaining to be released after day 56 (Table 3).

A study of dose dependence of suppression was performed in women with endometriosis in the range of 1.65–6.6 mg buserelin. The study showed that implants containing a dose of 1.65 mg are suitable for a dose interval of 1 month (Table 2). This was subsequently confirmed for controlled release injections of other LHRH agonists of similar biological activity, which showed efficacy of the goserelin implant at 1.8 mg every 28 days and leuprorelin microcapsules at 1.88 mg every 28 days[24–27,29,30]. A range of options remain for dose selection in endometriosis, depending on the clinical concept of obtaining profound estrogen suppression for long-lasting regression of lesions or transient relief from the disease symptoms[28,32]. For a predictable return to ovulation in treatment of infertility nasal spray treatment remains the method of choice[11,17]. Microparticle injections have a narrower range of suppression periods at a lower dose (Table 4), whereas implants have a much longer suppression period with a wide range for return to ovulation.

TREATMENT OF PROSTATE CARCINOMA

The suppression of testosterone to the castrate range must be maintained throughout the remaining lifetime of the patient[4]. It is therefore necessary to maintain a release rate considerably above the minimum therapeutic requirement, including a safety interval at the end of the dose interval in case of delayed injection of the next dose (release reserve, Figure 2). For the indication of prostate carcinoma, the MTR to maintain serum testosterone suppression was derived from study results with implants of dose size 6.6 mg buserelin in men with BPH. A daily release of 5 µg/24 hours was considered to be fully effective[28,31]. In therapeutic studies of prostate carcinoma, two dose sizes of implants were evaluated with different dose intervals (buserelin 3.3 mg every 28 days and buserelin 6.6 mg every 56 days). In each study the release rates R_{min} at the end of the dose interval were significantly higher than the limit of 5 µg/24 hours established to maintain testosterone suppression in men with BPH. The release reserve for slow degrading PLG 75:25 at the end of a 56-day interval was 18–20% (determined by single injection studies at two dose sizes in postmenopausal women) in normal young men substituted with testosterone to avoid deficiency symptoms, and in women of reproductive age[19]. In each case, the buserelin excretion for a study period of more than 180 days was monitored after single injection of implants (3.3 mg and 6.6 mg buserelin) until it had reached the limit of detection. The release rate R_{min} on day 56 in these studies was considerably higher than the MTR requirement for testosterone suppression of 5 µg/24 hours. The release rate at the end of 4 weeks at 3.3 mg and 8 weeks at 6.6 mg are similar (Table 1). The dose of 6.6 mg provided a safety period of 14–28 days in case of late dose renewal. This safety period was therefore defined as at least 14 days. This delay is compatible with full maintenance of testosterone suppression. In postmenopausal women the limits for use in estradiol suppression of premenopausal patients were explored by a study at two dose levels, confirming a sufficient release rate for more than 90 days at the implant dose of 6.6 mg (Figure 5). Such studies are of relevance for premenopausal mammary carcinoma and to estimate the safety interval in endometriosis patients.

Therapeutic serum concentrations

Therapeutic drug levels in serum are often determined for monitoring of drug efficacy. In the case of LHRH agonists this procedure is not as reliable as the estimate from urinary excretion data. In several studies, we calculated the correlation of serum buserelin concentrations (ng/

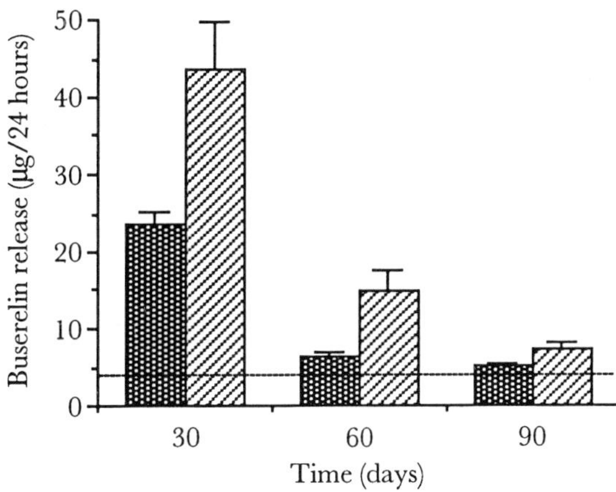

Figure 5 Release reserve of buserelin implants determined by biopharmaceutical study in postmenopausal women. The release rate on days 30, 60 and 90 after implantation of buserelin 6.6 mg is above the minimum therapeutic release (MTR) required for estradiol suppression in premenopausal women (e.g. mammary carcinoma and endometriosis). This limit was maintained by the dose 6.6 mg for more than 90 days. ■ , Dose 3.3 mg; ▨ , dose 6.6 mg; ⋯⋯, minimum therapeutic rate

ml) and buserelin excretion on the same day (buserelin µg/g CR). From these correlations it was determined that therapeutic serum concentrations at the end of the dose interval (C_{min}) are of the order of 0.4 ng/ml and may decrease to 0.05 ng/ml at the end of suppression. These concentrations are determined with careful blood sampling using enzyme inhibitors (bacitracin) during blood collection and centrifugation. Buserelin concentrations in urine remain in a much higher range so that monitoring by buserelin excretion became our preferred non-invasive method for long-term studies. At the time of the decrease to the MTR serum buserelin concentrations were of the order of 50 pg/ml and had often decreased below detection limits in several patients of the group investigated.

Therapeutic release rates (prostate carcinoma)

Pharmacokinetic studies with buserelin implants and the long duration of testosterone suppression confirmed major advantages of this new dosage

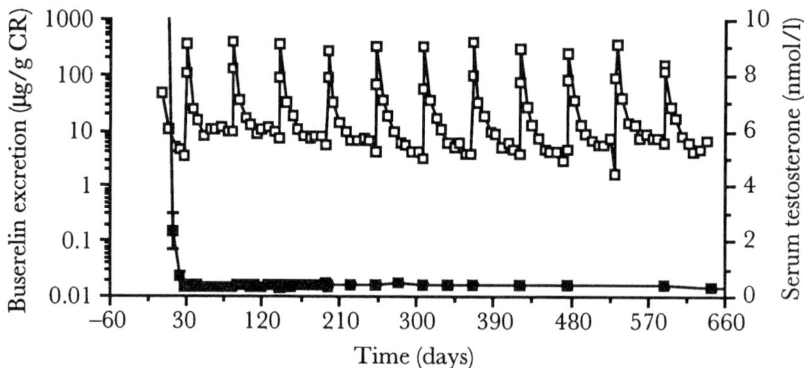

Figure 6 Treatment of prostate carcinoma with buserelin implants. Dose 6.6 mg, dose interval two months. Relation of pharmacokinetics and pharmacodynamics. At the start of treatment, testosterone secretion is stimulated requiring protective medication with an anti-androgen for 2 weeks. Subsequently, serum testosterone is retained in the castrate range as long as medication is continued. □, excretion; ■, testosterone

form in patient convenience and compliance. Consistent testosterone suppression is achieved with 6.6 mg buserelin at 2-month intervals. The release of buserelin has an extended plateau phase from days 14–42 after injection. The maximum therapeutic serum concentration C_{max} on the first day of implantation is 8.24 ng/ml (range 5.74–10.1) and the minimum therapeutic concentration C_{min} at the end of 56 days is 0.41 ng/ml serum (range 0.33–0.62). The maximum release rate on day 1 (R_{max}) is 1157 µg/24 hours (range 985–1487), and the minimum release at the end of the dose interval (day 56) is 33.7 µg/24 hours (range 14.9–48.24). Serum testosterone concentrations are consistently suppressed to the low castrate range with buserelin implants for up to 3 years of treatment[30]. In biopharmaceutical studies in rats and dogs it was shown that 70–80% of the dose is released after 56 days, and biodegradation of the implant material is complete after 180–240 days[12]. Buserelin concentrations in the serum and in the urine were monitored. The buserelin/CR ratio is closely correlated with the serum concentration; buserelin excretion data were therefore preferred for monitoring of long-term studies and for calculation of release R_{min} at the end of each dose interval (Table 1). The percentage of dose released during each dose interval was calculated from the cumulative area under the curve (AUC) of buserelin excretion data (Table 3).

Four studies with implants were performed using a dose size of 3.3 mg (dose interval 28 days) and two studies included a dose size of 6.6 mg (dose interval 56 days)[4,15]. In each of the four studies serum testosterone was consistently suppressed to the low castrate range, confirming full efficacy of testosterone suppression. The release profile after each implant injection was highly reproducible. In the four studies, serum concentration and urinary buserelin/CR ratio were closely related; the average conversion factor was × 20 for the relation of serum concentration (ng/ml) to buserelin excretion (µg/g CR). The measured serum concentration (C_{min}) at the end of the dose interval was 0.41 ng/ml (range 0.33–0.62), and the calculated serum concentration obtained by conversion from buserelin excretion E_{min} of 6.78 µg/g CR (range 3.02–9.74) on the last day of each treatment period was C_{min} 0.31 ng /ml serum (range 0.15–0.49). Biopharmaceutical studies in normal male test controls, in postmenopausal women and in women of reproductive age, established that more than 70% of the dose is released after 56 days (Table 3).

From the four studies with buserelin PLG 75:25 implants it is concluded that dose sizes of 3.3 mg every 28 days and dose size 6.6 mg every 56 days maintain consistent therapeutic release rates above the MTR requirement of 5 µg/day at the end of each treatment period. Testosterone secretion is consistently and reliably suppressed when the implants are administered at the appropriate dose intervals (Figure 6). Slow degrading implant material is suitable for a dose interval of 56 days at an appropriate dose size of 6.6 mg buserelin.

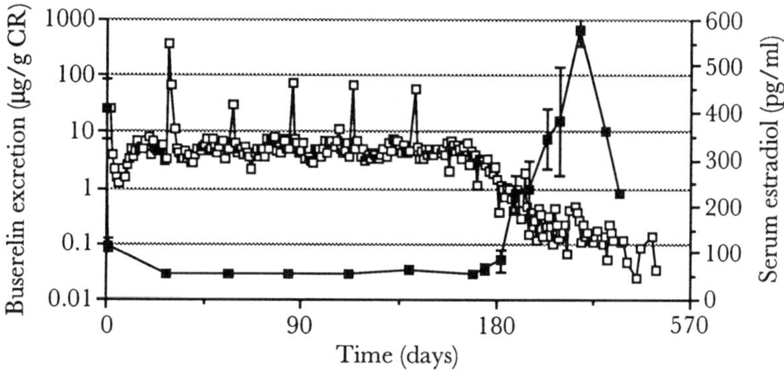

Figure 7 Treatment of endometriosis. Buserelin microparticles of PLG 50:50 dose of 3.6 mg, dose interval 1 month. Relation of pharmacokinetics and estradiol suppression. Consistent estradiol suppression is obtained for 180 days with a predictable return to ovulation after the last dose within 70 days

Nasal spray and implant treatment

The minimum therapeutic release rate (MTR) of 5 μg/24 hours required for testosterone suppression in prostate carcinoma patients was estimated from buserelin excretion data and testosterone suppression in patients with benign prostate hyperplasia (BPH). In BPH a transient suppression of testosterone may improve urinary outflow after involution of the testosterone-dependent hyperplasia tissue. A comparison was performed for the amount excreted every day during treatment with the buserelin nasal spray at a daily dose of 1200 μg, and the excretion during implant treatment. Both regimens achieve consistent testosterone suppression. The intranasal daily dose is equivalent to the subcutaneous injection of 30 μg buserelin (2.5% nasal absorption). The average excretion E_{av} (buserelin /CR ratio) in 24 hours urine specimens during treatment of prostate carcinoma patients with the nasal buserelin formulation was 5.89 μg/g CR[30], equivalent to an amount absorbed of 29.1 μg/24 hours. In the implant studies, the buserelin/CR ratio E_{min} on the last day of dose interval (day 56) was 6.77 μg/g CR, equivalent to an amount absorbed of 33.7 μg/24 hours. The two regimens were therefore considered bioequivalent when compared at the end of the implant dose interval.

Estimates of the MTE required for ovarian steroid suppression are also available from studies in women of reproductive age treated for endometriosis and gynecological disorders[3].

Estradiol secretion was consistently suppressed until reaching a buserelin/CR ratio of 0.4–0.6 μg/ g CR (MTE) equivalent to a minimum therapeutic release (MTR) of 3–4 μg/24 hours. The MTC in serum for maintaining estradiol suppression calculated from the MTR was 20–60 pg/ml serum, using a conversion factor of × 20 from serum buserelin (ng/ml) to buserelin excretion (μg/g CR). Further repeated studies with microparticles confirmed that the average MTR is in the range of 1.6–2.4 μg/24 hours independent of the preceding duration of suppression (Table 4).

Future perspectives

There are now several LHRH agonists in clinical use with high suppressive activity for which long-acting dosage forms (implants and microparticles) are available[23,24,26–33]. This facilitates clinical disease management and becomes an essential part of a therapy plan, for example in endometriosis. In our studies with microparticles we found that the dose interval of 28 days with a dose of 3.6 mg buserelin is preferable if predictable return of ovulation is required (Figure 7). The dose increment to 5.4 or 7.2 mg buserelin with an interval of 42 days does not prolong the duration of action to the same extent as that seen with implants. There is a dose-related average release R_{min} at the end of the dose interval (Table 5). However, due to individual variability a dose

Table 5 Buserelin microparticles, release rates R_{min} at end of dose interval in endometriosis patients, average of five clinical studies. The minimum therapeutic release (MTR) for maintaining estradiol suppression is a daily release rate of 1.7–2.5 µg/24 hours (see Table 4)

Treatment microparticles dose size (mg)	Release rate on day 28 (µg/24 hours)			Release rate on day 42 (µg/24 hours)		
	Mean	SE	n	Mean	SE	n
3.6	20.61	0.69	337	6.58	0.69	135
5.4	39.23	1.91	168	12.06	1.06	134
7.2	50.35	2.63	148	20.50	1.22	127

SE, standard error; n, number of determinations in patients

interval of 28 days is recommended for consistent estradiol suppression. In contrast to the long-lasting suppression by implants of PLG 75:25 (2-month and 3-month implants), microparticles have a terminal half-life of release of 10–11 days.

With the conveniently spaced treatment intervals, supporting medication can be explored. One example is the introduction of bone-sparing agents to prolong the suppression periods in endometriosis, to obtain more lasting involution of the endometriosis lesions but at the same time to maintain normal bone mineral content and biomechanical competence of bone. In a study in rats we found that ovariectomy and treatment with buserelin implants induces similar changes in bone morphology, bone density and biochemical parameters. There is a loss of trabecular structure, an increased excretion of bone-specific collagen cross links[37] and an increase in serum osteocalcin. These changes are related to estrogen deficiency and they are prevented by treating the animals with alendronate, a highly specific bone-sparing agent also used in the treatment of postmenopausal osteoporosis. This indicates that treatment periods with LHRH agonists and antagonists can be extended considerably when the bone is protected from the effects associated with estrogen deficiency.

There is considerable scope for the improvement of release profiles using surface modification of implants and new polymer materials with a reduced initial release (Figure 8). We are currently exploring microparticles of

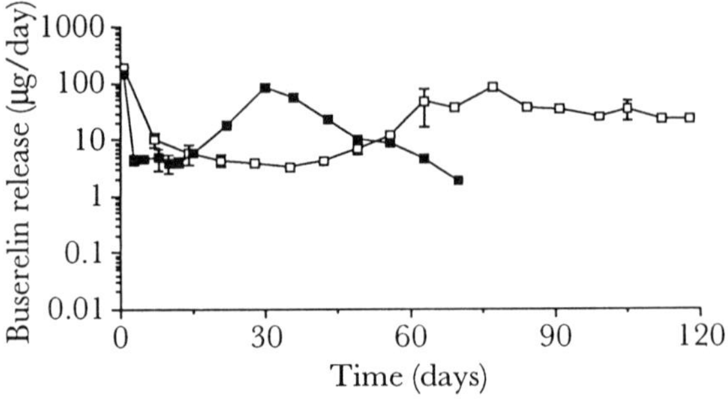

Figure 8 Advanced release systems: long-acting implants of PLG 75:25 and controlled release from microparticles of polytartrate (PTA). This new polymer offers release periods of 2–3 months in rats due to a significantly reduced initial release rate. The tissue tolerance of PTA is excellent, biodegradation is complete within 6 weeks after reaching the minimum therapeutic release rate MTR. □, Implant 9.9 mg; ■, PTA microparticles 7.2 mg

polytartrate, a new polymer which restricts the initial release to less than 20% of the dose on days 1–3 in relation to more than 40% of the dose using PLGA microparticles. Release periods of more than 4 months after a single injection are obtained with modified implant technology in rats and dogs, and release periods of 3 months are obtained with modified PTA microparticles.

The steady release rates provided by such preparations are, of course, dependent on using LHRH agonists of very high biological activity and superior biological tolerance. To avoid the initial stimulation observed (e.g. when implants are used for testosterone suppression in prostate carcinoma), LHRH antagonists are good candidates for the next generation of controlled release injections. In our experience, release periods of 1 month can be obtained using the LHRH antagonist ramorelix[36]. Clearly, there remains considerable potential for such new dosage forms which alternately will include other therapeutic peptides following the example set by the LHRH agonists.

Development of microparticle injections

Microparticle suspensions which can be injected subcutaneously have considerable attraction for gynecology, because the duration of suppression is more predictable than with long-acting implants and injections are more easily administered. Currently polylactide–glycolide microcapsules and microparticles (PLG 50:50) are in clinical use, with a release profile which differs from implants by a wider range of drug concentrations released during the dose interval. The comparative pharmacology of microparticles and implants in animal models shows that similar inhibition of target organs in the reproductive system can be obtained, but at the expense of increasing the dose or reducing the dose interval of microparticles. However, microparticle injections are an attractive alternative provided that similar drug loads can be obtained in the future, as with implants[34]. A major advantage of this approach is that thermal stress is avoided in the production process so that microencapsulation of polypeptides and proteins can be envisaged with less restrictions than those imposed by the implant technology.

Clinical studies have confirmed the efficacy and convenience of controlled release injections of LHRH agonists. Retrospective comparison of the animal models has established their predictive value in selecting suitable polymers for dose intervals up to 3 months, and has provided estimates of the release rate closely related to those found in clinical studies. Clinical research can now focus on optimal regimens using these dosage forms for reversible suppression of ovarian testicular function and its efficacy as part of a therapy plan for disease conditions.

References

1. Sandow, J. (1987). Pharmacology of LHRH Agonists. In Furr, B. J. A. and Wakeling, A. E. (eds.) *Pharmacology and Clinical Uses of Inhibitors of Hormone Secretion and Action*, pp. 365–84. (London: Baillière Tindall)

2. Sandow, J., Seidel, H. R., Krauss, B. and Jerabek-Sandow, G. (1987). Pharmacokinetics of LHRH agonists in different delivery systems and the relation to endocrine function. In Klijn, J. G. M., Paridaens, R. and Foekens, J. A. (eds.) *Hormonal Manipulation of Cancer: Peptides, Growth Factors, and New (Anti) Steroidal Agents*, pp. 203–12. (New York: Raven Press)

3. Fraser, H. M., Sandow, J., Cowen, G. M., Lumsden, M. A., Haining, R. and Smith S. K.(1989). Long-term treatment of endometriosis with a luteinizing hormone-releasing hormone agonist implant. *Fertil. Steril.*, **53**, 62–8

4. Waxman, J., Sandow, J., Abel, P., Farah, N., O'Donoghue, E., Fleming, J., Cox, J., Sikora, K. and Williams, G. (1989). Two-monthly depot gonadotropin releasing hormone agonist (buserelin) for treatment of prostatic cancer. *Acta Endocrinol. Copenh.*, **120**, 315–18

5. Lewis, D. (1993). Biodegradable polymers as drug delivery systems. *Pharm. Manufact. Int.*, **3**, 99–105

6. Furr, B. J. and Hutchinson, F. G. (1992). Biodegradable delivery system for peptides: preclinical experience with the gonadotrophin-releasing hormone agonist Zoladex . *J. Controlled Rel.*, **21**, 117–27

7. Goldspiel, B. R. and Kohler, D. R. (1991). Goserelin acetate implant: depot luteinizing hormone-releasing hormone analog for advanced prostate cancer. *DICP Ann. Pharmacother.*, **25**, 796–804

8. Reichel, R. P. and Schweppe, K. W. (1992). Goserelin (Zoladex) depot in the treatment of endometriosis. *Fertil. Steril.*, **57**, 1197–202

9. Sandow, J., v. Rechenberg, W., Seidel, H. and Keil, M. (1989). Experimental studies on tissue tolerance and on biodegradation of polylactide/

glycolide-buserelin implants in rats. In Aumüller, G., Krieg, M. and Senge, Th. (eds.) *New Aspects in the Regulation of Prostatic Cancer*, pp. 157–160. (Munich: Klinische und Experimentelle Urologie 20, Urological Research, Zuckschwerdt Verlag)

10. Mauduit, J. and Vert, M. (1993). Polymers based on lactic and glycolic acids and controlled drug delivery. *STP Pharm. Sci.*, **3**, 197–212

11. Sandow, J. (1990). The clinical use of LHRH agonists. In Edwards, B. (ed.) *Establishment of a Successful Human Pregnancy*, pp. 11–31. (New York: Raven Press)

12. Sandow, J. and Donnez, J. (1990). Clinical pharmacokinetics of LHRH analogues. In Brosens, I., Jacobs, H. S. and Runnebaum, B. (eds.) *LHRH Analogues in Gynaecology*, pp. 17–34. (Carnforth, UK: Parthenon Publishing)

13. Lemay, A., Sandow, J., Bureau, M., Maheux, R., Fontaine, J.-Y. and Merat, P. (1988). Prevention of follicular maturation in endometriosis by s.c. infusion of luteinizing hormone-releasing hormone (LHRH) agonist started in the luteal phase. *Fertil. Steril.*, **49**, 410–17

14. Klijn, J. G. M., Van Geel, B., De Jong, F. H., Sandow, J. and Krauss, B. (1991). The relation between pharmacokinetics and endocrine effects of buserelin implants in patients with mastalgia. *Clin. Endocrinol.*, **34**, 253–8

15. Blom, J. H. M., Hirdes, W. H., Schroeder, F. H., de Jong, F. H., Kwekkeboom, D. J., van't Veen, A. J., Sandow, J. and Krauss, B. (1989). Pharmacokinetics and endocrine effects of the LHRH analogue buserelin after subcutaneous implantation of a slow release preparation in prostatic cancer patients. *Urol. Res.*, **17**, 43–6

16. Waxman, J., Sandow, J., Abel, C., Barton, C., Keane, P. and Williams, G. (1990). Three-monthly GnRH agonist (buserelin) for prostatic cancer. *Br. J. Urol.*, **64**, 43–54

17. Donnez, J., Nisolle-Pochet, M., Clerckx-Braun, F., Sandow, J. and Casanas-Roux, F. (1989). Administration of nasal buserelin as compared with subcutaneous buserelin implant for endometriosis. *Fertil. Steril.*, **52**, 27–30

18. Donnez, J., Schrurs, B., Gillerot, S., Sandow, J. and Clerckx, F. (1989). Treatment of uterine fibroids with implants of gonadotropin-releasing hormone agonist: assessment by hysterography. *Fertil. Steril.*, **51**, 947–50

19. Fraser, H. M., Haining, R., Cowen, G. M., Sandow, J., Smith, K. B. and Smith, S. K. (1992). Long acting gonadotrophin releasing hormone agonist implant causes variable duration of suppression of ovarian steroid and inhibin secretion. *Clin. Endocrinol.*, **36**, 97–104

20. Fraser, H. M., Sandow, J., Seidel, H. and von Rechenberg, W. (1987). An implant of a gonadotropin releasing hormone agonist (buserelin) which suppresses ovarian function in the macaque for 3–5 months. *Acta Endocrinol. Copenh.*, **115**, 521–7

21. Behre, H. M., Sandow, J. and Nieschlag, E. (1992). Pharmacokinetics of the gonadotropin-releasing hormone agonist buserelin after injection of a slow-release preparation in normal men. *Arzneimittelforschung – Drug Res.*, **42**, 80–4

22. von Rechenberg, W., Sandow, J., Horstmann, G., Weinbauer, G. and Engelbart, K. (1989). Reversible inhibition of sexual maturation in male monkeys. *Acta Endocrinol. Copenh.*, **120** (Suppl. 1), 54–5

23. Healy, D. L., Lawson, S. R., Abbot, M., Baird, D. T. and Fraser, H. M. (1986). Towards removing uterine fibroids without surgery: subcutaneous infusion of a luteinizing hormone-releasing hormone agonist. *J. Clin. Endocrinol. Metab.*, **63**, 619–23

24. Chrisp, P. and Goa, K. L. (1991). Goserelin. A review of its pharmacodynamic and pharmaco-kinetic properties, and clinical use in sex hormone-related conditions. *Drugs*, **41**, 254–88

25. Plosker, G. L. and Brogden, R. N. (1994). Leuprorelin. A review of its pharmacology and therapeutic use in prostatic cancer, endometriosis and other sex hormone-related disorders. *Drugs*, **48**, 930–67

26. Friedman, A. J., Lobel, S. M., Rein, M. S. and Barbieri, R. L. (1990). Efficacy and safety considerations in women with uterine leiomyoma treated with gonadotropin-releasing hormone agonists: estrogen threshold hypothesis. *Am. J. Obstet. Gynecol.*, **163**, 1114–19

27. Toguchi, H., Ogawa, Y., Yamamoto, M. and Okada, H. (1991). Once-a-month injectable microcapsules of leuprorelin acetate. *J. Pharm. Soc. Jpn.*, **111**, 397–409

28. Sandow, J. (1994). Controlled release injections of buserelin in malignancy and gynaecological disorders. *Releaser*, **9**, 9–15

29. Ogawa, Y., Yamamoto, M., Okada, H. and Shimamoto, T. (1988). *In vivo* release profiles of leuprolide acetate from microcapsules prepared with polylactic acids or copoly (lactic/glycolic) acids and *in vivo* degradation of these polymers. *Chem. Pharm. Bull.*, **36**, 2576–81

30. Okada, H., Heya, T., Ogawa, Y., Toguchi, H. and Shimamoto, T. (1991). Sustained

pharmacological activities in rats following single and repeated administration of once-a-month injectable microspheres of leuprolide acetate. *Pharm. Res.*, **8**, 584–7

31. Sandow, J., Stoeckemann, K. and Jerabek-Sandow, G. (1990). Pharmacokinetics and endocrine effects of slow release formulations of LHRH analogues. *J. Steroid. Biochem. Mol. Biol.*, **37**, 925–31

32. Barradell, L. B. and McTavish, D. (1993). Histrelin. A review of its pharmacological properties and therapeutic role in central precocious puberty. *Drugs*, **45** , 570–88

33. Broekmans, F. J., Bernardus, R. E., Broeders, A., Berkhout, G. and Schoemaker, J., (1993). Pituitary responsiveness after administration of a GnRH agonist depot formulation: Decapeptyl CR. *Clin. Endocrinol.*, **38**, 579–87

34. Devisaguet, J. P., Drieu, K., Dray, F. and Ezan, E. (1988). Pharmacokinetic study of a sustained-release form, poly-(dl-lactide co-glycolide) microcapsules, of triptorelin (DTRP6-LHRH) in humans. *Pharm. Weekbl. Sci. Ed.*, **10**, 56–57

35. Lumsden, M. A., West, C. P. and Baird, D. T. (1987). Goserelin therapy before surgery for uterine fibroids. *Lancet*, **i**, 36–7

36. Van Leusden, H. A. (1994). Impact of different GnRH analogs in benign gynecological disorders related to their chemical structure, delivery systems and dose. *Gynecol. Endocrinol.*, **8**, 215–22

37. Stoeckemann, K. and Sandow, J. (1993). Effects of the luteinizing-hormone-releasing hormone (LHRH) antagonist ramorelix (Hoe013) and the LHRH agonist buserelin on dimethylbenz(a)-anthracene-induced mammary carcinoma: studies with slow-release formulations. *J. Cancer Res. Clin. Oncol.*, **119**, 457–62

38. Arshady, R. (1991). Preparation of biodegradable microspheres and microcapsules: 2. polylactides and related polyesters. *J. Control. Rel.*, **17**, 1–22

39. Dijkman, G. A., del Moral, P. F., Plasman, J. W., Kums, J. J., Delaere, K. P., Debruyne, F. M., Hutchinson, F. J. and Furr, B. J. (1990). A new extra long acting depot preparation of the LHRH analogue Zoladex. First endocrinological and pharmacokinetic data in patients with advanced prostate cancer. *J. Steroid Biochem. Mol. Biol.*, **37**, 933–6

40. Uebelhart, D., Schlemmer, A., Johansen, J., Gineyts, E., Christiansen, C. and Delmas, P. D. (1991). Effect of menopause and hormone replacement therapy on the urinary excretion of pyridinium crosslinks. *J. Clin. Endoc. Metab.*, **72**, 369–73

Sustained release formulations for long-term LHRH antagonist administration 7

J. Engel, Th. Reissmann, Th. Klenner, R. Hermann, E. Nieschlag, H. M. Behre, P. Hilgard, W. Deger and A. Sarlikiotis

INTRODUCTION

In 1971 luteinizing hormone releasing hormone (LHRH) was isolated from hypothalamic extracts and its amino acid sequence was established by Schally and co-workers[1]. Subsequently, amino acid modifications within the molecule resulted in the development of superagonists which are now widely used clinically[2,3]. To achieve suppression of gonadotropins, chronic administration of these compounds is necessary in order to induce down-regulation of pituitary receptors. Preceding this effect is an initial stimulation of luteinizing hormone (LH) and follicle stimulating hormone (FSH) secretion and desensitization of gonadotropic cells.

Avoidance of this initial gonadotropin release represents an advantage of LHRH antagonistic analogs, which are able to induce immediate suppression of gonadotropins and sex steroids by competitive binding to the LHRH receptors[4]. Based on a different mode of action, higher dosages of antagonist are needed to achieve these hormone-suppressive effects. Therefore new concepts for the development of an LHRH antagonist depot formulation for long-term treatment need to be established.

One of the LHRH antagonists currently under clinical evalution is Cetrorelix, which compared to former antagonists[5,6] is free of anaphylactoid effects[7], shows strong suppression of gonadotropins (and subsequently sex steroids) in animals and human beings[8–11] and, hence, was selected for further development. The LHRH agonists currently available are applied as nasal sprays, subcutaneous implants or intramuscular depot formulations based on polylactide/polyglycolide matrices. The monthly dose of these formulations is 3.8 mg, whereas the anticipated initial dose for Cetrorelix is approximately 30–60 mg. Together with other attempts such as, for example, the use of polylactide/polyglycolide (the pamoate salt of Cetrorelix), was tested. This chapter summarizes experimental results with Cetrorelix pamoate towards the development of a depot formulation.

PHARMACOLOGICAL EXPERIMENTS

Experiments in rats bearing the DMBA-induced mammary tumor

Using female rats with dimethylbenzanthracene (DMBA)-induced mammary tumor, single doses of pamoate salt of Cetrorelix (CP) produced a profound and long-lasting suppression of tumor growth, which, when compared to Cetrorelix acetate salt (CA), showed prolonged duration of action. In addition, in terms of reduction in tumor weight, the efficacy of CP treatment was superior to that with CA. At the time of maximal tumor mass reduction the mean number of tumor nodules still present were significantly lower in the CP group than in CA-treated animals. The achievable duration of anti-tumor efficacy after single dose treatment corresponded well with the period of estrus cycle interruption in normal rats. Prolonged efficacy of CP might be explained by the strong stability of Cetrorelix against degrading enzymes (submitted for publication) and the poor solubility

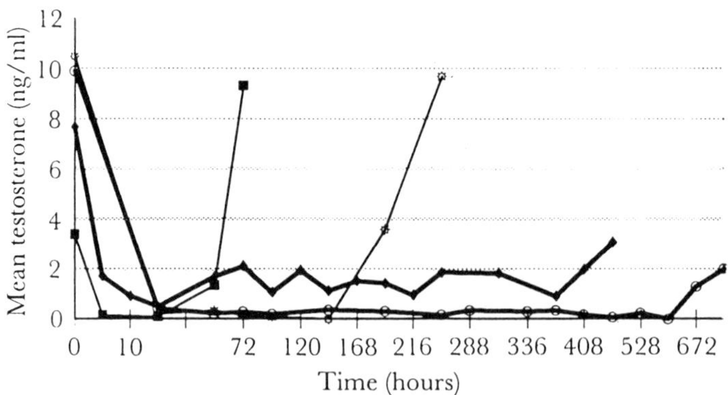

Figure 1 Cetrorelix pamoate in normal male rats. ■, acetate (0.5 mg/kg); ◆, pamoate (0.5 mg/kg); ●, pamoate (1.5 mg/kg); ▲, acetate (1.5 mg/kg)

of this salt (0.005 mg/mL in water). Based on first calculations, this salt has good bioavailability in rats.

Effects of Cetrorelix pamoate on testosterone levels in normal male rats

The prolonged anti-tumor activity of CP was obtained by using this salt not specifically formulated. Improvements were achieved by technical procedures which lead to more uniform material and, subsequently, to formulations without a carrier matrix but with defined particle sizes. In experimental animal studies, it was found that the most effective and long-lasting testosterone suppression was observed with pamoate particles of up to 125 μm. This was shown in experiments in which single doses of CP were injected subcutaneously into the right flank of male rats using doses of 0.5 mg/kg and 1.5 mg/kg, related to the peptide base. Blood samples were taken at different time intervals and testosterone was measured using an enzyme-linked immunoassay (EIA). Cetrorelix plasma levels were determined by using a radioimmunoassay originally developed by Csernus et al.[12]. After injection of 0.5 mg/kg, testosterone measurement revealed complete suppression for approximately 15 days. Using the higher dose of 1.5 mg/kg, the rats were completely suppressed with regard to testosterone levels for at least 30 days (Figure 1). Compared to CA the duration of action was extended by 5 days (0.5 mg) and 15 days (1.5 mg), respectively.

With regard to Cetrorelix plasma levels, it transpired that the duration of testosterone suppression did not correlate with the amount of Cetrorelix measured: although plasma level curves for CA and those for CP meet at 96 hours after injection, testosterone levels returned to normal values in the acetate group as early as 48 hours after injection (Figures 2,3).

Since the effective plasma levels measured for the depot fomulation are low in comparison to those of aqueous solution of CA, accumulation may occur within a pituitary compartment. Another possible mechanism could involve receptor down-regulation at the pituitary, as described by Srkalovic et al.[13] who also used Cetrorelix in their experiments. Subsequently, this inhibition can be maintained by low doses of the antagonist liberated from the depot formulation.

The homogeneity of pamoate formulation could be shown effectively for different laboratory batches, which produced a very similar pattern of testosterone suppression (Figure 4); the same applies for Cetrorelix plasma levels measured in these experiments.

Approximately 1% of the animals responded to treatment with Cetrorelix only for a short period of time. In one experiment the authors re-treated two animals 6 weeks after the first treatment and again observed a relatively short period of suppression. This can be based on a genetic alteration of the animals, different pharmacokinetics, a different sensibility of the

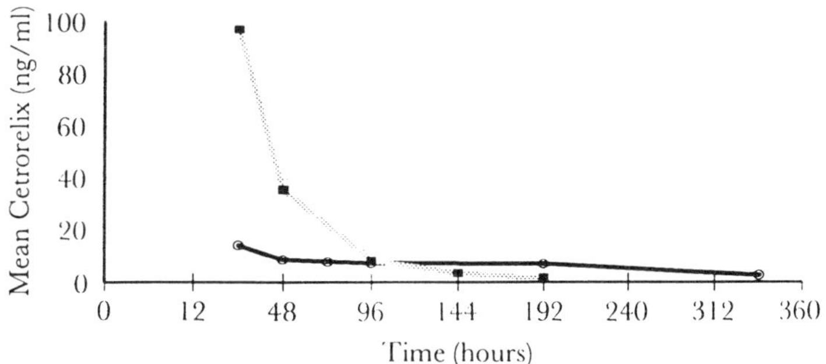

Figure 2   Cetrorelix depot in normal male rats, with 5 rats in each group. ■, Acetate (1.5 mg/kg); ●, pamoate (1.5 mg/kg)

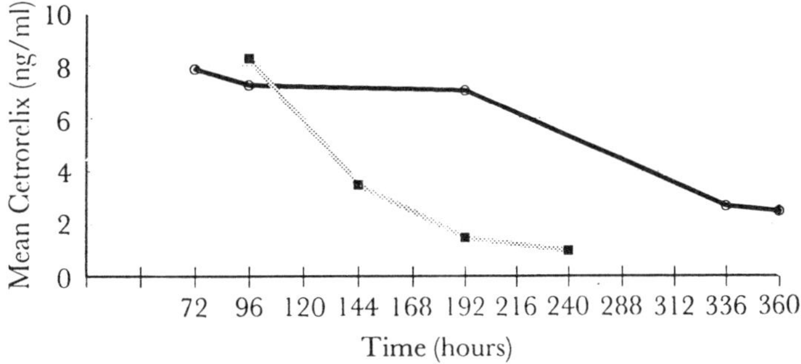

Figure 3   Cetrorelix plasma levels in normal male rats. ■, Acetate (1.5 mg/kg); ●, pamoate (1.5 mg/kg)

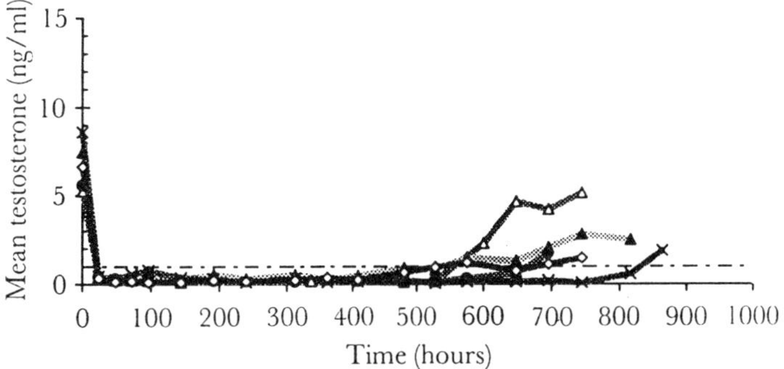

Figure 4   Testosterone suppression after single-dose treatment of male rats with different batches of Cetrorelix pamoate. △, DJ4; ●, DJ5; ▲, DJ8; ✕, DJ9; ◇, DJ10

gonadotropin releasing hormone (GnRH) receptor or a combination of these possibilities. In further experiments this phenomenon will be investigated in more detail.

Tolerability and clinical trials

Local tolerability of the new Cetrorelix pamoate microparticle formulation was tested in toxicological studies after intramuscular and subcutaneous injection. The results revealed no clinical signs of local intolerance at the injection sites. This was true for both the intramuscular and subcutaneous administration routes and also applies for the control animals, which had received the suspension medium only. No systemic toxic effects occurred in any of the animals. Therefore, there were no objections against the subcutaneous and intramuscular administration of this formulation in man and it was tested in four,

71

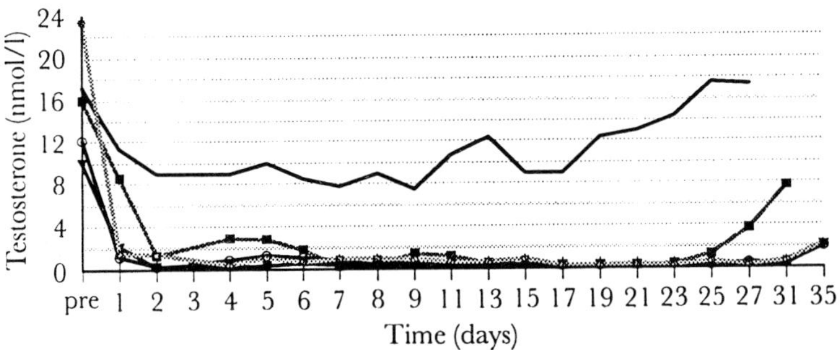

Figure 5 Treatment of male volunteers with Cetrorelix pamoate (60 mg on days 1 and 2). ▲, Volunteer 1; ─▲─, volunteer 2; ─●─, volunteer 3; ─■─, volunteert 4; ──, volunteer 5

placebo-controlled, phase-I studies in which a total of 47 healthy male individuals were injected intramuscularly

When single doses of 30 mg and 60 mg were tested, 12 hours after administration in all groups of treatment mean plasma testosterone (T) levels beneath 2 nmol/l were observed and demonstrated a clear dose relationship with a duration of T-suppression of 18–24 days in some, but not all, volunteers. On the basis of these results and from previous experience with CA, the duration of action of CP should also be investigated as maintenance therapy after an initial T-suppression by means of 5-day pretreatment with CA (also known as 'loading dose concept'). In a corresponding study, treatment started with daily subcutaneous injections of 10 mg CA for 5 days followed by a single administration of 60 mg CP intra-muscularly on day 6. Using this treatment schedule a reliable maintenance of T-suppression to castration level could be achieved for several weeks[14].

To simplify the 'loading dose concept', a further study was performed using only two administrations of CP, 24 hours apart. From all tested dose schedules the highest dosage group of 60 mg + 60 mg showed the most pronounced duration of action (Figure 5). T was suppressed to castration levels for a mean of 32 days (25–35 days) in four of five volunteers. The intramuscular route of administration was clearly well tolerated. Decreased libido and hot flushes were reported in two of five subjects after 22 days of T-suppression. Based on preliminary

calculations of the areas under the curve (AUC), a dose linearity is given from 10 mg to 60 mg.

CONCLUSIONS

The results described clearly indicate that the pamoate salt of Cetrorelix, due to its poor solubility, acts as a slow release formulation. Plasma level measurements of this formulation revealed short-term initial liberation and a subsequent long period of release. Therefore, the liberation of active peptide needed for the continuous suppression of testosterone in rats seems to be achievable in the most suitable way by the use of the pamoate itself. Compared to the acetate salt, the pamoate salt showed a remarkable prolongation of hormone suppressive effects in rats and a long-lasting anti-tumor efficacy in autochthonous DMBA-induced mammary tumors in rats. The range of variation within the hormone suppression of individual animals could be improved further by using pamoate salt of Cetrorelix in a defined particle size of up to 125 μm. The data presented, resulting from three phase-I studies with Cetrorelix pamoate, demonstrate effective suppression of gonadotropin and subsequently T-secretion in healthy male volunteers. With respect to the duration T-suppression, adequate pharmacodynamic action was observed in several subjects after a 60 mg single dose. A more reliable suppression of T to the level of castration for about 4 weeks could be demonstrated when the same dose of CP was administered either after a 5-day pretreatment with CA (maintenance therapy after loading dose) or when two injections of 60 mg of CP were administered 24 hours apart. Thus, the observed high intersubject variability in response after single doses and, in particular, in the lower dosage groups may be decreased with the availability of initial higher amounts of substance, which then facilitate maintenance of the pharmacodynamic effects with much lower plasma levels.

Cetrorelix pamoate was safe and well tolerated when administered intramuscularly in single doses of up to 60 mg and multiple doses of up to 2×60 mg in healthy males. This formulation is currently being investigated in further phase I and II trials in order to reproduce established dose schedules and to investigate the depot dosage needed for maintenance therapy. As well as indications of hormone dependent cancers[15,16], it is planned that benign indications in the field of gynecology and urology[17,18] will also be investigated.

References

1. Schally, A. V., Kastin, A. J. and Arimura, A. (1971). Hypothalamic FSH and LH-regulating hormone: structure, physiology and clinical studies. *Fertil. Steril.*, **22**, 703–21

2. Mansfield, M. J., Beardsworth, D. E. and Loughlin, J. S. (1983). Long-term treatment of central precocious puberty with a long-acting analogue of luteinizing hormone-releasing hormone. *N. Engl. J. Med.*, **309**, 1286–92

3. Furr, B. J. A. and Milsted, R. A. V. (1982). Use of analogues of LH-RH for treatment of cancer. *Endocr. Management Cancer*, **2**, 17–27

4. Wynn, P. C., Suarez-Quian, C., Childs, G. V. and Catt, K. J. (1986). Pituitary binding and internalization of radioiodinated gonadotropin-releasing hormone agonist and antagonist ligands *in vitro* and *in vivo*. *Endocrinology*, **119**, 1852–63

5. Schmidt, F., Sundaram, K., Thau, R. B. and Bardin, C. W. (1984). (Ac-D-Nal(2)1, 4FD-Phe2, D-Trp3, D-Arg6)-LH-RH, a potent antagonist of LH-RH, produces transient edema and behavioral changes in rats. *Contraception*, **29**, 283–9

6. Smith, R. D. and Edgren, R. A. (1982). Elevated blood pressure following LH-RH antagonists in rats. *Contraception*, **25**, 395–403

7. Bajusz, S., Kovacs, M., Gazdag, M., Bokser, L., Karashima, T., Csernus, V. J., Janaky, T., Guoth, J. and Schally, A. V. (1988). Highly potent antagonists of luteinizing hormone-releasing hormone free of edematogenic effects. *Proc. Natl. Acad. Sci. USA*, **85**, 1637–41

8. Szende, B., Srkalovic, G., Groot, K., Lapis, K. and Schally, A. V. (1990). Growth inhibition of mouse MXT mammary tumor by the luteinizing hormone-releasing hormone antagonist SB-75. *J. Natl. Cancer Inst.*, **82**, 513–17

9. Reismann, T., Hilgard, P., Harleman, J. H., Engel, J., Schally, A. V. and Comaru-Schally, A. M. (1992). Treatment of experimental DMBA induced mammary carcinoma with Cetrorelix (SB-75): a potent antagonist of luteinizing hormone-releasing hormone. *J. Cancer Res. Clin. Oncol.*, **118**, 44–9

10. Behre, H. M., Bockers, A., Schlingheider, A. and Nieschlag, E. (1994). Sustained suppression of serum LH, FSH and testosterone and increase of high-density lipoprotein cholesterol by daily injections of the GnRH antagonist Cetrorelix (SB-75) in normal men. *Clin. Endocrinol.*, **40**, 241–8

11. Gonzales-Barcena, D., Vadillo-Buenfil, M., Guerra-Arguero, E., Carenno, J., Comaru-Schally, A. M. and Schally, A. V. (1990). Potent antagonistic analog of LH-RH (SB-75) inhibits LH, FSH and testosterone levels in human beings. *The Endocrine Society Meeting*, Atlanta, Ga., p. 354, abstr. 1318

12. Csernus, V. J., Szende, B., Groot, K., Redding, T. W. and Schally, A. V. (1990). Development of radioimmunoassay for a potent luteinizing hormone-releasing hormone antagonist. *Drug Res.*, 40, 111–18

13. Srkalovic, G., Bokser, L., Radulovic, S., Korkut, E. and Schally, A. V. (1990). Receptors for luteinizing hormone-releasing hormone (LHRH) in Dunning R3327 prostate cancers and rat anterior pituitaries after treatment with a sustained delivery system of LHRH antagonist SB-75. *Endocrinology*, **127**, 3052–60

14. Behre, H. M., Kliesch, S., Bock, W., Hermann, R., Reissmann, Th., Engel, J. and Nieschlag, E. (1995). Suppression of serum testosterone in normal men by Cetrorelix pamoate, a GnRH antagonist depot preparation. *Exp. Clin. Endocrinol. Diabetes*, **103** (Suppl.1), 141

15. Schally, A. V., Bajusz, S., Redding, T. W., Zalatnai, A. and Comaru-Schally, A. M. (1989). Analogs of LHRH: the present and the future. In Vickery, B. H. and Lunenfeld, V. (eds.) *GnRH Analogs in Cancer and in Human Reproduction. Basic Aspects,* Vol. 1, pp. 5–31. (Dordrecht: Kluwer Academic Publishers)

16. Gonzalez-Barcena, D., Vadillo-Buenfil, M., Cortez-Morales, A., Fuentes-Garcia, M., Cardenas-Cornejo, I., Comaru-Schally, A. M. and Schally, A. V. (1995). Luteinizing hormone-releasing-hormone antagonist Cetrorelix as primary single therapy in patients with advanced prostatic cancer and paraplegia due to metastatic invasion of spinal cord. *Urology,* **45**, 275–81

17. Gonzalez-Barcena, D., Vadillo-Buenfil, M., Gomez-Orta, F., Fuentes-Garcia, M., Cardena-Cornejo, I., Graef-Sanchez, A., Comaru-Schally, A. M. and Schally, A. V. (1994). Responses to the antagonistic analog of LHRH (Cetrorelix) in patients with benign prostatic hyperplasia and prostatic cancer. *Prostate,* **24**, 84–92

18. Reissmann, T., Felberbaum, R., Diedrich, K., Engel, J., Comaru-Schally, A. M. and Schally, A. V. (1995). Development and applications of luteinizing hormone-releasing hormone antagonists in the treatment of infertility: an overview. *Hum. Reprod.,* **10** (8), 1974–81

Section 3

Characteristics of GnRH antagonists

Potential clinical applications of GnRH antagonists

8

H. J. T. Coelingh Bennink

INTRODUCTION

Gonadotropin releasing hormone (GnRH) antagonists are capable of immediate inhibition of pituitary gonadotropin secretion by competing with the stimulatory effect of GnRH. GnRH antagonists are likely to offer several advantages over the currently available GnRH agonists, such as the absence of an initial gonadotropin stimulation (flare) and the dose proportional efficacy[1]. GnRH antagonists are not yet available for clinical use. The development of these compounds has been hampered by: (1) histamine-release inducing properties; and (2) the depot formation after injection due to 'gelling' resulting in unreliable and unpredictable release from the injection site. The most recent generation of GnRH-antagonists, such as azaline B, Cetrorelix and Ganirelix, however, seem to have overcome these problems and are in phase II of clinical development. Therefore, only limited data on the clinical use of GnRH antagonists are available, so the potential clinical application of these compounds is still largely based on theoretical and pharmacological considerations.

The common denominator of the clinical use of GnRH antagonists is the aim to suppress endogenous gonadotropins and/or sex steroids. This suppression may be required for either short periods of time (e.g. during infertility treatment) or for long periods (e.g. during the treatment of endocrine cancers). Depending on the specific indication, short-term treatment varies from 1–6 weeks, whereas long-term treatment may last from several months to many years. A subdivision in short- and long-term treatment has a practical background too because the presently available pharmaceutical formulations of GnRH antagonists allow for daily subcutaneous administration only. Long-term treatment requires long-acting sustained release formulations. Such formulations are even at an earlier stage of pharmaceutical development.

POTENTIAL SHORT-TERM TREATMENT INDICATIONS

Short GnRH antagonist treatment (1–6 weeks) is anticipated to be effective in the following situations:

(1) Prevention of luteinizing hormone (LH) surges in controlled ovarian hyperstimulation (COH) for assisted reproductive techniques (ART);

(2) Suppression of increased LH levels during induction of ovulation in polycystic ovarian disease (PCOD) to decrease the incidence of spontaneous abortion;

(3) Treatment of threatening ovarian hyper-stimulation syndrome (OHSS);

(4) Preparation for surgery of leiomyoma;

(5) Functional menometrorrhagia;

(6) Male contraception by (initiating the) suppression of gonadotropins;

(7) Protection of the gonads during cytostatic treatment for cancer; and

(8) Interval treatment of endometrial cancer between diagnosis and surgery.

Prevention of LH surges in COH for ART such as *in vitro* fertilization (IVF) or intracytoplasmatic sperm injection (ICSI) is the most developed clinical indication for GnRH antagonists. The objective of this treatment is not to suppress gonadotropins, but to interfere with the estradiol-induced positive feedback on LH, thereby preventing premature LH surges and premature luteinization. Pioneer work has been performed in this area by the group of Bouchard and Frydman, who have tested several GnRH antagonists[2-4]. They have focused on single, or if necessary dual administration of the GnRH antagonist with a first dose on day 8 of the COH cycle. Continuous, low-dose GnRH antagonist treatment has been investigated by Diedrich *et al.*[5], starting treatment on day 7 and continuing until the day of human chorionic gonadotropin (hCG). These studies and others[6,7] have shown that GnRH antagonists are capable of preventing LH surges during COH. In addition, compared to GnRH agonist down-regulation for COH, the treatment duration with GnRH antagonists was much shorter and the required gonadotropin dose of follicle stimulating hormone (FSH) was significantly less. Pavlou's group[7] even showed more mature oocytes and better quality embryos with a GnRH antagonist when compared with a GnRH agonist. Appropriate dose finding studies have to establish the lowest effective dose of GnRH antagonists for COH, which should then be tested in large phase III clinical trials.

Of special concern in infertility treatment is the potential carry-over effect of a GnRH antagonist on the corpus luteum and, even more importantly, on an established pregnancy. Depending on factors such as elimination half-life of the GnRH antagonist and its depot formation at the injection site, carry-over may occur, stressing the importance of finding the lowest effective dose. When carry-over does occur, luteal support may be required and the pregnancy may be at risk. However, the group led by Siler-Khodr[8] has isolated a chorionic peptidase (C-ase-1) from trophoblast that actively degrades GnRH analogs at the 9–10 postproline site of the molecule. All GnRH antagonists in clinical development have preserved proline at position 9 and are, therefore, expected to be metabolised by trophoblast tissue, thus probably preventing exposure of the embryo to the compound.

When GnRH antagonists are shown to be safe and effective for routine use in COH to prevent LH surges, COH treatment may be simplified to a regimen of a rather low, fixed dose of recombinant FSH starting on day 2 of the cycle, a single, dual or continuous low dose of GnRH antagonist starting on day 7 or 8 and, instead of hCG, a final injection of recombinant LH, a GnRH agonist, or even GnRH. Such a simple regimen would be easier, shorter, less expensive and more acceptable for women and could, therefore, be repeated more frequently. The rather vigorous stimulation of ovaries practised nowadays could then be replaced by more careful limited controlled hyperstimulation aiming at just two or three follicles. Combined with ICSI, a high fertilisation rate could be obtained. This approach would minimize the risk of OHSS and might also appear to be safer at long-term follow-up.

Suppression of increased LH levels during ovulation induction (OI) in PCOD to decrease the incidence of spontaneous abortion after *in vivo* fertilization is the second infertility indication for GnRH antagonists. However, this is far more speculative than the COH indication. This is because there is no consensus on the reported correlation between increased LH levels in women with PCOD and an increased early pregnancy loss[9]. Appropriate studies with GnRH agonists to test this hypothesis are difficult to perform due to the mechanism of action of GnRH agonists which, initially, even further stimulate LH secretion. GnRH antagonists provide an easier tool to investigate this clinical problem. After establishing the dose needed to normalize LH, a placebo-controlled, randomised OI-study in PCOD could be performed with, as the primary end-point, the incidence of spontaneous abortion. A significant decrease of abortions would confirm the indication. An interesting theoretical consideration is whether normalization of LH would be required only during the gonadotropin-dependent phase of follicular development when LH receptors are present (the last 10–12 days before ovulation) or whether LH should be normalized for the full period of follicular development (about 80 days).

GnRH antagonists may be useful for the treatment of threatening OHSS when too many follicles are developing and/or estradiol is rising too quickly. Also, when OHSS has developed, elimination of stimulation by endogenous LH may be useful. Since vascular endothelial growth factor (VEGF) has been implicated in the pathogenesis of OHSS[10] and VEGF production by granulosa cells is dose- and time-dependently enhanced by hCG (and most likely also by LH), the effect of GnRH antagonists on VEGF production would be relevant to study.

The following short-term indications for GnRH-antagonist treatment are discussed in more detail by other authors in these proceedings:

(1) Preparation for surgery of uterine fibroma (leiomyoma) by reducing the size of the fibromas with GnRH antagonists may be faster and therefore more effective compared to GnRH agonists due to the absence of the 'flare' effect. For the same reason, treatment of functional menometrorrhagia may be more effective with GnRH antagonists.

(2) A GnRH antagonist might be particularly suitable to induce azoospermia followed by maintenance treatment with a testosterone preparation for male hormonal contraception. The efficacy of this concept has still to be proven in man. For long-term treatment, a GnRH antagonist depot preparation would be required, although a continuous combination of a GnRH antagonist and testosterone may not be cost-effective.

(3) Short-term treatment with a GnRH antagonist may also be useful as an adjunctive therapy in two cancer indications. The first one is the protection of the gonads during cytostatic treatment for cancer in fertile-age individuals for the preservation of endocrine and reproductive function of the gonads. The second indication might be interval treatment between the diagnosis of endometrial cancer and final surgery which sometimes lasts several weeks, although rapid surgery would certainly

be preferable from both a clinical and psychological point of view.

POTENTIAL LONG-TERM TREATMENT INDICATIONS

Long-term GnRH-antagonist treatment (several months to many years) is expected to be effective in the following situations:

(1) Prostate cancer;

(2) Breast cancer;

(3) Endometrial cancer;

(4) Ovarian cancer;

(5) Benign prostatic hypertrophia;

(6) Precocious puberty;

(7) Endometriosis; and

(8) Hyperandrogenism.

In view of the long period of treatment these indications require a sustained release GnRH antagonist depot preparation. Daily subcutaneous injections would only be acceptable when efficacy would be significantly superior to, for example, GnRH agonists, in addition to the initial advantage of no 'flare'. Linkage of GnRH analogs to cytotoxic radicals, as discussed by Schally in the proceedings, may increase the efficacy of cancer treatment with these compounds with a concomitant decrease of general toxicity.

When GnRH antagonists do not show convincing advantages over GnRH agonists for these long-term indications, cost/benefit ratios and health–economic considerations may be decisive for further clinical development.

For more details on the long-term indications the reader is referred to the respective chapters in these proceedings.

References

1. Gordon, K., Danforth, D. R., Williams, R. F. and Hodgen, G. D. (1992). New trends in combined use of gonadotropin-releasing hormone antagonists with gonadotropins or pulsatile

gonadotropin-releasing hormone in ovulation induction and assisted reproductive technologies. *Curr. Sci.*, **4**, 690–6

2. Frydman, R., Cornel, C., De Ziegler, D., Taieb, J., Spitz, I. M. and Bouchard, P. (1991). Prevention of premature luteinizing hormone and progesterone rise with a gonadotropin-releasing hormone antagonist, Nal-Glu, in controlled ovarian hyperstimulation. *Fertil. Steril.*, **56**, 923–7

3. Olivennes, F., Fanchin, R., Bouchard, P., De Ziegler, D., Taieb, J., Selva, J. and Frydman, R. (1994). The single or dual administration of the gonadotropin-releasing hormone antagonist Cetrorelix in an *in vitro* fertilization-embryo transfer program. *Fertil. Steril.*, **62**, 468–76

4. Olivennes, F., Fanchin, R., Bouchard, P., Taieb, J., Selva, J. and Frydman, R. (1995). Scheduled administration of a gonadotrophin-releasing hormone antagonist (Cetrorelix) on day 8 of *in vitro* fertilization cycles: a pilot study. *Hum. Reprod.*, **10**, 1382–6

5. Diedrich, K., Diedrich, C., Santos, E., Zoll, C., Al-Hasani, S., Reissmann, T., Krebs, D. and Klingmüller, D. (1994). Suppression of the endogenous luteinizing hormone surge by the gonadotrophin-releasing hormone antagonist Cetrorelix during ovarian stimulation. *Hum. Reprod.*, **9**, 788–91

6. Cassidenti, D. L., Sauer, M. V., Paulson, R. J., Ditkoff, E. C., Rivier, J., Yen, S. S. C. and Lobo, R. A. (1991). Comparison of intermittent and continuous use of a gonadotropin-releasing hormone antagonist (Nal-Glu) in *in vitro* fertilization cycles: a preliminary report. *Am. J. Obstet. Gynecol.*, **165**, 1806–10

7. Minaretzis, D., Alper, M. M., Oskowitz, S. P., Lobel, S. M., Mortala, J. F. and Pavlou, S. N. (1995). Gonadotropin-releasing hormone antagonist versus agonist adminstration in women undergoing controlled ovarian hyperstimulation: cycle performance and *in vitro* steroidogenesis of granulosa-lutein cells. *Am. J. Obstet. Gynecol.*, **172**, 1518–25

8. Siler-Khodr, T. M., Kang, I. S., Kuehl, T. J., and Khodr, G. S. (1994). Potential for embryo damage of GnRH analogs. In Filicori, M. and Flamigni, C. (eds.) *Ovulation Induction: Basic Science and Clinical Advances*, pp. 297–306. (Amsterdam: Elsevier)

9. Homburg, R., Armar, N. A., Eskel, A., Adams, J. and Jacobs, H. S. (1988). Influence of serum LH concentrations on ovulation, conception and early pregnancy loss in polycystic ovary syndrome. *Br. Med. J.*, **297**, 1024–6

10. Neulen, J., Yan, Z., Raczek, S., Weindel, K., Keck, C., Weich, H. A., Marmé, D. and Breckwoldt, M. (1995). Human chorionic gonadotropin-dependent expression of vascular endothelial growth factor/vascular permeability factor in human granulosa cells: importance in ovarian hyperstimulation syndrome. *J. Clin. Endocrinol. Metab.*, **80**, 1967–71

LHRH antagonist Cetrorelix (INN): biological and clinical characteristics

9

Th. Reissmann, J. Engel, P. Hilgard, W. Deger, H. M. Behre, E. Nieschlag, R. Felberbaum, K. Diedrich, A. M. Comaru-Schally and A. V. Schally

INTRODUCTION

The clinical interference with sex hormone production is based on analogs of the hypothalamic hormone which controls the secretion of luteinizing hormone (LH) and follicle, stimulating hormone (FSH) from the anterior pituitary gland. This peptide hormone named luteinizing hormone releasing hormone (LHRH) was isolated from hypothalamic extracts and its amino acid sequence was established by Matsuo and co-workers[1]. Replacement or deletion of different amino acids within the parent molecule resulted in analogs with higher receptor binding affinities. This led to the discovery of superagonists. Given in frequent intervals these agonistic analogues are highly potent in inducing the secretion of LH and FSH, whereas the chronic administration of these compounds results in a down-regulation of pituitary receptors and subsequent inhibition of gonadotropin and sex steroid secretion, which can be used clinically[2,3]. The mechanism underlying these phenomena is a desensitization of the gonadotropic cells followed by a down-regulation of pituitary receptors leading to a selective medical hypophysectomy. However, in those situations where an immediate suppression of the gonadotropins is desired, the major disadvantage of agonists is their initial stimulatory effect on hormone secretion. The use of antagonists which produce an immediate inhibition of gonadotropin release by competitive blockade of the receptors is, therefore, more desirable. However, severe side effects such as edematogenic reactions due to histamine release were observed with some antagonists and have hampered their clinical development[4,5].

Today, new antagonists have been synthesized whose safety profile seems to warrant their clinical development[6,7]. One of the most advanced antagonists is Cetrorelix (SB-75), which has been shown to inhibit LH and testosterone secretion effectively in a variety of animal models as well as in clinical studies, including normal young men and women as well as patients suffering from advanced carcinoma of the prostate or benign prostatic hyperplasia. Recently, Cetrorelix has also been tested in combination with human menopausal gonadotropin (hMG) for ovarian hyperstimulation in *in vitro* fertilization regimens[8,9].

SUMMARY OF PRECLINICAL RESULTS

Chemistry

The natural LHRH, Cetrorelix, is a decapeptide (see Table 1) which originally was synthesized by

Table 1 Sequence of amino acids

Ac-D-Nal(2)	*-D-Phe(4Cl)*	*-D/PAL*	*-SER*	*-TYR*	*-D/CIT-*	*LEU-*	*ARG-*	*PRO*	*-D-Ala-NH²*
1	2	3	4	5	6	7	8	9	10

Molecular weight: 1431.07

Bajusz *et al.* (Tulane University, New Orleans). Within the molecule five amino acids were replaced by unnatural D-amino acids[6].

The chemical and physical stability of Cetrorelix has been well characterized. In general, peptides are considered 'not stable' and are subject to hydrolysis, oxidation, photo decomposition and other side reactions. However, when the aqueous stability of Cetrorelix was investigated in the range of pH 1.0–13.0, the peptide was found to be surprisingly stable at pH 7.0 for a period of 21 days and is resistant to oxidative attack with H_2O_2 under neutral conditions; peptides and proteins usually undergo proteolysis by enzymes, with striking consequences for the bioavailability of peptidic drugs. Cetrorelix is highly resistant to degrading enzymes such as chymotrypsin, pronase and nargase for several days, which is in sharp contrast to LHRH agonists which undergo almost complete degradation within several hours[10].

Cetrorelix showed a high binding affinity to rat pituitary receptors[11], leading to a pronounced suppressive effect on the gonadotropins (LH, FSH) and, subsequently, on sex-hormones in various experimental animal models. The strong suppression of sex steroids resulted in a complete tumor regression in the dimethylbenzanthracene (DMBA)-induced mammary carcinoma of rats[12] and similar growth inhibitory effects were found in the MXT mammary carcinoma of mice[13], the Dunning prostate carcinoma of rats and on different human ovarian cancer cell lines[14,15].

Compared to other antagonists, much lower doses proved to be sufficient and a prolonged duration of action was observed. Figure 1 shows the dose-dependent efficacy of Cetrorelix in DMBA-induced mammary tumors of rats. The dose range tested was 10 µg/kg to 316 µg/kg. The dose of 10 µg/kg was not effective in reducing tumor weight. These dose groups were not significantly different from the control data. However, doses of 100 µg/kg and 316 µg/kg gave an anti-tumor response, with 100 µg/kg being an optimal dose in the DMBA-tumor model. Microscopically, the effects of Cetrorelix on this tumor were characterized by a loss of mitotic activity, marked atrophy with apoptosis

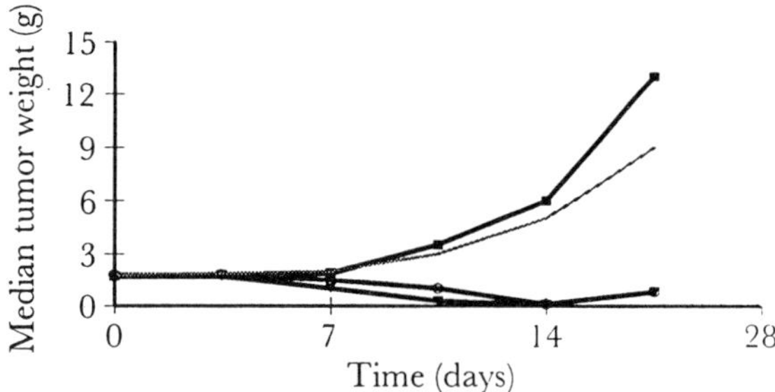

Figure 1 Treatment of DMBA-tumor bearing rats eith Cetrorelix in different doses. —— , control; —■— , 10 µg/kg; —●— , 100 µg/kg; —▲— , 316 µg/kg

and normalization and differentiation towards a normal mammary architecture[12].

Interestingly, a significant anti-tumor activity was also found in ovarian cancer xenografts and hormone-independent animal tumor models, such as the Dunning prostate cancer of rats[16,17]. In both tumor models a decrease in tumor weight and a prolongation in survival time of the animals was found. For both tumor models direct cytostatic/ cytotoxic effects can be assumed, since the measurement of epidermal growth factor (EGF) revealed a loss of the corresponding receptor as well as a decrease in EGF levels in the tumor tissues after treatment with Cetrorelix. Thus, an interference of the antagonist with growth factors might contribute to the observed effects[18]. Preclinical studies are ongoing in order to clarify the phenomenon.

The immediate and strong suppression of testosterone within hours after administration of Cetrorelix was demonstrated in rats[19] and in monkeys, with Cetrorelix being more effective than other antagonists in these models[20].

In contrast to former antagonists, Cetrorelix was not very potent in inducing histamine release from mast cells *in vitro* and so no anaphylactoid reactions were seen in clinical phase I studies. In safety pharmacological, as well as in 6-month toxicological studies in rats and dogs, Cetrorelix exerted no systemic side effects. In addition, it was shown to be non-teratogenic and no mutagenic potential was observed. Those effects which are related to the pharmacological action of the compound (reduction in weight of testis, ovaries, uterus and sperm counts) were reversible,

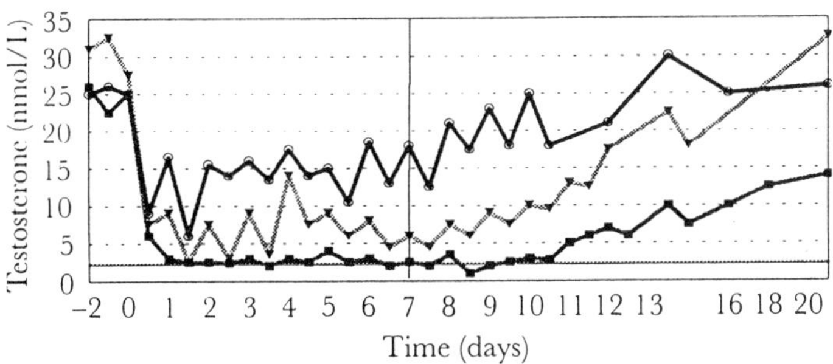

Figure 2 Phase I – daily (8 days) treatment of male volunteers. ⊸⊶ , 2 mg/day; ⊸▾⊷ , 5 mg/day; ⊸■⊷ , 10 mg/day; ⎯ , castration

with the time period needed for recovery being dependent on the treatment duration. Based on this favorable safety profile, clinical phase 1 studies were initiated in volunteers. In these studies a lyophilisate of Cetrorelix acetate was used.

SUMMARY OF CLINICAL RESULTS

Phase 1 studies

The safety of Cetrorelix was also confirmed in clinical trials in which more than 100 volunteers, male and female, received Cetrorelix. Even in supra-optimal doses, tolerability proved to be very good. Mild erythemas were observed at the injection site, which were not associated with pruritus or pain and vanished within a few minutes. The dose range tested for single doses was 0.25–5 mg[21].

Compared to the placebo group, the extent duration of suppression augmented with increasing doses. After the administration of 1.0 mg Cetrorelix, maximal testosterone suppression was seen 8 hours after injection and 12 hours after single doses of 2.0–5.0 mg of Cetrorelix. Twenty-four hours after administration of 1.0–2.0 mg of Cetrorelix, testosterone values were no longer different from those in the placebo group, whereas in the 5.0 mg dose group testosterone concentrations increased slightly and reached serum concentrations within the lower normal range after 48 hours. A linear kinetic relationship was found, with a calculated plasma half-life of 30 hours after single doses of 5 mg.

During daily doses for 8 days[22], a dose-dependent suppression was again found but,

interestingly, only a dosage as high as 10 mg/day was able to maintain testosterone levels within the castration range over the period of administration (Figure 2). With the use of lower doses an increase of testosterone levels was found between days 2–4 of treatment. Therefore, based on results from animal studies and pharmacokinetic considerations, tests were made to discover if the suppression of LH, FSH and testosterone could be achieved by initial high-dose Cetrorelix and maintained by continued low-dose injections. A loading-dose schedule which involved administering a 10 mg/day dose for 5 days followed by a maintenance dose of 1 mg/day was then tested in male volunteers[23] and resulted in a continuous suppression of testosterone. This finding opened technical possibilities for the development of a depot formulation. In addition, in these studies it was found that treatment with Cetrorelix induced a strong (approximately 40%), reversible reduction of the prostatic volume within 2 weeks of treatment. Whether a receptor down-regulation induced by Cetrorelix[24] is the basis for the efficacy of low maintenance dosages requires further investigation.

Benign prostatic hyperplasia (BPH) and prostate cancer

A beneficial effect was also found in patients suffering from BPH and prostate cancer who have been treated with Cetrorelix[25]. In BPH patients, the efficacy with regard to improvement in symptoms was independent of the degree of testosterone suppression[26,27]. It was established that testosterone withdrawal results in a decrease of prostate volume and weight, and so Cetrorelix is effective in the treatment of BPH. One of the standard therapies to achieve total testosterone suppression in prostate cancer is orchiectomy, with the occurrence of hormone-withdrawal symptoms such as hot flushes and impotence, but this is not acceptable for benign disease. Since total testosterone suppression may not be mandatory in BPH, it should be possible to develop a regimen in which the degree of testosterone suppression is limited to that which is necessary. In addition, according to recent results, a short-term treatment of about 4 weeks should result in an immediate relief of clinical symptoms, lasting for several months in some cases. Due to the high incidence of BPH with dysuric complaint in men above 50 years of age and the lack of an effective therapy, the investigation of new compounds which may have fewer side effects when treating patients with this disease is justified. The authors have, therefore, started a confirmative, placebo-controlled study with Cetrorelix for BPH. An intermittent treatment schedule, possibly in combination with an α blocker, should be elaborated in subsequent trials.

Controlled ovarian hyperstimulation (COH)

Clinical studies were initiated in women suffering from tubal infertility who were treated with hormones in order to induce multiple follicular maturation for assisted reproduction (COH). The classical stimulation procedure with gonadotropins such as hMG or human chorionic gonadotropin (hCG) has the disadvantage of an unpredictable ovarian reaction and the occurrence of premature LH surges. The endogenous LH surge can result in luteinization with a negative impact on the quality of the oocytes, which in turn result in the cancellation of the treatment cycle[28]. The introduction of LHRH agonists into the stimulation protocols increased the effectiveness of *in vitro* fertilization by achieving improved synchronization of follicular maturation and reduced frequency of premature luteinization. Currently, the so-called long protocol, in which the treatment with agonists starts at least 14 days

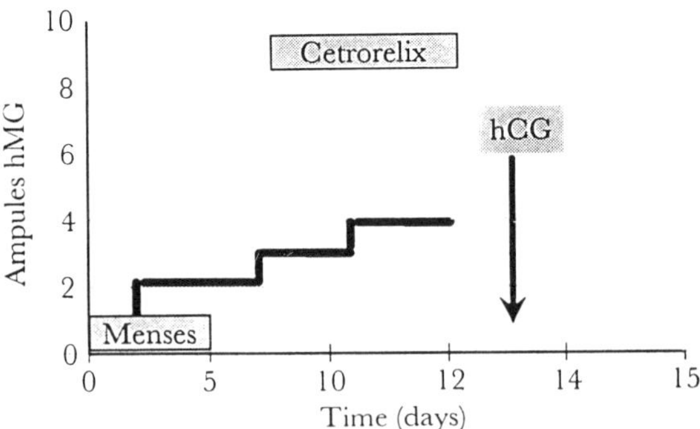

Figure 3 Treatment schedule for Cetrorelix in ovarian hyperstimulation for *in vitro* fertilization/embryo transfer

before the stimulation with gonadotropins, has proved to be the most effective procedure. However, disadvantages of this treatment schedule are the long treatment period and the high doses of gonadotropins necessary. In addition, there are individual fluctuations, until the suppressive phase is reached, so multiple hormone determinations are required to monitor each patient.

New uses may be possible with the introduction of the LHRH antagonist Cetrorelix into *in vitro* fertilization procedures (Figure 3). Due to the immediate suppression of gonadotropins, the unwanted stimulatory phase of the LHRH agonists can be avoided and the prolonged treatment duration can be reduced significantly. A short-term treatment with Cetrorelix has avoided these LH peaks in about 100 patients that have so far been treated with different dosages or dose schedules[8,9,29]. The pregnancy rate, so far, is comparable with standard treatment and there is a chance to reduce overall treatment costs by the possible reduction in the amount of hMG needed[30]. Currently, first feasibility studies have also been initiated in the treatment of uterine fibroma.

CONCLUSION

On the basis of the preclinical and clinical data from the treatment of more than 500 individuals, Cetrorelix has proved to be a safe LHRH antagonist and because of its hormone-suppressive effectiveness has the potential to be applied in a variety of clinical conditions[31–34]. Since the antagonist effectively inhibits spermatogenesis and ovulation it may, in addition to the 'classical' indications, be useful in male contraception and in the prevention of gonadal damage by cytostatic agents during chemotherapy, in which the efficacy of agonists was not satisfactory[35,36]. At present, daily injections of the lyophilisate are used. However, for long-term treatment a depot formulation is desirable and different approaches towards a clinically suitable depot formulation are being evaluated.

References

1. Matsuo, H., Baba, Y., Nair, R. M. G., Arimura, A. and Schally, A. V. (1971). Structure of porcine LH and FSH releasing factor, the proposed amino acid sequence. *Biochem. Biophys. Res. Commun.*, **43**, 1334–9

2. Lemay, A., Maheux, R., Faure, N., Jean, C. and Fazekas, A. T. A. (1984). Reversible hypogonadism induced by a luteinizing hormone-releasing hormone (LH-RH) agonist (buserelin) as a new therapeutic approach for endometriosis. *Fertil. Steril.*, **41**, 863

3. Mansfield, M. J., Beardsworth, D. E., Loughlin, J. S., Crawford, J. D., Bode, H. H., Rivier, J., Vale, W., Kushner, D. C., Crigler, J. F. and Crowley, W. F. Jr. (1983). Long-term treatment of central precocious puberty with a long-acting analogue of luteinizing hormone-releasing hormone. *N. Engl. J. Med.*, **309**, 1286

4. Schmidt, F., Sundaram, K., Thau, R. B. and Bardin, C. W. (1984). (Ac-D-Nal(2)1, 4FD-Phe2, D-TRP3, D-Arg6)-LH-RH, a potent antagonist of LH-RH, produces transient edema and behavioral changes in rats. *Contraception*, **29**, 283–9

5. Hahn, D. W., McGuire, J. L., Vale, W. W. and Rivier, J. (1985). Reproductive/endocrine and anaphylactoid properties of an LH-RH-antagonist, ORF-18260 (Ac-DNal1(2), 4FDPhe2, D-TRP3, D-Arg6)-GnRH. *Life Sci.*, **37**, 505–14

6. Bajusz, S., Kovacs, M., Gazdag, M., Bokser, L., Karashima, T., Csernus, V. J., Janaky, T., Guoth, J. and Schally, A. V. (1988). Highly potent antagonists of luteinizing hormone-releasing hormone free of edematogenic effects. *Proc. Natl. Acad. Sci. USA*, **85**, 1637–41

7. Rivier, J. (1993). Novel antagonists of GnRH: a compendium of their physiochemical properties, activities, relative potencies and efficacy in humans. In Lunenfeld, B. and Insler, V. (eds.) *GnRH Analogues. The State of the Art, 1993.* pp. 13–26. (London: Parthenon Publishing Group)

8. Diedrich, K., Diedrich, C., Santos, E., Zoll, C., Al-Hasani, S., Reissmann, T., Krebs, D. and Klingmüller, D. (1994). Suppression of the endogenous luteinizing hormone surge by the gonadotropin-releasing hormone antagonist Cetrorelix during ovarian stimulation. *Hum. Reprod.*, **9**, 788–91

9. Olivennes, F., Fanchin, R., Bouchard, P., De Ziegler, D., Taieb, J., Selva, J. and Frydman, R. (1994). The single or dual administration of the gonadotropin-releasing hormone antagonist Cetrorelix in an *in vitro* fertilization–embryo transfer program. *Fertil. Steril.*, **62**, 468–76

10. Deger, W. Presented at the *2nd European Medical Chemistry Conference*, 31 March 1993, Bad Nauheim, Germany

11. Fekete, M., Bajusz, S., Groot, K., Csernus, V. J. and Schally, A. V. (1989). Comparison of different agonists and antagonists of luteinizing hormone-releasing hormone for receptor-binding ability to rat pituitary and human breast cancer membranes. *Endocrinology*, **124**, 946–55

12. Reissmann, T., Hilgard, P., Harleman, J. H., Engel, J., Schally, A. V. and Comaru-Schally, A. M. (1992). Treatment of experimental DMBA induced mammary carcinoma with Cetrorelix (SB-75): a potent antagonist of luteinizing hormone-releasing hormone. *J. Cancer Res. Clin. Oncol.*, **118**, 44–9

13. Szende, B., Srkalovic, G., Groot, K, Lapis, K. and Schally, A. V. (1990). Growth inhibition of mouse MXT mammary tumor by the luteinizing hormone-releasing hormone antagonist SB-75. *J. Natl. Cancer Inst.*, **82**, 513–17

14. Korkut, E., Bokser, L., Comaru-Schally, A. M., Groot, K. and Schally, A. V. (1991). Inhibition of growth of experimental prostate cancer with sustained delivery systems (microcapsules and microgranules) of the luteinizing hormone-releasing hormone antagonist SB-75. *Proc. Natl. Acad. Sci. USA*, **88**, 844–8

15. Emons, G. and Schally, A. V. (1994). The use of luteinizing hormone releasing hormone agonists and antagonists in gynaecological cancers. *Hum. Reprod. Update*, **9**, 1364–79

16. Shirahige, Y., Cook, C., Pinski, J., Halmos, G., Nair, R. and Schally, A. V. (1994). Treatment with luteinizing hormone-releasing hormone antagonist SB-75 decreases levels of epidermal growth factor receptor and its mRNA in OV-1063 human epithelial ovarian cancer xenografts in nude mice. *Int. J. Oncol.*, **5**, 1031–5

17. Pinski, J., Reile, H., Halmos, G., Groot, K. and Schally, A. V. (1994). Inhibitory effects of luteinizing hormone-releasing hormone on the growth of the androgen-independent Dunning R-3327-AT-1 rat prostate cancer. *Int. J. Cancer*, **59**, 51–5

18. Sharoni, Y., Bosin, E., Miinster, A., Levy, J. and Schally, A. V. (1989). Inhibition of growth of human mammary tumor cells by potent antagonists of luteinizing hormone-releasing hormone. *Proc. Natl. Acad. Sci. USA*, **86**, 1648–51

19. Bokser, L., Bajusz, S., Groot, K. and Schally, A. V. (1990). Prolonged inhibition of luteinizing hormone and testosterone levels in male rats with the luteinizing hormone-releasing hormone antagonist SB-75. *Pro. Natl. Acad. Sci. USA*, **87**, 7100–4

20. Weinbauer, G. F. and Nieschlag, E. (1990). Evaluation of the antigonadotropic activity of different GnRH antagonists in the non-human primate. Proceedings of the 2nd International Symposium on GnRH Analogues in Cancer and Human Reproduction, Geneva. *Gynecol. Endocrinol.*, **4**, abstr. 21

21. Behre, H. M., Klein, B., Steinmeyer, E., McGregor, G. P., Voigt, K. and Nieschlag, E. (1992). Effective suppression of luteinizing hormone and testosterone by single doses of the new gonadotropin-releasing hormone antagonist Cetrorelix (SB-75) in normal men. *J. Clin. Endocrinol. Metab.*, **75**, 393–8

22. Behre, H. M., Böckers, A., Schlingheider, A. and Nieschlag, E. (1994). Sustained suppression of serum LH, FSH and testosterone and increase of high-density lipoprotein cholesterol by daily injections of the GnRH antagonist Cetrorelix (SB-75) in normal men. *Clin. Endocrinol.*, **40**, 241–8

23. Behre, H. M., Kliesch, S., Pühse, G. and Nieschlag, E. (1994). Initial high doses of a GnRH antagonist followed by low maintenance doses suppress serum LH, FSH and testosterone effectively in normal men. *Exp. Clin. Endocrinol.*, **102**, 53

24. Srkalovic, G., Bokser, L., Radulovic, S., Korkut, E. and Schally, A. V. (1990). Receptors for luteinizing hormone-releasing hormone (LHRH) in Dunning R3327 prostate cancers and rat anterior pituitaries after treatment with a sustained delivery system of LHRH antagonist SB-75. *Endocrinology*, **127**, 3052–60

25. Schally, A. V., Srkalovic, G., Szende, B., Redding, T. W., Korkut, E., Szepeshazi, K., Bokser, L., Pinski, J., Groot, K., Serfozo, P., Comaru-Schally, A. M., Bajusz, S., Gonzalez-Barcena, D., Reissmann, T., Hilgard, P. and Engel, J. (1990). New antagonistic analogs of LH-RH: experimental oncological and clinical studies. International Symposium on GnRH Analogues in Cancer and Human Reproduction; Geneva, November 6–10, 1990. *Gynecol. Endocrinol.*, **4**, 92

26. Gonzalez-Barcena, D., Vadillo-Buenfil, M., Cortez-Morales, A., Fuentes-Garcia, M., Cardenas-Cornejo, I., Comaru-Schally, A. M. and Schally, A. V. (1995). Luteinizing hormone-releasing-hormone antagonist Cetrorelix as primary single therapy in patients with advanced prostatic cancer and paraplegia due to metastatic invasion of spinal cord. *Urology*, **45**, 275–81

27. Gonzalez-Barcena, D., Vadillo-Buenfil, M., Gomez-Orta, F., Fuentes-Garcia, M., Cardenas-Cornejo, I., Graef-Sanchez, A., Comaru-Schally, A. M. and Schally, A. V. (1994). Responses to the antagonistic analog of LHRH (Cetrorelix) in patients with benign prostatic hyperplasia and prostatic cancer. *Prostate*, **24**, 84–92

28. Stanger, J. D. and Yovich, J. L. (1985). Reduced *in vitro* fertilization of human oocytes from patients with raised basal luteinizing hormone levels during the follicular phase. *Br. J. Obstet. Gynaecol.*, **92**, 385–93

29. Olivennes, F., Fanchin, R., Bouchard, Ph., Taieb, J., Selva, J. and Frydman, R. (1994). A simple administration protocol of a new GnRH antagonist (Cetrorelix) was able to prevent premature LH surges in an IVF programme. *Hum. Reprod.*, **9** (Suppl. 4), 87

30. Felberbaum, R., Reissmann, T., Zoll, C., Al-Hasani, S., Küpker, W., Diedrich, C. and Diedrich, K. (1995). Fertilization rate and amount of human menopausal gonadotropin needed in controlled ovarian hyperstimulation under low-dose gonadotropin-releasing-hormone antagonist treatment. In *Abstracts of the 11th Annual Meeting of the ESHRE*, Hamburg, 1995. p. 8, abstr. 15

31. Schally, A. V. and Redding, T. W. (1987). Use of LH-RH analogs for the treatment of prostate

cancer: combination therapy and direct effects. In Klijn, J. G. M. *et al.* (eds.) *Hormonal Manipulation of Cancer: Peptides, Growth Factors, and New (Anti) Steroidal Agents*, p. 273. (New York: Raven Press)

32. Schally, A. V., Bajusz, S., Redding, T. W., Zalatnai, A. and Comaru-Schally, A. M. (1989). Analogs of LHRH: the present and the future. In Vickery, B. H. and Lunenfeld, V. (eds.) *GnRH Analogs in Cancer and in Human Reproduction, Basic Aspects*, Vol. 1, pp. 5–31. (Dordrecht: Kluwer Academic Publishers)

33. Reissmann, T., Felberbaum, R., Diedrich, K., Engel, J., Comaru-Schally, A. M. and Schally, A. V. (1995). Development and applications of luteinizing hormone-releasing hormone antagonists in the treatment of infertility: an overview. *Hum. Reprod.*, **10** (in press)

34. Bouchard, P., Dubourdieu, S., Hajri, S., Le Nestour, E., d'Acremont, M. F., Leroy, I., Spitz, I. M., Frydman, R. and Charbonnel, B. (1993). Perspectives of the use of GNRH antagonists in gynecology. In Bouchard P., Caraty A., Coelingh Bennink H. J. T. and Pavlou S. N. (eds.) *GnRH, GnRH-Analogs and Gonadal Peptides*, pp. 265–83. (London: Parthenon Publishing Group)

35. Weinbauer, G. F., Behre H. M. and Nieschlag, E. (1993). Gonadotrophin releasing hormone analog-induced regulation of testicular function in monkeys and men. In Bouchard P., Caraty A., Coelingh-Bennink H. J. T. and Pavlou S. N. (eds.) *GnRH, GnRH-Analogs, Gonadotrophins and Gonadal Peptides*, pp. 211–27. (London: Parthenon Publishing Group)

36. Ataya, K. M., Palmer, K. C., Blacker, C. M., Moghissi, K. S. and Mohammad, S. H. (1988). Inhibition of rat ovarian (3H)thymidine uptake by luteinizing hormone-releasing hormone agonists: a possible mechanism for preventing damage by cytotoxic agents. *Cancer Res.*, **48**, 7252–6

Antarelix™   10

R. Deghenghi

INTRODUCTION

Antarelix™ *[1] is an effective gonadotropin releasing hormone (GnRH) antagonist of the structure:

Ac-D-Nal-D- pCl-Phe-D-Pal-Ser-Tyr-D-Hci-Leu-Lys(iPr)-Pro-D-Ala-NH$_2$

which has been extensively studied in animals in recent years. Free-flowing solutions of Antarelix in water, 5% aqueous mannitol and saline can be obtained at concentrations up to 10 mg/ml and higher. In presence of electrolytes (saline, NaCl 0.9%) its solutions are, however, opalescent and there is a tendency for gel to form on standing, particularly at low temperature.

PHYSICO-CHEMICAL ASPECTS

This 'glassy' behavior is common to most, if not all, GnRH antagonists reported to date and indeed to many polypeptides and proteins[2]. However, GnRH antagonists differ in various degrees in exhibiting this property, undoubtedly related to their structure, but in a way which is poorly understood.

Antide is poorly soluble in water, whereas Antide B (which has a Cis-PzACala or 3-(4-pyrazinylcarbonylaminocyclohexyl)alanine in position 5 instead of NicLys (Nε-nicotinoyllysine) has 'excellent solubility'[3]. Cetrorelix, which differs from Antarelix in positions 6 and 8, is soluble in water, but 'quickly becomes gelatinous in this solvent'[4] whereas Antarelix, at the same concentrations, does not. Azaline B can be dissolved (≥ 20 mg/ml) in 3% aqueous mannitol – 5% ethanol[5], but it forms a gel when injected subcutaneously in rats in 5% aqueous mannitol solutions at concentrations from 5 to 20 mg/ml[6].

---

*The proposed international non-proprietary name (INN) is Teverelix

Ganirelix forms a gel when solutions in saline (≥ 10 mg/ml) are stored at 25°C for > 12 hours[7]. Detirelix at 4–8 mg/ml in water forms liquid crystals (aggregation) which can be disrupted by addition of propylene glycol[8].

These physico-chemical aspects of GnRH antagonists are obviously very important for formulation work, such as stability of their solutions, filterability, adsorption on surfaces (including filters), syringeability and problems connected to their lyophilization, pharmacokinetics, *in vivo* potency and *in vitro/in vivo* safety determinations.

HISTAMINE RELEASE DETERMINATION

We are indebted to Dr M. J. Karten and his colleagues at National Institutes of Health for pointing out that freshly prepared aqueous solutions of Antarelix gave an ED$_{50}$ of 81 in the usual histamine release determination on peritoneal rat mast cell preparations *in vitro*[1], but that higher values (i.e. *less* histamine releasing) were obtained when the stock solution, kept at − 20°C, was assayed 1 and 2 weeks later. Since Antarelix is 'chemically' stable under these conditions a plausible explanation is that an intervening 'physical' change, such as formation of liquid crystals, may have been responsible for this loss of activity. Since practically all histamine-liberating values (ED$_{50}$) reported in the literature for GnRH antagonists do not specify how promptly their respective solutions have been tested, these values may not be comparable if obtained with solutions of different 'age'.

MEASUREMENT OF PLASMA LEVELS

Gel formation, including *in situ* upon subcutaneous injection, is concentration-dependent. To study the effect of concentration on pharmacokinetic parameters of Antarelix *in vivo* (using beagle dogs) we have measured the plasma levels of Antarelix, with a radio-immunological assay, following subcutaneous injections of solutions in 5% aqueous mannitol of identical doses (100 µg/kg) but at two different concentrations (1 mg/ml and 5 mg/ml) as shown in Figure 1.

There is a striking difference in bioavailability between the two concentrations, the lower giving a peak of 80 pm/ml at 3 hours, the higher a near zero-order release with a peak of 20 pm/ml. The relevance of this concentration-dependent effect to safety and efficacy in a clinical situation is obvious.

SUMMARY

We have established that:

(1) *In vitro*-derived histamine release values, in order to be comparable, must take into account the 'freshness' of the antagonist solution;

(2) Solubility values, in whichever solvent, must be determined at different times (e.g. 1 and 24 hours) at a given temperature; and

(3) The effect of concentration at a given dose must be determined, particularly as is most common, if the product is injected subcutaneously.

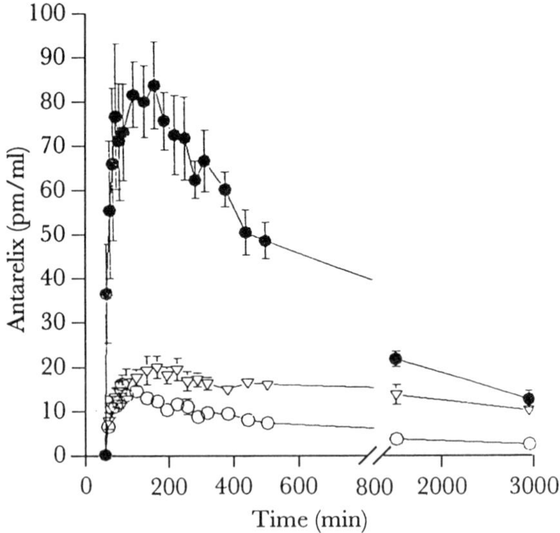

Figure 1 Plasma levels of Antarelix injected subcutaneously with solutions in 5% aqueous mannitol (three dogs per study). ●, 100 µg/kg (1 mg/ml, $n = 3$); ▽, 100 µg/kg (5 mg/ml, $n = 3$); ○, 10 µg/kg (1 mg/ml, $n = 3$)

ACKNOWLEDGEMENTS

I am indebted to Dr Marvin J. Karten of the NIH for having pointed out the relevance of freshness of solutions on histamine-release determinations, to Professor Huy Ong of the University of Montreal for the kinetic determinations of Figure 1, and to Dr François Boutignon who measured solubility parameters of Antarelix in our laboratories.

References

1. Deghenghi, R., Boutignon, F., Wüthrich, P. and Lenaerts, V. (1993). Antarelix (EP24332) a novel water soluble LHRH antagonist. *Biomed. Pharmacother.*, **47**, 107–10

2. Angell, C. A. (1995). Formation of glasses from liquids and biopolymers. *Science*, **267**, 1924–35

3. Janecka, A., Janecki, T., Bowers, C. and Folkers, K. (1995). Antide B, an antagonist of LHRH with *cis*-3-(4-pyrazinylcarbonylaminocyclohexyl)alanine in position 5. *Aminoacids*, **8**, 89–96

4. Müller, A., Busker, E., Engel, J., Kutscher, B., Bernd, M. and Schally, A. V. (1994). Structural investigation of Cetrorelix, a new potent and long-acting LH-RH antagonist. *Int. J. Peptide Protein Res.*, **43**, 264–70

5. Rivier, J., Porter, J., Hoeger, C., Theobald, P., Grey Craig, A., Dykect, J., Corrigan, A., Perrin, M., Hook, W. A., Siraganian, R. P., Vale, W. and Rivier, C. (1992). Gonatrophin-releasing hormone antagonists with N$^\omega$-triazolylornithine, -lysine, or-p-aminophenylalanine residues at positions 5 and 6. *J. Med. Chem.*, **35**, 4270–8

6. Gray, R. A., Wong, G. K., Lai, M. T., Corbo, D. C. and Igbal, K. (1994). Dissolution studies in the

sustained-release characteristics of a gel-forming decapeptide. *Pharm. Res.*, **11**, Suppl. 10, *Biotech*, 2069

7. Wan, J., Trimble, K., Lidgate, D., Floy-Laidlow, B. and Sanders, L. (1994) Pseudo-zero order sustained release of a decapeptide from an injectable liquid crystal gel under physiologically relevant conditions. *Pharm. Res.*, **11** (Suppl. 10), PDD 7275

8. Powell, M. F., Sanders, L. M., Rogerson, A. and Si, V. (1991). Parenteral peptide formulations: chemical and physical properties of native LHRH and hydrophobic analogues in aqueous solution. *Pharm. Res.*, **8**, 1258–63

Reproductive pharmacology and safety of azaline B: an overview of preclinical studies

11

G. A. Shangold, C. A. Campen, A. Phillips, M. T. Lai, T. Kirchner, R. Williams and G. D. Hodgen

INTRODUCTION

Azaline B (RWJ 47428) [Ac-DNal-DCpa-DPal-Ser-Aph(atz)-DAph(atz)-Leu-Lys(Ipr)-Pro-DAla-NH_2] is a potent gonadotropin releasing hormone receptor antagonist, synthesized in the laboratories of Jean Rivier at the Salk Institute. The potency of this compound in inhibiting ovulation in the rat and suppressing the pituitary–gonadal axis in both rat and primate models has been the subject of previous reports[1–3], as has been the extremely low anaphylactoid activity of this molecule. The studies that support these observations are reviewed herein, along with previously unpublished data which demonstrate the activity of this compound during and after 2-week administration to cycling cynomolgus monkeys. Where relevant, evaluations comparing azaline B to other gonadotropin releasing hormone (GnRH) antagonists currently in development are presented.

MATERIALS AND METHODS

Peptides

The amino acid sequences of the GnRH analogs used in these studies are shown in Table 1.

Animal assays

All rats were housed at The R.W. Johnson Pharmaceutical Research Institute (PRI) vivarium facility and treated in accordance with the US Laboratory Animal Welfare Act and all its subsequent revisions and amendments. Room

Table 1 Amino acid sequences of GnRH and GnRH analogs used in these studies

Peptide	Sequence
GnRH	pGlu^1-His^2-Trp^3-Ser^4-Tyr^5-Gly^6-Leu^7-Arg^8-Pro^9-Gly^{10}-NH$_2$
Histrelin	[DHis(N-Im-bzl)^6-Pro^9-NH-C$_2$H$_5$]-GnRH
Azaline B	[Ac-DNal^1-DCpa^2-DPal^3-Ser-Aph^5(atz)-DAph^6(atz)-Ilys8-DAla^{10}]-GnRH
Antide	[Ac-DNal^1 -DCpa^2-DPal^3-NicLys^5-DNicLys^6-ILys^8-DAla^{10}]-GnRH
N-Me-Tyr^5-antide	[Ac-DNal^1-DCpa^2-DPal^3-N-MeTyr^5-DNicLys^6-ILys^8-DAla^{10}]-GnRH
[Nal-Glu]-GnRH	[Ac-DNal^1-DCpa^2-DPal^3-Arg^5-DGlu^6(AA)-DAla^{10}]-GnRH
Cetrorelix	[AcDNal^1 -DCpa^2-DPal^3-DCit^6-IIys^8-DAla^{10}]-GnRH

AA, anisole adduct; Aph, amino-phenylalanine; atz, 5'-(3'-amino-1 *H*-1',2',4'-triazolyl); Cit, citrullyl; Cpa, 4-chloro-phenylalanine; DGlu (AA), D-4-(*p*-[methoxy-benzoyl]-2-aminobutyric acid; ILys, N$^\varepsilon$ isopropyl-lysine; Nal, 3-(2'-naphthyl)-alanine; Nic, nicotinyl; Pal, 3-(3'-pyridyl)-alanine

temperature was kept at 25 °C with a 12 hours light : 12 hours dark cycle (lights on at 06.30). Standard food and water were available *ad libitum*.

Monkey studies were performed in the primate research facilities at the Jones Institute for Reproductive Medicine, wherein all animals are treated in accordance with the above guidelines and statutes.

Primary rat pituitary cell culture studies

Hemisected rat pituitaries from immature male rats (Wistar, Charles River, Wilmington, MA, USA) were enzymatically dispersed using collagenase followed by viokase. All tissue culture supplies were purchased from GIBCO BRL (Grand Island, NY, USA) unless otherwise specified. Aliquots of a single cell suspension in DMEM/F12 medium supplemented with 8% fetal bovine serum (FBS, HyClone, Logan, UT, USA), 0.52 µg/ml transferrin (Sigma Chemical Co., St Louis, MO, USA), 0.5 ng/ml parathyroid hormone (CalBioChem, La Jolla, CA, USA), 1 ng/ml basic fibroblast growth factor, 0.29 mg/ml glutamine, 5 µg/ml insulin (Sigma Chemical Co., St Louis, MO, USA) and penicillin, streptomycin and nystatin were plated in a 24-well tissue culture plate and placed in a 5% CO_2 incubator at 37°C for 3 days. On the fourth day, the wells were washed with and reincubated in the nutrient medium. At this time the cultures were treated with 0.1 nmol/l histrelin alone or in combination with various concentrations of the appropriate GnRH antagonist. For the recovery experiments, cultures were treated with 10 nmol/l of each antagonist alone or in combination with histrelin. After 4 hours at 37°C, the media were removed and stored at −20°C until assayed for gonadotropin release by radioimmunoassay (RIA). Gonadotropin levels in tissue culture media were determined by standard RIA techniques using NIDDK kits for rat follicle stimulating hormone (FSH) (RP-2) and rat luteinizing hormone (LH) (RP-3).

Rat anti-ovulatory activity

Female Wistar rats (175–225 g, Charles River, Wilmington, MA, USA) with predictable 4-day estrous cycles were injected subcutaneously with a GnRH antagonist between 13.00 and 14.00 hours on the day of proestrus. The vehicle was 8 nmol/l HCl in normal saline (acidified saline, pH 3, 299 mOsm/kg, µOsmette Precision Systems, Natick, MA, USA). The animals were sacrificed the following morning and the presence or absence of ova in the oviduct was determined by microscopic inspection. The animals were scored as ovulating if one or more ova were present in the oviduct. ED_{50} was calculated using the SAS probit analysis program (SAS Institute Inc., Cary, NC, USA).

Ovariectomized rat studies

Female Wistar rats (175–225 g, Charles River, Wilmington, MA, USA) were ovariectomized using Metofane (Pitman–Moore, Mundelein, IL, USA) anesthesia. After 2–3 weeks, one jugular vein was cannulated. The following day, the GnRH antagonists dissolved in either 5% mannitol or acidified saline (vehicle kept constant within each experiment) were injected subcutaneously. Blood samples were then collected through the cannulae. Approximately 350 µl of plasma was obtained from each sampling and the red blood cells, resuspended in sterile saline, were replaced through the cannula into each rat. This blood collection procedure was followed for studies lasting less than 15 days. For the 15–30-day time course studies, jugular vein cannulations were not performed, but instead 1.0 ml or less of blood was collected by heart puncture after Metofane anesthesia. All blood samples were then centrifuged using an IEC HN-SII centrifuge at 1500 r.p.m. for 10 min at room temperature, and the resulting supernatant (plasma fraction) was stored at −20°C until assayed by RIA for gonadotropin levels. Gonadotropin levels in plasma samples were determined by standard RIA techniques using NIDDK kits for rat FSH (RP-2) and rat LH (RP-3).

Castrate monkey studies

Ovariectomized cynomolgus monkeys were utilized in these studies. A pretreatment femoral blood sample (3.5 ml) was collected on day 0, followed by daily blood collections for 4 consecutive days. All blood collections were made under ketamine-induced anesthesia (10 mg/kg, intramuscularly). The GnRH antagonist was administered subcutaneously on day 0, following the zero-time blood collection. All serum samples were analyzed for LH by RIA. The treatment groups were: azaline B 1.5, 5.0, 15 and 45 μg/kg; [Nal-Glu]-GnRH 5.0 and 45 μg/kg; N-Me-Tyr^5-antide 5.0 and 45 μg/kg; Cetrorelix 5.0 and 45 μg/kg.

Studies in intact rats

Intact male Wistar rats (175–225 g, Charles River, Wilmington, MA, USA) were injected subcutaneously for 14 days with the indicated GnRH antagonist at the following doses: 7, 21, 63, 189 and 567 μg/kg per day. The vehicle was 5% mannitol in water (Baxter Healthcare Corp., Deerfield, IL, USA). On the day following the last injection, animals were sacrificed and the testes, ventral prostate and seminal vesicles were extracted, trimmed free of any surrounding fatty tissue and weighed. Intact rats treated with vehicle served as intact controls. Rats castrated on the first day of treatment served as castrate controls.

Subacute studies in cycling monkeys

Normally cycling female cynomolgus monkeys were utilized for these studies. On menstrual cycle days 20–22 in the pretreatment cycle, an evaluation of serum progesterone concentrations was undertaken. If the serum progesterone concentration was greater than 1.0 ng/ml, the monkey was assigned to a treatment group at the start of the next menstrual cycle. The four treatment groups with azaline B were 5.0, 15, 25 and 40 μg/kg per day. Azaline B was administered daily as a subcutaneous injection from cycle days 2 to 15. Femoral blood samples were collected daily from cycle days 2 to 16 in all treatment groups and were collected on alternate days from days 18 to 42 from monkeys in the two higher dosage groups. Estradiol concentrations were analyzed in all serum samples using a commercial RIA kit.

Cutaneous and pulmonary anaphylactoid activity

Male Hartley guinea pigs (450–550 g) were anesthetized with urethane (2.0 g/kg intraperitoneally) and placed in a whole-body plethysmograph. A jugular vein and a carotid artery were cannulated for compound administration and monitoring of blood pressure, respectively. The trachea was also cannulated for ventilation at a constant volume via a miniature Starling pump. Transpleural pressure was measured with a Validyne differential pressure transducer ($\pm$ 20 cm H$_2$O) bridged between the pleural cavity and a side arm on the tracheal cannula. Tidal volume was recorded from pressure changes occurring inside the plethysmograph with another Validyne differential pressure transducer ($\pm$ 2.0 cm H$_2$O). An on-line Buxco pulmonary mechanics computer calculated dynamic lung compliance and airway resistance from the tidal volume and transpleural pressure. Blood pressure was also monitored with the pulmonary mechanics computer. The guinea pigs were pretreated with succinylcholine (1.2 mg/g intravenously) to arrest spontaneous respiration. After a 5 min stabilization period one of the GnRH antagonists was administered in a volume of 0.1 ml intravenously over 30 s. Percentage change from baseline was monitored over 30 min for all parameters and recorded at 1, 3, 5 and 30 min after administration. Statistical evaluation of the pulmonary data was conducted using SAS (version 5). At each time point, analysis of variance (ANOVA) was performed for each of the three transformed variables, airway resistance, dynamic lung compliance and mean arterial blood pressure (MABP). Multiple comparisons were performed if the ANOVAs detected differences.

Male Wistar rats (500–750 g, Charles River, Wilmington, MA, USA) were injected intravenously with 1.0 ml of 0.5 % solution of Evan's blue dye. Various concentrations of GnRH antagonists in acidified saline as well as vehicle control were injected intradermally into a shaved section on the back of the animal. Five injections at separate sites were made into each animal, and were used for determining a dose–response relationship. At 15 min after the intradermal injection, the animals were sacrificed and the area of each wheal (as indicated by the intradermal presence of the Evan's blue dye) was measured as the product of the longest perpendiculars.

RESULTS

Inhibition of LH release in rat pituitary cell culture

The GnRH superagonist histrelin (0.1 nmol/l) induced a sixfold increase in LH secretion and a four- to fivefold increase in FSH secretion, over a 4-hours incubation period in static cultures. This stimulation was inhibited completely, in a dose-dependent fashion, by co-incubation with any of three different GnRH antagonists. The dose–inhibition curves for azaline B, [Nal-Glu]-GnRH and antide were superimposable, with all compounds showing an ED_{50} of approximately 0.6 nmol/l.

Inhibition of ovulation in proestrus rats

Subcutaneous administration of a GnRH antagonist to female rats on the afternoon of proestrus was effective in reducing the percentage of rats ovulating ($n = 10$/group), in a dose-dependent manner. In this model, the dose–response curves were parallel, but azaline B showed the greatest potency in anti-ovulatory activity. The ED_{50}s were 5.6 µg/kg for antide, 2.4 µg/kg for [Nal-Glu]-GnRH and 1.4 µg/kg for azaline B.

Inhibition of LH levels after a single injection to ovariectomized rats and monkeys

The potency of azaline B in suppressing gonadotropins in the castrate female rat was examined via single subcutaneous administrations in a 5% mannitol vehicle. Azaline B at 1 µg/kg was indistinguishable from vehicle. At 3 µg/kg, LH suppression of about 50% was evident within 2 hours, and a nadir (> 90%) was reached by 6 hours; recovery was complete within 24 hours. Higher doses induced even more rapid suppression

of LH, with near-maximal inhibition in evidence by 2 hours after injection. Speed of recovery proceeded inversely with dose, with a return to baseline occurring between 30 and 48 hours at 10 and 30 µg/kg, respectively. To explore the limits of duration of this inhibitory action on gonadotropins, higher doses of azaline B were examined in experiments that were extended in time. At 200 µg/kg, gonadotropins returned to baseline at approximately 3 days, whereas at 2000 µg/kg both LH and FSH remained maximally suppressed for at least 15 days following administration of azaline B. Thereafter recovery proceeded gradually, and was complete by 30–35 days.

The dose-dependency of the duration of action of azaline B in this model was compared to that of several other GnRH antagonists which are currently in development. In one such experiment, GnRH antagonists were dissolved in a 5% mannitol vehicle; sampling was performed at 2, 6 and 24 hours, and daily thereafter. At 2 µg/kg (Figure 1A), all compounds induced similar and maximal LH inhibition within 2–6 hours. A return to baseline was complete by 6 hours after injection for N-Me-Tyr[5]-antide and Cetrorelix, but suppression remained maximal at that time point for [Nal-Glu]-GnRH and azaline B. Escape from suppression by the latter two compounds was complete by 24 hours. Increasing the dose to 20 µg/kg (Figure 1B) enabled both N-Me-Tyr[5]-antide and Cetrorelix to maintain suppression at 6 hours, with return to baseline now being effected by 24 hours for both, as well as for [Nal-Glu]-GnRH. At this dose, azaline B sustained maximal inhibition at 24 hours, and complete escape occurred by 48 hours. Further separation occurred at a dose of 200 µg/kg (Figure 1C), at which LH returned to baseline by 24 hours for N-Me-Tyr[5]-antide and by 48 hours for [Nal-Glu]-GnRH. The suppression induced by Cetrorelix was returning toward baseline (about 60 % of maximal) by 72 hours, while remaining maximal for azaline B at that time. At a dose of 2000 µg/kg (Figure 1D), all antagonists maintained maximal LH suppression for 96 hours. By 120 hours following injection of N-Me-Tyr[5]-antide, LH had returned to baseline,

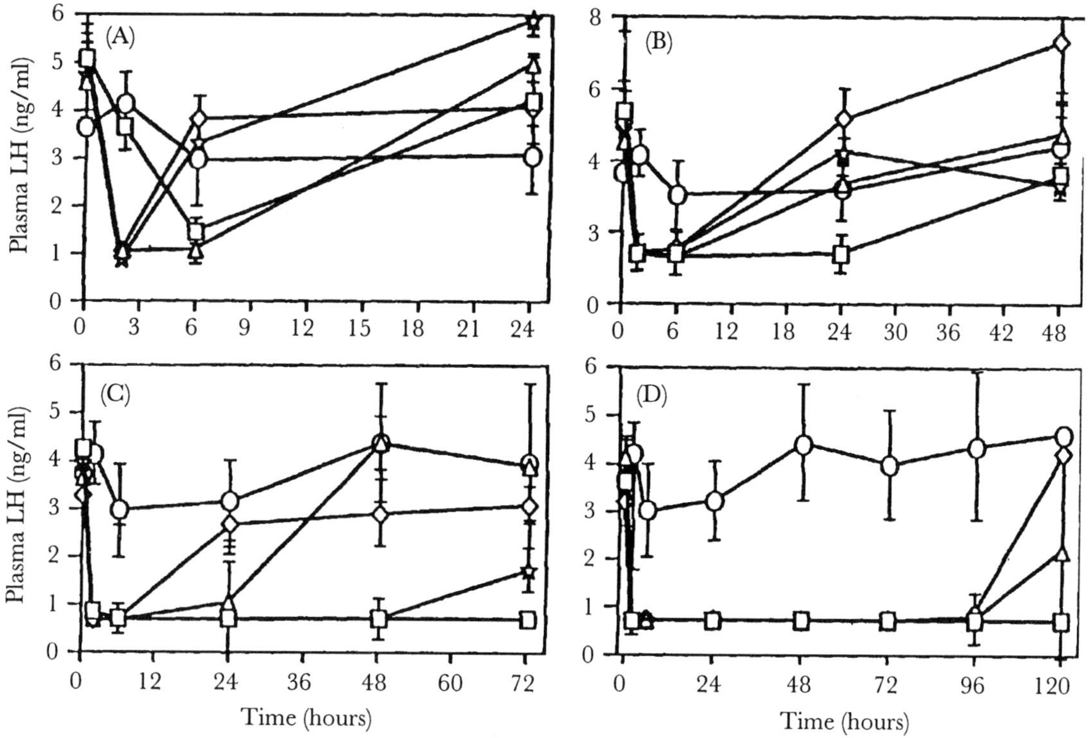

Figure 1 Suppression of plasma LH levels after a single subcutaneous injection of a GnRH antagonist to ovariectomized cannulated rats: (A) 2 μg/kg (*n* = 3); (B) 20 μg/kg (*n* = 3); (C) 200 μg/kg (*n* = 3); and (D) 2000 μg/kg (*n* = 3). ○, Vehicle: □ azaline B; △, [Nal-Glu]-GnRH; ◇ , N-MeTyr⁵-antide; ☆, Cetrorelix

whereas [Nal-Glu]-GnRH maintained about 50% inhibition at this time point. Maximal suppressive effects were still in evidence at 120 hours for both Cetrorelix and azaline B at this high dose. In a separate experiment, where acidified saline was the vehicle, azaline B was compared to antide and [Nal-Glu]-GnRH at a dose of 2000 mg/kg. Here the sampling intervals were daily up to day 4, and then every other day thereafter. As in the previously described investigation, [Nal-Glu]-GnRH maintained suppression of LH and FSH for no more than 4 days. Antide sustained this inhibition maximally for 6 days, but escape toward baseline was evident for both hormones by day 8. As before, gonadotropins remained maximally suppressed 8 days after administration of azaline B at this dose.

In ovariectomized cynomolgus monkeys, a single subcutaneous administration of azaline B in 5 % mannitol at a dose of 1.5 μg/kg had no

effect on LH levels, whereas doses of 5, 15 and 45 μg/kg induced maximal (80–90 %) LH suppression between 6 and 24 hours. The duration of this suppression was again dose-dependent. At 5 μg/kg, return toward baseline was evident by day 2 and complete by day 3; at 15 μg/kg, complete suppression was sustained on day 2 but by day 3 LH had returned to baseline levels. At the 45 μg/kg dose, significant (>70%) suppression was still in effect 4 days after administration.

When other GnRH antagonists were compared in the same system, stratification of the dose-duration characteristics was seen as it was in the rat model. At 5 μg/kg, [Nal-Glu]-GnRH, N-Me-Tyr⁵-antide, and cetrorelix all had induced > 75% suppression of LH within 6 hours of administration; resolution of this inhibition had begun by 24 hours for all three compounds, but was complete at 24 hours for [Nal-Glu]-GnRH, by 48 h for N-Me-Tyr⁵-antide, and between 72 and

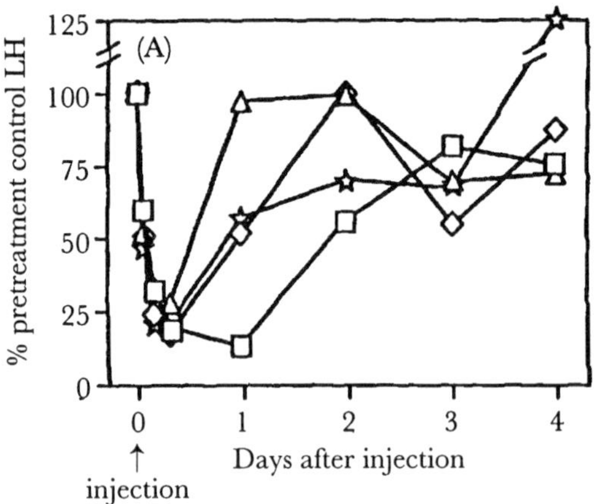
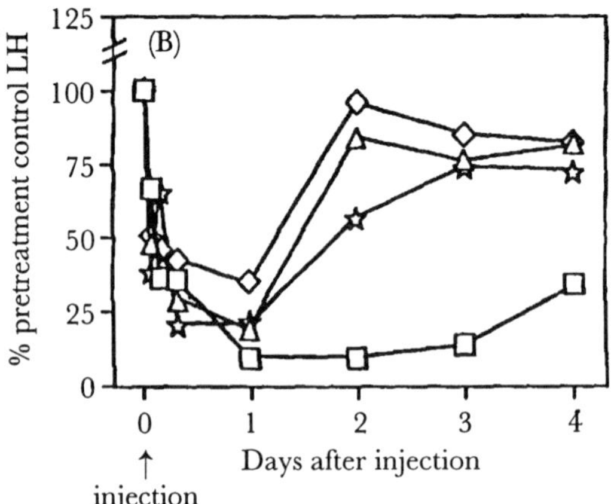

Figure 2 Effect of single subcutaneous injection of a GnRH antagonist in a 5% mannitol on serum LH levels in ovariectomized cynomolgus monkeys: (A) 5 μg/kg; and (B) 45 μg/kg. □, Azaline B ($n = 3$); △, [Nal-Glu]-GnRH; ◇, N-Me-Tyr[5]-antide; ☆, Cetrorelix

96 hours for Cetrorelix (Figure 2A). Following administration of a higher dose of 45 μg/kg, LH levels had re-turned to pre-treatment levels by day 2 after both N-Me-Tyr[5]-antide and [Nal-Glu]-GnRH, and by day 3 with Cetrorelix. At least 70% suppression was still in evidence by the fourth day following injection of this dose of azaline B (Figure 2B).

Potency relative to other GnRH antagonists during and after 2 weeks of daily administration to intact rats

The effect of daily administration of GnRH antagonists over an extended (2-week) treatment period was evaluated in intact male rats; change in testicular, ventral prostate, and seminal vesicle weight after 14 days of dosing was compared with that observed following surgical castration. While decreases of approximately 30 and 50 % were seen with N-Me-Tyr[5]-antide and [Nal-Glu]-GnRH, respectively at the highest dose tested (567 μg/kg per day), castrate values were not achieved with either of these two compounds. Cetrorelix was ineffective at 63 μg/kg per day, but induced castrate organ weights at a dose of 189 μg/kg per day. Azaline B demonstrated the greatest potency in this model, with about 25 % suppression following a dose of 21 μg/kg per day and near-maximal (about 90 %) suppression at 63 μg/kg per day; castrate values were seen at 189 μg/kg per day.

Similar studies were performed in intact female rats, using changes in vaginal cytology to document dose-dependent lengthening of the estrous cycle and ultimately induction of constant diestrus. These data, which were recently presented[3], revealed a similar order of potency when the same GnRH antagonists were compared in'the female rat model.

Inhibition and recovery of estradiol levels during and after 2 weeks of daily administration to cycling monkeys

To determine its potency in suppressing estradiol secretion, azaline B was administered subcutaneously to cycling cynomolgus monkeys via daily injection for 2 weeks (cycle days 2 to 15). At 5 μg/kg per day, suppression of estradiol was inconsistent, with mean levels varying between approximately 20 and 50 pg/ml. At doses of 15, 25 and 40 μg/kg per day, mean estradiol levels remained in the castrate range, below 20 pg/ml, for the duration of treatment. Following cessation of antagonist administration, estradiol recovery began within 1 to 5 days, even at the highest dose, with ovulation occurring in all monkeys by cycle day 30–35, i.e. within 15–20 days of discontinuing azaline B.

Assessment of anaphylactoid potential

The potential of azaline B and several other GnRH antagonists to induce anaphylaxis was assessed using whole-body plethysmography to measure changes in lung compliance and airway resistance following intravenous administration of 10 mg of drug to guinea pigs. At this dose of [Nal-Glu]-GnRH, a significant 80% diminution in lung compliance was seen; this was accompanied by a reciprocal > 1000% increase in airway resistance. Virtually no changes in these parameters were encountered with similar injections of 10 mg of either antide or azaline B.

Further analysis of comparative histaminic potential was undertaken via the intradermal injection of 1, 3, 6 or 10 µg of several antagonists to male rats. In this model, dose-related increases in wheal response were observed with [Nal-Glu]-GnRH, N-Me-Tyr^5-antide and Cetrorelix, in that order of potency. Azaline B at all doses tested was ineffective in eliciting any wheal response greater than control (Figure 3).

DISCUSSION

The above studies evaluated the activity of azaline B, alone and in comparison to several other GnRH antagonists now in development, in pituitary cell culture and in both intact and castrate animal models. The gonadotroph remains the principal target tissue for the action of GnRH antagonists, which renders suppression of gonadotropins in pituitary cultures and in the castrate model a critical measure of the activity of these compounds. Nonetheless, the therapeutic benefits offered by this class of drug are obtained almost exclusively via indirect suppressive effects on gonadal steroids brought about by this inhibition of gonadotropin secretion. As such, meaningful assessments of the utility of these compounds must of necessity include investigations of their ability to sustain gonadal steroid suppression over time and/or to render the expected attendant changes in sex steroid-dependent organs. The intact male and cycling female animal are thus also essential models for the evaluation of these GnRH analogs.

In cell culture, [Nal-Glu]-GnRH, antide, and azaline B exhibited similar potency, though in the

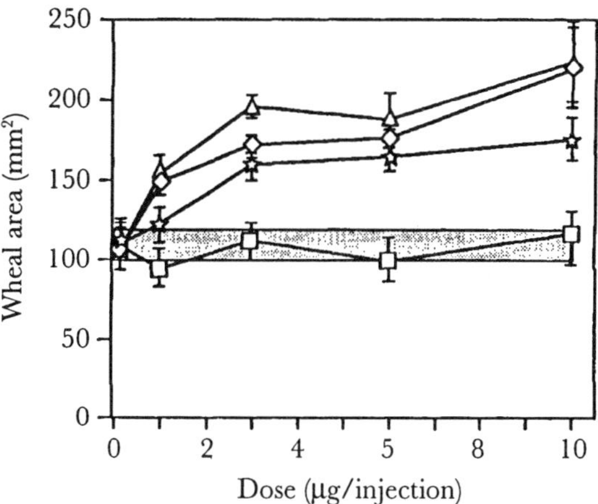

Figure 3 axis labels:

Figure 3 Wheal response after intradermal injection of GnRH antagonists in male rats. ▓, Control; □, azaline B; △, [Nal-Glu]-GnRH; ◇, N-Me-Tyr^5-antide; ☆, Cetrorelix

anti-ovulatory assay in rats these same antagonists were clearly separable, with azaline B demonstrating greater potency. In castrate rats and monkeys, the minimally effective dose of azaline B in suppressing LH below castrate levels was between 2 and 5 µg/kg. Increasing the dose of azaline B beyond this did not further enhance the degree of suppression achieved, but did extend the duration of this inhibition. This same phenomenon was evident with the other antagonists studied. In comparative studies, the duration of action of a single injection of a given dose of antagonist was greatest for azaline B, followed generally in order by antide, cetrorelix, [Nal-Glu]-GnRH and, lastly, N-Me-Tyr^5-antide.

In intact male rats, these same compounds given daily for 2 weeks appeared to rank in a similar order of potency in regard to their ability to suppress testicular, ventral prostate and seminal vesicle weights to castrate levels. This presumably reflected their relative impact at a given dose on circulating testosterone levels.

The minimal dose of azaline B required to suppress ovarian estradiol secretion reliably in the cycling monkey appears to lie between 5 and 15 µg/kg per day. Even at higher doses (40 µg/kg per day), however, ovarian follicular activity quickly resumed after cessation of treatment, with ovulation occurring within approximately 2 weeks. Reversibility of suppression after chronic treatment thus appears assured, as one would wish for a therapy which induces a medical castration.

The prolongation of gonadotropin suppression which was achieved by increasing the dose of these antagonists may have several underlying mechanisms. In theory, these could involve changes in gonadotropin synthesis, receptor occupancy time, protein binding, or plasma clearance of the antagonist. However, it is probably more likely that these differential dose-duration characteristics are explicable on the basis of differences in the solubility of these compounds, and the resultant potential for spontaneous depot formation and delayed absorption. Resolution of these possible mechanisms will await other studies, most importantly pharmacokinetic analyses. It is intriguing to speculate as to whether the propensity for some of these compounds to gel subcutaneously will remain problematic or whether this can be exploited for the purposes of developing drugs with intrinsically extended release profiles over time.

A critical obstacle to the successful development of GnRH antagonists as useful therapeutic agents has been the propensity of this class of peptides to induce histamine release. The avoidance of anaphylaxis observed previously in response to administration of earlier compounds in this class has been a major goal of efforts by peptide chemists in synthesizing newer generations of GnRH antagonists. Anaphylaxis is the result of multiple cascading immunological and inflammatory events, only one of which is the degranulation of mast cells and attendant release of histamine. For this reason, we have elected to study changes in pulmonary airway dynamics and wheal formation, rather than simply *in vitro* histamine release itself, in our characterization of the anaphylactoid potential of various GnRH antagonists. In the foregoing studies, we have demonstrated that azaline B, of all compounds tested, remains the most selective for the GnRH receptor, in exhibiting the least potential for inducing anaphylactoid responses in these animal models.

The preclinical studies presented herein have elucidated the doses of azaline B that produce gonadotropin suppression and castration in rats and monkeys, its high relative potency and prolonged duration of action with respect to other antagonists in these animal models, and the minimal anaphylactoid potential of azaline B compared to other antagonists. These parameters of potency, duration of action and ultimate safety are now being validated in humans with azaline B. The foregoing studies would lead one to predict that azaline B will have a wide therapeutic index relative to other GnRH antagonists. The potential impact of formulation, route of administration and delivery system on these properties is likely to be critical in the development and commercialization of this and other GnRH antagonists.

References

1. Campen, C. A., Lai, M. T., Kraft, P., Kirchner, T., Phillips, A., Hahn, D. W. and Rivier, J. (1992). Characterization of a new selective GnRH antagonist with potent antiovulatory activity and extremely low anaphylactoid activity (Abstr. 869), *74th Annual Meeting of The Endocrine Society*, San Antonio, TX
2. Campen, C. A., Lai, M. T., Kraft, P., Kirchener, T., Phillips, A., Hahn, D. W. and Rivier, J. (1985). Potent pituitary–gonadal axis suppression and extremely low anaphylactoid activity of a new gonadotropin releasing hormone (GnRH) antagonist: azaline B. *Biochemical Pharmacol.*, **49**, 1313
3. Campen, C. A., Lai, M. T. and Phillips, A. (1995). The potency of azaline B, a new GnRH antagonist, in female and male rat models (Abstr. P2-50), *77th Annual Meeting of The Endocrine Society*, Washington, D.C.

Section 4

Steroid replacement during analog treatment

12

Steroid supplementation of GnRH analog treatment in women with leiomyomas

A. J. Friedman

INTRODUCTION

Uterine leiomyomas, the most common pelvic tumor in women during their reproductive years, are a major public health problem. It is estimated that 20–30% of women will have clinically recognizable tumors[1]. Of these women, approximately 20–50% will experience symptoms due to an enlarged pelvic mass (e.g. pelvic pressure, pelvic discomfort, urinary frequency and bloating), excessive menstrual flow (e.g. menorrhagia, hypermenorrhea, inconvenience and anemia) and/or reproductive dysfunction (e.g. infertility, pregnancy wastage, premature labor, abruptio placenta and postpartum hemorrhage).

Surgical treatment, the mainstay of leiomyoma therapy, usually involves hysterectomy or myomectomy. For at least 20–30 years leiomyomas have been the single largest diagnostic category for women undergoing hysterectomy in the United States, accounting for one-third of all cases[2]. Myomectomy may be performed when uterine preservation is an important goal of therapy but is done far less frequently than hysterectomy.

Although surgical treatment is usually highly successful, some women may benefit from long-term medical therapy. Long-term medical therapy may be prescribed to avoid or postpone more definitive surgical treatment in selected cases. Examples of situations in which women may benefit from long-term medical therapy include symptomatic perimenopausal women, women at high risk for surgical or anesthetic complications and women wishing to postpone surgical treatment for more than 6 months.

Currently, there is no long-term (i.e. > 6 months) medical therapy for leiomyomas approved by the Food and Drug Administration in the United States. Accordingly, any long-term medical treatment for this purpose must be considered experimental and appropriate consent should be obtained before initiating therapy.

GnRH AGONIST AND LOW-DOSE STEROID SUPPLEMENTATION

One long-term medical treatment for leiomyomas that has received much attention is the combination of a gonadotropin releasing hormone (GnRH) agonist and low-dose steroid supplementation. By eliminating ovarian hormone production, GnRH agonist treatment results in uterine and leiomyoma shrinkage and menstrual suppression leading to a reduction in symptom severity. Maximal size reduction of the uterus and tumors is often achieved after 2–3 months of treatment[3–8]. Menstrual suppression is usually achieved after 1 month of treatment with significant improvement in hemoglobin (Hgb) concentration and hematocrit (Hct) often noted after 2–3 months[9,10]. The goal of long-term medical treatment of women with leiomyomas is to achieve symptom suppression with a GnRH agonist before adding steroids to avoid the adverse sequelae of prolonged hypoestrogenemia (e.g. rapid bone loss, increased risk of cardiovascular disease, vasomotor symptoms and vaginal epithelial atrophy). This type of combination medical therapy is usually administered in a stepwise fashion, with the patient receiving a GnRH agonist initially for 1–3 months before steroids are added[11]. Recommended doses of estrogen and progestin added to GnRH agonist therapy are comparable to those used for postmenopausal women. Estrogen is usually administered continuously (i.e. daily), whereas the progestin may be administered either continuously or cyclically (i.e. for 10–14 days each month). Calcium supplementation (1000–1500 mg elemental calcium daily) is also recommended to reduce the risk of osteoporosis.

Although it is unlikely that women will achieve additional uterine/leiomyoma shrinkage or further menstrual suppression following the addition of steroid hormones, it is hoped that the degree of symptomatic improvement experienced after 1–3 months of GnRH agonist therapy will be sustained. The possibility exists that the addition of steroids may lead to uterine/leiomyoma regrowth and/or abnormal (rarely heavy) vaginal bleeding[12,13].

ADDITION OF ESTROGEN AND PROGESTIN

Some preliminary studies have shown that addition of estrogen and progestin, in doses typically used for hormone replacement therapy in postmenopausal women, will often, but not always sustain the beneficial effects of GnRH agonist therapy which are achieved after 3 months[14]. In addition, the use of steroids is usually highly successful in eliminating or diminishing the frequency and intensity of hot flushes, the occurrence of vaginal dryness, and will provide significant bone-sparing effects when compared with GnRH agonist therapy alone.

In a prospective, randomized clinical trial[15], 51 premenopausal women with symptomatic uterine fibroids were treated with 3.75 mg of the GnRH agonist leuprolide acetate depot (Lupron depot, TAP Pharmaceuticals Inc., Deerfield, IL, USA) intramuscularly every 4 weeks for 12 weeks before being randomized to receive either low-dose estrogen/progestin or a high-dose progestin supplementation for a 2-year treatment period. Twenty-six women received 0.75 mg of estropipate (Ogen 0.625, Abbott Laboratories, Chicago, IL, USA) daily plus 0.7 mg of norethindrone (Micronor, Ortho Pharmaceutical Corporation, Raritan, NJ, USA) on days 1–14 each month from treatment week 12 to 104; 25 women received 10 mg of norethindrone (Norlutate, Parke-Davis, Morris Plains, NJ, USA)

daily from treatment week 12 to 104. Calcium supplementation was not prescribed. The mean decrease in uterine volume was 40% during the first 12 weeks of treatment when the women received only leuprolide acetate depot. Women receiving low-dose estrogen/progestin supplementation had no significant change in mean uterine volume during the final 92 weeks of treatment. In contrast, women in the high-dose progestin group had an increase in mean uterine volume to 92% of the mean pretreatment volume. All women experienced regrowth of their uterus to pretreatment size 6 months after completion of treatment. These findings suggest that progestins, not just estrogens, modulate growth of the myometrium and/or leiomyomas either directly or through changes in local growth factor concentrations, receptors or binding proteins. Other studies have reported that addition of a progestin to GnRH agonist therapy will block uterine shrinkage observed when women are treated with a GnRH agonist alone[16,17]. Another study[18] reported a mean decrease in leiomyoma volume of 49% after 12 weeks of treatment with the antiprogestin RU-486, giving further support to the hypothesis that progestins modulate uterine/leiomyoma growth.

In the 2-year study reported above[15] all women had significant increases in mean Hct and Hgb concentration during the first 12 weeks of treatment. The improvement in these hematological parameters was sustained in both treatment groups during the last 92 weeks of treatment. A greater proportion of women in the high-dose progestin group had irregular and, on occasion, heavy vaginal bleeding compared to women receiving estrogen/progestin supplementation. Pretreatment menstrual patterns returned within 6 months after completion of the study, with a corresponding return of mean Hct and Hgb concentration to pretreatment levels.

HIERARCHICAL RESPONSIVENESS TO ESTROGEN

Lumbar spine bone density, assessed by dual X-ray absorptiometry, decreased by a mean of 2.6% during the first 12 weeks of treatment. Neither group had a significant change in bone density during the final 92 weeks of treatment; the estrogen/progestin and high-dose progestin groups had decrements of 1.4% and 0.7%, respectively. These findings suggest that there exists a hierachy of tissue responsiveness to circulating levels of estrogen. Women rendered profoundly hypoestrogenemic while on GnRH agonist therapy will experience regression of all estrogen sensitive tissues (e.g. uterine leiomyoma shrinkage, vaginal epithelial and endometrial atrophy, rapid bone loss, etc.). Addition of low doses of estrogen may protect some tissues (e.g. block rapid bone loss) whereas other tissues (e.g myometrium and/or leiomyomas) may require higher circulating concentrations of estrogen to modulate tissue responsiveness. This hypothesis of hierarchical responsiveness to estrogen has been referred to as the estrogen threshold hypothesis[19].

In the above clinical trial[15], mean high-density lipoprotein cholesterol concentrations decreased by 37% in the group receiving high-dose progestin supplementation whereas no significant change was noted in the estrogen/progestin group. These findings suggest that 10 mg of norethindrone daily is not a safe or totally efficacious steroid supplementation regimen.

THE NEED FOR CAREFUL MONITORING

Since dose–response studies have not been performed, the ideal steroids and doses of steroids used in combination with a GnRH agonist, if they exist, are not known. It is likely that women may benefit from different combinations and doses of steroids while on GnRH agonist treatment. Consequently, each women treated with a GnRH agonist plus steroid supplementation should be monitored closely by periodically assessing safety (e.g. bone density measurements, lipid profiles, etc.) and efficacy (e.g. uterine/leiomyoma volume changes, symptom relief, menstrual suppression and change in hematological values) parameters.

Finally, in addition to the potential clinical usefulness of this treatment strategy, treatment with a GnRH agonist followed by steroid supplementation will allow researchers to study the steroid sensitivities of a number of gynecological diseases (e.g. leiomyomas, endometriosis, hirsutism, etc.). This treatment strategy mimics the classic endocrine experiments in which endocrine organs were ablated (usually surgically) and the missing hormones were then added back to elucidate the action of these hormones on various target tissues.

References

1. Buttram, V. C. and Reiter, R. C. (1981). Uterine leiomyomata: etiology, symptomatology, and management. *Fertil. Steril.*, **36**, 433–45
2. National Center for Health Statistics (1987). *Hysterectomies in the United States 1965–1984*, pp. 88–1753. National Health Survey Series 13, No. 92. (Bethesda, MD: DHHS Publication (PHS))
3. Friedman, A. J., Barbieri, R. L., Benacerraf, B. R. and Schiff, I. (1987). Treatment of leiomyomata with intranasal or subcutaneous leuprolide, a gonadotropin releasing-hormone agonist. *Fertil. Steril.*, **48**, 560–4
4. Friedman, A. J., Harrison-Atlas, D., Barbieri, R. L., Benacerraf, B., Gleason, R. E. and Schiff, I. (1989). A randomized, placebo-controlled, double-blind study evaluating the efficacy of leuprolide acetate depot in the treatment of uterine leiomyomata. *Fertil. Steril.*, **51**, 251–6
5. Friedman, A. J., Hoffman, D. I., Comite, F., Browneller, R. W. and Miller, J. D. (1991). Treatment of leiomyomata uteri with leuprolide acetate depot: a double-blind, placebo-controlled, multicenter study. *Obstet. Gynecol.*, **77**, 720–5
6. Schlaff, W. D., Zerhouni, E. A., Huth, J. A. M., Chen, J., Damewood, M. D and Rock, J. A. (1989). A placebo-controlled trial of a depot gonadotropin-releasing hormone analogue (leuprolide) in the treatment of uterine leiomyomata. *Obstet. Gynecol.*, **74**, 856–62
7. Maheux, R., Guilloteau, C., Lemay, A., Bastide, A. and Fazekas, A. T. A. (1985). Luteinizing hormone-releasing hormone agonist and uterine leiomyoma: a pilot study. *Am. J. Obstet. Gynecol.*, **152**, 1034–8
8. Kessel, B., Liu, J., Mortola, J., Berga, S. and Yen, S. S. C. (1988). Treatment of uterine fibroids with

agonist analogs of gonadotropin-releasing hormone. *Fertil. Steril.*, **49**, 538–41

9. Candiani, G. B., Vercellini, P., Fedele, L., Arcaini, L., Bianchi, S. and Candiani, M. (1990). Use of goserelin depot, a gonadotropin-releasing hormone agonist, for the treatment of menorrhagia and severe anemia in women with leiomyomata uteri. *Acta Obstet. Gynecol. Scand.*, **69**, 41–5

10. Fedele, L., Bianchi, S., Baglioni, A., Arcaini, L., Marchini, M. and Bocciolone, L. (1990). Intranasal buserelin versus surgery in the treatment of uterine leiomyomata: long-term follow-up. *Eur. J. Obstet. Gynecol. Reprod.*, **38**, 53–7

11. Friedman, A. J. (1993). Treatment of uterine myomas with GnRH agonists. *Semin. Reprod. Endocrinol.*, **11**, 154–61

12. Friedman, A. J. (1989). Vaginal hemorrhage associated with degenerating submucous leiomyomata during leuprolide acetate treatment. *Fertil. Steril.*, **52**, 152–4

13. Friedman, A. J. (1993). Combined oestrogen–progestin treatment of vaginal haemorrhage following gonadotropin-releasing hormone agonist therapy of uterine myomas. *Hum. Reprod.*, **8**, 540–2

14. Friedman, A. J. (1989). Treatment of leiomyomata uteri with short-term leuprolide followed by leuprolide plus estrogen–progestin hormone replacement therapy for two years: a pilot study. *Fertil. Steril.*, **51**, 526–8

15. Friedman, A. J., Daly M., Juneau-Norcross, M., Gleason, R., Rein, M. S. and LeBoff, M. (1994). Long-term medical therapy for leiomyomata uteri: a prospective, randomized study of leuprolide acetate depot plus either estrogen–progestin or progestin 'add-back' for two years. *Hum. Reprod.*, **9**, 1618–25

16. Friedman, A. J., Barbieri, R. L., Doubilet, P. M., Fine, C. and Schiff, I. (1988). A randomized, double-blind trial of a gonadotropin releasing-hormone agonist (leuprolide) with or without medroxyprogesterone acetate in the treatment of leiomyomata uteri. *Fertil. Steril.*, **49**, 404–9

17. Carr, B. R., Marshburn, P. B., Weatherall, P. T., Bradshaw, K. D., Breslau, N. A., Byrd, W., Roark, M. and Steinkampf, M. P. (1993). An evaluation of the effect of gonadotropin-releasing hormone analogs and medroxyprogesterone acetate on uterine leiomyomata volume by magnetic reasonance imaging: a prospective, randomized, double blind, placebo-controlled, crossover trial. *J. Clin. Endocrinol. Metab.*, **76**, 1217–23

18. Murphy, A. A., Kettel, L. M., Morales, A. J., Roberts, V. J. and Yen, S. C. C. (1993). Regression of uterine leiomyomata in response to the antiprogesterone RU-486. *J. Clin. Endocrinol. Metab.*, **76**, 513–8

19. Friedman, A. J., Lobel, S., Rein, M. S. and Barbieri, R. L. (1990). Efficacy and safety considerations in women with uterine leiomyomata treated with gonadotropin-releasing hormone agonists: the estrogen threshold hypothesis. *Am. J. Obstet. Gynecol.*, **163**, 1114–9

13

Steroid supplementation of GnRH analog treatment in endometriosis

E. S. Surrey

INTRODUCTION

Highly potent gonadotropin releasing hormone (GnRH) agonists have been consistently shown to reduce the painful symptoms and extent of implants associated with endometriosis[1-3]. The secondary hypoestrogenic state induced by these agents commonly results in vasomotor symptoms and reversible bone mineral density loss which may limit compliance and safety for long-term use[3-7]. Prolonged hypoestrogenism has been associated with an increase in risk factors for cardiovascular disease in menopausal women[8,9]. Extrapolation of such data to younger women receiving GnRH agonists for an extended period has not been established but is worrying. A subset of refractory endometriosis patients with symptoms responsive only to GnRH agonists administration would benefit from prolongation of therapy should these side effects be safely minimized or eliminated entirely.

'Add-back' therapy represents a means by which various steroidal and non-steroidal agents have been combined with GnRH agonists in an effort to ameliorate the impact of a hypoestrogenic state while preserving therapeutic efficacy. Short term ($\leq$ 6 months) add-back therapy is aimed primarily at elimination of vasomotor symptoms, whereas longer-term therapy must also eliminate progressive loss of bone mineral density and any deleterious effects on cardiac risk profiles.

Each of the regimens which have been investigated shall be described in this brief review. Unfortunately, the studies cited represent relatively small-scale clinical trials and so truly definitive recommendations cannot yet be made.

PROGESTIN SUPPLEMENTATION

Given that endometriosis is an estrogen-sensitive disorder, investigators have attempted to avoid estrogen supplementation by employing various progestins as add-back for endometriosis patients administered GnRH agonists. In the absence of exogenous estrogens, these compounds have been shown to suppress vasomotor symptoms and bone density loss in menopausal women[10,11]. The mechanism by which both natural and synthetic progestins exert this effect on bone has not been conclusively demonstrated. Direct interaction with progesterone, androgen or glucocorticoid receptors has been reported[12-14]. Others have suggested that progestin may stimulate such bone tropic agents as calcitonin, or transforming growth factor-β may play a more predominant role[15,16].

Medroxyprogesterone acetate (MPA) was assessed as a potential add-back agent by two sets of investigators. Five endometriosis patients self-administered intranasal buserelin daily during treatment courses of 7 to 24 months in an uncontrolled series[17]. MPA was added for 7 to 10 days of each month. Although pain relief was reported in all patients in conjunction with uniform suppression of estradiol levels, hot flushes were eliminated in all but one patient. A qualitative decrease in lumbar spine bone density was described. A larger 6-month clinical trial involving eight patients administered histrelin (100 µg) and MPA (20–30 mg) daily was subsequently reported by Cedars and co-workers[18]. Vasomotor symptoms and bone density loss at the levels of the distal radius and lumbar spine were virtually eliminated. Compared to historic controls receiving histrelin alone, the progestin-supplemented group experienced worsening of painful symptoms by the sixteenth week of therapy and lack of resolution of implants at follow-up laparoscopy.

Norethindrone, a 19-nortestosterone-derived progestin, is structurally dissimilar to MPA (a 17α-hydroxyprogestin). However, this progestin has also been reported to inhibit bone density loss and hot flushes when administered to menopausal women in the absence of exogenous estrogens[19–21].

Surrey *et al.*[22] have reported upon the effects of norethindrone supplementation in a 6-month prospective trial of ten patients with symptomatic endometriosis. All patients received 100 mg of the GnRH agonist histrelin subcutaneously each day and norethindrone in 0.35 mg minimal daily doses. Patients were allowed to increase norethindrone doses in 0.35 mg increments up to a maximal daily allowable dose of 3.5 mg to eliminate persistent vasomotor symptoms. Employing a maximal mean daily dose of 2.04 mg, hot flushes were suppressed when compared to historic controls receiving the agonist alone. Dramatic suppression of symptoms and endometriotic implants was noted (Figure 1). No change in bone density at the level of the distal radius was noted after a 24-week treatment course. However, a significant but reversible loss in primarily trabecular bone at the level of the lumbar spine was appreciated. There were no changes in triglyceride, cholesterol or lipoprotein subfractions with the norethindrone doses employed in this investigation.

These findings contrast to some extent with those reported by Riis and co-workers[23]. Norethindone in 1.2-mg daily doses was administered to 17 endometriosis patients in conjunction with an intranasal preparation of the GnRH agonist nafarelin. Suppression of bone mineral density loss of the lumbar spine and radius as compared to historic controls receiving agonist alone was reported. Interestingly, the effects of this regimen on painful symptoms, disease extent or hot flushes were not described.

This discrepancy in bone density findings between the two studies was partially resolved by the results of an investigation reported by Eldred and co-workers[24]. Employing nafarelin acetate in combination with various norethindrone doses in a 6-month randomized double-blind trial, these investigators noted significant but reversible lumbar spine bone loss with daily supplemental doses as high as 2.45 mg. Others have shown that only 5–10 mg daily norethindrone doses are sufficient to prevent

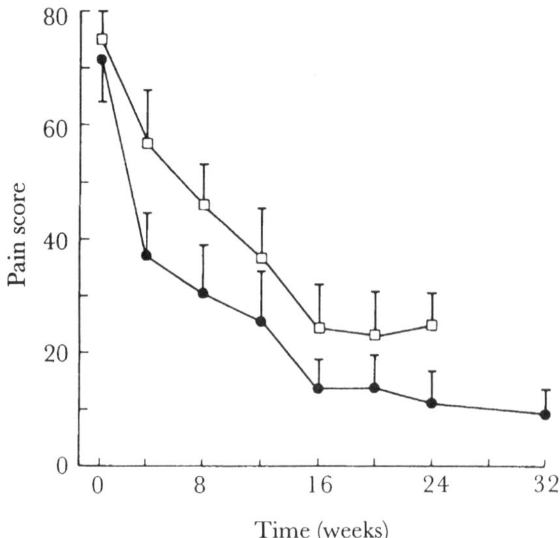

Figure 1 Monthly pain scores (mean ± SEM) in patients receiving GnRH agonist and norethindrone (closed circles) and historic controls receiving GnRH agonist only (open squares). From Surrey, E., Gambone, J., Lu, J. and Judd, H. (1990). The effects of combining norethindrone with a gonadotropin-releasing hormone agonist in the treatment of symptomatic endometriosis. *Fertil. Steril.*, **53**, 620–6[22]. Reproduced with permission of the publisher, the American Society for Reproductive Medicine (formerly The American Fertility Society)

bone loss in otherwise untreated menopausal women[19,20].

The author and co-workers have therefore administered higher norethindrone doses to symptomatic endometriosis patients receiving a depot preparation of the GnRH agonist leuprolide acetate in two prospective randomized trials[3,25]. During an initial 6-month trial, ten control patients were administered depot leuprolide acetate alone[3]. Another ten patients received the agonist plus norethindrone in 5-mg daily doses for 4 weeks and then 10-mg daily doses for the subsequent 20 weeks. Suppression of symptoms, circulating serum estrone and estradiol levels, as well as extent of disease at second-look laparoscopy, were equivalent between the two groups. However, vasomotor and vaginal symptoms were nearly eliminated in the add-back group (Figure 2). A significantly greater degree of lumbar spine bone density loss as measured by dual X-ray

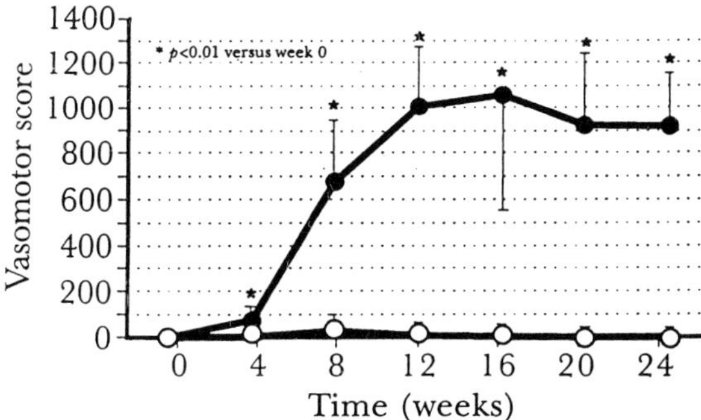

Figure 2 Vasomotor symptom scores (mean ± SEM) throughout therapy based on daily documentation of subjective hot flush frequency and intensity for patients receiving GnRH agonist alone or GnRH agonist and 10 mg of norethindrone (NEt) 10 mg daily. ●, GnRH agonist only; ○, GnRH agonist + NEt; p <0.01 versus week 0. From Surrey, E. and Judd, H. (1992). Reduction of vasomotor symptoms and bone mineral density loss with combined norethindrone and long-acting gonadotropin-releasing hormone agonist therapy of symptomatic endometriosis: a prospective randomised trial. *J. Clin. Endocrinol. Metab.*, **75**, 558–63[3]. Reproduced with permission of the Endocrione Society

absorptiometry (DEXA) was noted in control patients (–5.6% versus –2.5%, respectively). By increasing the daily norethindrone dose to 10 mg throughout the course of a more recent 1-year clinical trial, the author and his co-workers noted that all significant lumbar spine bone density loss was eliminated[25,26]. Undesirable but reversible increases in the low-density lipoprotein (LDL) : high-density lipoprotrein (HDL) ratio and decreases in circulating HDL-cholesterol levels were noted in both studies.

PROGESTIN ± ORGANIC BISPHOSPHONATE SUPPLEMENTATION

In an effort to reduce the undesirable effect of higher norethindrone doses on circulating lipoproteins while maintaining the beneficial effects of this progestin on inhibiting vasomotor symptoms induced by GnRH agonist, other agents have been added. The author and his co-workers have recently described the effects of an add-back regimen comprised of low-dose norethindrone combined with cyclic sodium etidronate in a prospective randomized 48-week clinical trial of symptomatic endometriosis patients administered a depot preparation of leuprolide acetate[25,26]. Sodium etidronate is in a class of organic bisphosphonate compounds which inhibit osteoclast-mediated bone resportion when administered in a cyclic fashion. The efficacy of this agent in the retardation of osteoporotic fractions in postmenopausal women untreated with estrogens has been demonstrated during 2 years of cyclic therapy[27].

In the author and co-workers' series, sodium etidronate (400 mg daily) was self-administered for 2 weeks followed by calcium carbonate (500 mg daily) for 6 weeks. This 8-week treatment course was repeated six times during the 48-week trial. Norethindrone (2.5 mg daily) was administered to effectively suppress vasomotor symptoms. Although persistent hypoestrogenism was induced without escape during the clinical trial, no bone density loss as recorded by serial DEXA scans of the lumbar spine was noted (Table 1). The significant reductions in painful symptoms recorded in daily diaries and extent of disease

Table 1 Lumbar spine bone mineral density changes (DEXA scans) in endometriosis patients receiving norethindrone (NEt) ± etidronate add-back (results expressed as mean ± SEM percentage change from week 0)

Group	n	Week 24	Week 48

Group I: GnRH agonist + NEt 2.5 mg
    + sodium etidronate 400 mg (14/42 days)
    + calcium carbonate 500 mg (28/42) days)
	10	–0.44 ± 0.79*	–0.76 ± 0.94*

Group II: GnRH agonist + NEt 10 mg	8	–0.45 ± 1.40*	–1.10 ± 1.30*
Group III: Untreated matched controls	18	–0.22 ± 0.86	–0.32 ± 0.77

*NS versus Group III; NEt, norethindrone. Modified from Surrey *et al.* 1995[25]

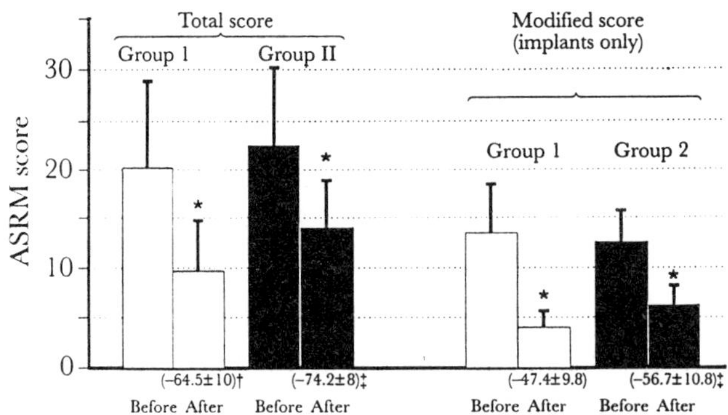

Figure 3 Changes in revised American Society of Reproductive Medicine (ASRM) endometriosis scores (mean ± SEM) derived from independent observers' review of coded videotapes before and 4 weeks after completion of 48 weeks of therapy. Group I patients received GnRH agonist plus cyclic etidronate plus low-dose norethindrone. Group II patients received GnRH agonist plus high-dose norethindrone. $*p < 0.05$ versus pre-therapy; †percentage change in scores from pre-therapy laparoscopies; ‡$p > 0.2$ versus group I. From Surrey, E., Voight, B., Fournet, N. and Judd, H. (1995). Prolonged gonadotropin releasing hormone agonist treatment of symptomatic endometriosis: the role of cyclic sodium sodium etidronate and low dose norethindrone 'add-back' therapy. *Fertil. Steril.*, **63**, 747–55. Reproduced with permission of the publisher, the American Society for Reproductive Medicine (formerly The American Fertility Society)

detected at second-look laparoscopy after 48 weeks of therapy were noted (Figure 3). No significant changes in the ratio of LDL to HDL cholesterol subfractions could be detected.

SUPPLEMENTAL ESTROGEN REPLACEMENT

An alternative approach to avoid the undesirable changes in circulating lipids induced by high-dose progestin add-back is the use of estrogen-dominant regimens in conjunction with a GnRH agonist. Previous investigators have reported suppression of both vasomotor symptoms and bone loss in menopausal women administered a variety of estrogen replacement regimens[28,29]. The primary concern regarding the use of these hormones is stimulation of the underlying estrogen-sensitive disorder for which the patient had been treated in the first place. The 'estrogen threshold hypothesis' suggests that an ideal circulating estradiol level can be reached which would be sufficient to suppress hypoestrogenic side effects while avoiding stimulation of disease[30]. Little information exists to allow accurate determination of this level. If one were to accept this hypothesis, however, it must also be assumed that the estrogen level which is sufficient to prevent side effects must be lower than that which would result in disease stimulation. Unfortunately, there are little data to confirm this assumption.

A paucity of clinical trials assessing the efficacy of estrogen add-back in endometriosis patients has been reported. Most investigators have employed progestins in conjunction with estrogens. The largest series to date has been a 6-month prospective trial of 50 symptomatic endometriosis patients reported by Edmonds and Howell[31]. Subjects were randomized to receive 3.6 mg goserelin subcutaneously monthly for 6 months with or without twice-weekly transdermal 17β-estradiol (25 μg) and daily oral MPA (5 mg). Pain relief and resolution of disease at second-look laparoscopy were similar between the two groups. Hot flushes were significantly decreased, but not eliminated in the add-back group (96% versus 46% of patients, respectively). Bone mineral density loss as measured by serial DEXA scans of the lumbar spine and femoral neck was reduced by 50% to 2.5% overall in the supplemented group. It is interesting to note that the density failed to return to baseline in either group 6 months after therapy. A smaller 2-year uncontrolled retrospective series recently reported by Friedman and Hornstein[32] described eight patients treated with leuprolide acetate for 12 weeks then supplemented with daily oral conjugate equine estrogens (0.625 mg) and MPA (2.5 mg) for the subsequent 92 weeks. Symptoms and extent of disease were suppressed in the six patients who completed the trial. Vasomotor symptoms and lumbar spine bone density loss were minimized. In a case report, Reid and co-workers described a single patient treated for 1 year with goserelin and a similar add-back regimen with favorable results[33]. Sugimoto *et al.*[34] have questioned the ability of these doses of conjugated equine estrogens to prevent bone loss uniformly in patients administered leuprolide acetate over 1 year of therapy. Only higher (1.25 mg) daily doses consistently preserved bone in this retrospective series, a dose which may be more prone to stimulate disease. The use of estrogens alone as supplementation was described in a case report of a single endometriosis patient administered goserelin in conjunction with transdermal 17β-estradiol (25 μg) during a 6-month period[35]. Although bone density was not assessed, pain, disease and hot flushes were minimized. A variety of supplemental estrogen replacement regimens are currently being evaluated in prospective multicenter trials.

CONCLUSIONS

Prolonged administration of a GnRH agonist beyond the currently accepted 6-month interval may be appropriate for those endometriosis patients with refractory pelvic pain unresponsive to other means. The ideal add-back regimen would suppress undesired aspects of the hypoestrogenic state induced by the GnRH agonist while preserving their efficacy. In appropriate doses, MPA and norethindrone can both suppress vasomotor symptoms and bone density loss induced by the GnRH agonist. Unfortunately, MPA appears to reverse the beneficial effects of these agents on suppressing extent of disease and painful symptoms. Low norethindrone doses do achieve this effect, but fail to prevent some reversible bone loss. This strategy is effective for shorter (≤ 6 months) courses of therapy. Prolonged therapy with higher norethindrone doses has been shown to be highly effective in the treatment of the symptoms and implants associated with endometriosis while suppressing vasomotor symptoms and bone density changes. Nevertheless, undesirable but reversible changes in lipoprotein subfractions resulted. The combination of sodium etidronate with lower norethindrone doses may be more ideally suited for safe and effective long-term GnRH agonist therapy. The onset of second- and third-generation organic bisphosphonates may further enhance the safety of these regimens. Little data exist regarding the efficacy of estrogen replacement regimens as a supplemental therapy in these patients, although preliminary studies established their potential. Issues of cost-effectiveness must also be addressed. Larger scale multicenter trials are currently under way to provide more standardized approaches.

References

1. Henzl, M. R., Corson, S. L., Moghissi, K., Buttram, V. C., Berquist, C. and Jacobson, J. (1988). Administration of nasal nafarelin as compared with oral danazol for endometriosis: a randomized placebo-controlled, double-blind study. *Fertil. Steril.*, **318**, 485–9

2. Steingold, K. A., Cedars, M., Lu, J. K. H., Randle, D., Judd, H.L. and Meldrum, D.R. (1989). Treatment of endometriosis with a long-acting gonadotropin releasing hormone agonist. *Obstet. Gynecol.*, **69**, 403–11

3. Surrey, E. and Judd, H. (1992). Reduction of vasomotor symptoms and bone mineral density loss with combined norethindrone and long-acting gonadotropin-releasing hormone agonist therapy of symptomatic endometriosis: a prospective randomized trial. *J. Clin. Endocrinol. Metab.*, **75**, 558–63

4. DeFazio, J., Meldrum, D., Laufer, L., Vale, W., Rivier, J., Lu, J. and Judd, H. (1983). Induction of hot flushes in premenopausal women treated with a long-acting GnRH agonist. *J. Clin. Endocrinol. Metab.*, **56**, 445–8

5. Gallagher, J. (1993). Effect of gonadotropin-releasing hormone agonists on bone metabolism. *Semin. Reprod. Endocrinol.*, **11**, 201–8

6. Fogelman, I., Fentiman, I., Hamed, H., Studd, J. W. W. and Leather, A. T. (1994). Goserelin (Zoladex) and the skeleton. *Br. J. Obstet.*, **101** (Suppl. 10), 19–23

7. Surrey, E. S. (1995). Steroidal and nonsteroidal 'add-back' therapy: extending safety and efficacy of GnRH agonists in the gynecologic patient. *Fertil. Steril.* **64**, 673–85

8. Stampfer, M., Willett, W., Colditz, G., Rosner, B., Speizer, F. and Hennekens, C. (1985). A prospective study of postmenopausal oestrogen therapy and coronary heart disease. *N. Engl. J. Med.*, **313**, 1044–9

9. Matthews, K., Meilahn, E., Kuller, L., Kelsey, S., Cagguila, A. and Wing, R. (1989). Menopause and risk factors for coronary heart disease. *N. Engl. J. Med.*, **321**, 641–6

10. Paterson, M. (1982). A randomized double-blinded cross-over trial into the effects of norethindrone on climacteric symptoms and biochemical profiles. *Br. J. Obstet. Gynaecol.*, **89**, 464–72

11. Gallagher, J., Kable, W. and Goldgar, D. (1975). Effect of progestin therapy on cortical and trabecular bone: comparison with estrogen. *Am. J. Med.*, **90**, 171–8

12. Colvard, D. S., Eriksen, E. F., Keeting, P. E., Wilson, E. M., Lubahn, D. B., French, F. S., Riggs, B. L. and Spelsberg, T. C. (1989). Identification of androgen receptors in normal human osteoblast-like cells. *Proc. Natl. Acad. Sci. USA.*, **86**, 854–7

13. Erikson, E. F., Colvard, D. S., Berg, N. J., Graham, M. L., Mann, K. G., Spelsberg, T. C. and Riggs, B. L. (1988). Evidence of estrogen receptors in normal human osteoblast-like cells. *Science*, **241**, 84–6

14. Mangolas, S. and Anderson, D. (1975). Detection of high affinity glucocorticoid binding in rat bone. *J. Endocrinol.*, **7**, 379–80

15. Greenberg, C., Kukreja, S. C., Bowser, E. N., Hargis, G. K., Henderson, W. J. and Williams, G. A. (1986). Effects of estradiol and progesterone on calcitonin secretion. *Endocrinology*, **118**, 2594–8

16. Kasperk, C., Fitzsimmons, R., Strong, D., Subburman, M., Jennings, J., Wergedal, J. and Baylink, D. (1990). Studies of the mechanism by which androgens enhance mitogenesis and differentiation in bone cells. *J. Clin. Endocrinol. Metab.*, **71**, 1322–9

17. Lemay, A., Dodin, S. and Dewailly, S. (1989). Long-term use of the low dose LHRH analogue combined with monthly medroxy-progesterone administration. *Horm. Res.*, **32** (Suppl. 1), 141–5

18. Cedars, M., Lu, J., Meldrum, D. and Judd, H. (1990). Treatment of endometriosis with a long-acting gonadotropin-releasing hormone agonist plus medroxyprogesterone acetate. *Obstet. Gynecol.*, **75**, 641–5

19. Abdalla, H., Hart, D., Lindsay, R., Leggate, I. and Hooke, A. (1985). Prevention of bone mineral density loss in postmenopausal women by norethisterone. *Obstet. Gynecol.*, **66**, 789–92

20. Horowitz, M., Wishart, J., Need, A., Morris, H., Philcox, J. and Nordin, C. (1987). Treatment of postmenopausal hyperparathyroidism with norethindrone: effects on biochemistry and forearm mineral density. *Arch. Intern. Med.*, **147**, 681–5

21. Nordin, B., Jones, M., Crilly, R., Marshall, D. and Brook, R. (1980). A placebo-controlled trial of ethinyl estradiol and norethisterone in climacteric women. *Maturitas*, **2**, 247–51

22. Surrey, E., Gambone, J., Lu, J. and Judd, H. (1990). The effects of combining norethindrone with a gonadotropin-releasing hormone agonist in the treatment of symptomatic endometriosis. *Fertil. Steril.*, **53**, 620–6

23. Riis, B., Christiansen, C., Johansen, J. and Jacobson, J. (1990). Is it possible to prevent bone loss in young women treated with luteinizing hormone-releasing hormone agonists? *J. Clin. Endocrinol. Metab.*, **70**, 920–4

24. Eldred, J., Haynes, P. and Thomas, C. (1992). A randomized double-blind placebo controlled trial of the effects on bone metabolism of the combination of nafarelin acetate and norethisterone. *Clin. Endocrinol.*, **37**, 354–9

25. Surrey, E., Voigt, B., Fournet, N. and Judd, H. (1995). Prolonged gonadotropin releasing hormone agonist treatment of symptomatic endometriosis: the role of cyclic sodium etidronate and low dose norethindrone 'add-back' therapy. *Fertil. Steril.*, **63**, 747–55

26. Surrey, E., Fournet, N., Voigt, B. and Judd, H. (1993). Effects of sodium etidronate in combination with low-dose norethindrone in patients administered a long-acting GnRH agonist: a preliminary report. *Obstet. Gynecol.*, **81**, 581–6

27. Storm, T., Thamsborg, G., Steiniche, T., Genant, H. and Sorenson, O. (1990). Effect of intermittent

cyclic etidronate therapy on bone mass and fracture rate in women with postmenopausal osteoporosis. *N. Engl. J. Med.*, **322**, 1265–71

28. Ettinger, B., Genant, H. and Cann, C. (1985). Long-term estrogen therapy prevents bone loss and fracture. *Ann. Intern. Med.*, **102**, 319–24

29. Ravnikar, V. (1990). Physiology and treatment of hot flushes. *Obstet. Gynecol.*, **75**, 3S–8S

30. Barbieri, R. (1992). Hormone treatment of endometriosis: the estrogen threshold hypothesis. *Am. J. Obstet. Gynecol.*, **166**, 740–5

31. Edmonds, D. K. and Howell, R. (1994). Can hormone replacement therapy be used during medical therapy of endometriosis. *Br. J. Obstet. Gynaecol.*, **101** (Suppl. 10), 24–6

32. Friedman, A. and Hornstein, M. (1993). Gonadotropin-releasing hormone agonist plus estrogen progestin 'add-back' therapy for endometriosis-related pelvic pain. *Fertil. Steril.*, **60**, 236–41

33. Reid, B. A., Gangar, K. F. and Beard, R. W. (1992). Endometriosis treated with gonadotropin releasing hormone agonist and continuous hormone replacement therapy. *Br. J. Obstet. Gynaecol.*, **99**, 344–8

34. Sugimoto, A., Hodsman, A. and Nisker, J. (1993). Long-term gonadotropin-releasing hormone agonist with standard postmenopausal estrogen replacement failed to prevent vertebral bone loss in premenopausal women. *Fertil. Steril.*, **60**, 672–4

35. Maouris, P., Dowsett, M., Rose, G. and Edmonds, D. (1989). A new treatment for endometriosis. *Lancet*, **ii**, 1018–9

Steroid supplementation of GnRH analog in ovarian hyperandrogenism

14

E. Carmina and R. A. Lobo

INTRODUCTION

Hirsutism due to ovarian hyperandrogenism is commonly treated by oral contraceptives and/or antiandrogens[1]. Although the results are generally good in terms of improvement of hirsutism during drug administration, hirsutism and hyperandrogenism return quickly after drug withdrawal. Moreover, in a few patients conventional treatment of hirsutism is disappointing, because of only a minimal reduction of excess hair[1]. Therefore, the search for new approaches continues.

Several years ago it was shown that gonadotropin releasing hormone (GnRH) agonists are able to reduce androgen secretion in women with ovarian hyperandrogenism[2]. Later, several studies using the GnRH agonist showed that hirsutism markedly improved in women with ovarian hyperandrogenism and severe insulin resistance[3–5]. However, the application to clinical practice of these observations was largely limited by the findings that GnRH agonists induce amenorrhea, and concerns emerged concerning the possible side effects of prolonged hypoestrogenism including bone loss, vasomotor symptoms, urethral and vaginal atrophy[6–8]. Recently, we have shown that supplementation by low doses of estrogens and progestins enhances the effects of GnRH agonist treatment of patients with severe ovarian hyperandrogenism while preventing most side effects[9]. After our report, many other studies, using different methods of steroid supplementation, have confirmed and extended our observations, although some controversy has arisen on the difference in efficacy between the effects of GnRH agonists alone or with the addition of estrogens and progestins[10–13].

In this paper we review our experience of the treatment of ovarian hyperandrogenism with GnRH agonists with supplemental estrogen and progestins and we compare our results with those of other research groups. While doing so, we attempt to answer to some important and practical questions:

(1) Is steroid supplementation of GnRH agonists useful in the treatment of ovarian hyperandrogenism?

(2) What is the best method for steroid supplementation?

(3) How does treatment with GnRH agonists and estrogens plus progestins compare with other conventional treatments of ovarian hyperandrogenism?

EFFECTS OF GnRH AGONISTS AND ESTROGEN SUPPLEMENTATION ON OVARIAN HYPERANDROGENISM

In our pilot study[9], we evaluated the effects of combining a long-acting GnRH agonist with low doses of estrogens, as used after menopause. All patients presented with a severe form of hirsutism due to ovarian hyperandrogenism, which had been previously treated with oral contraceptives, cyproterone acetate or spironolactone with unsatisfactory results. They were treated for 1 year with a long-acting GnRH agonist (Decapeptyl, Ipsen, France) at a dose of 3.75 mg intramuscularly every 28 days, starting on day 1 of spontaneous or progestin-induced menses. After the first month of GnRH agonist treatment, estrogens plus progestins were added. Conjugated equine estrogens 0.625 mg were administered on days 1–21 of each month. In addition, medroxyprogesterone acetate (10 mg) was administered on days 12–21 of each month.

During treatment with the combination regimen, both gonadotropins (luteinizing hormone, LH, and follicle stimulating hormone, FSH) were significantly suppressed, suggesting a more complete pituitary suppression than that obtained by GnRH agonists alone. In all patients serum estradiol was reduced to less than 30 pg/ml, but because it has been shown that androgen secretion is less sensitive than estradiol secretion to GnRH agonists[14], LH was suppressed to levels lower than 1.5 mIU/ml. In order to suppress LH to these levels, in some patients the dose of GnRH agonists was increased by administering the drug every 21 days.

A significant decrease of total testosterone, unbound testosterone and androstenedione was obtained while mean serum dehydroepiandrosterone sulfate DHEA-S levels were unchanged (Figure 1). Interestingly, ovarian morphology was reversed in most patients with normalization of ovarian size and disappearance of microcysts. The polycystic appearance of the ovary returned gradually after withdrawal of treatment, suggesting that polycystic ovary morphology is a dynamic process linked to the endocrine abnormalities. Hirsutism progressively improved, with a significant decrease occurring in the Ferriman–Gallwey–Lorenzo scores after 6 months. After 1 year of treatment most patients had normal scores (Figure 2). Normal menstrual cycles were maintained in almost all patients and there were no vasomotor symptoms, changes in lipids or alterations in bone metabolism markers (Table 1).

Although in our initial study we used low doses of estrogens, other methods of estrogen supplementation (transdermal estradiol, estradiol valerate, oral contraceptives) have been used with similar results[10–13,15]. As shown in Table 2, in most studies hirsutism scores decreased by about 25–30% after 6 months and by about 50% after 1 year. Testosterone and unbound testosterone

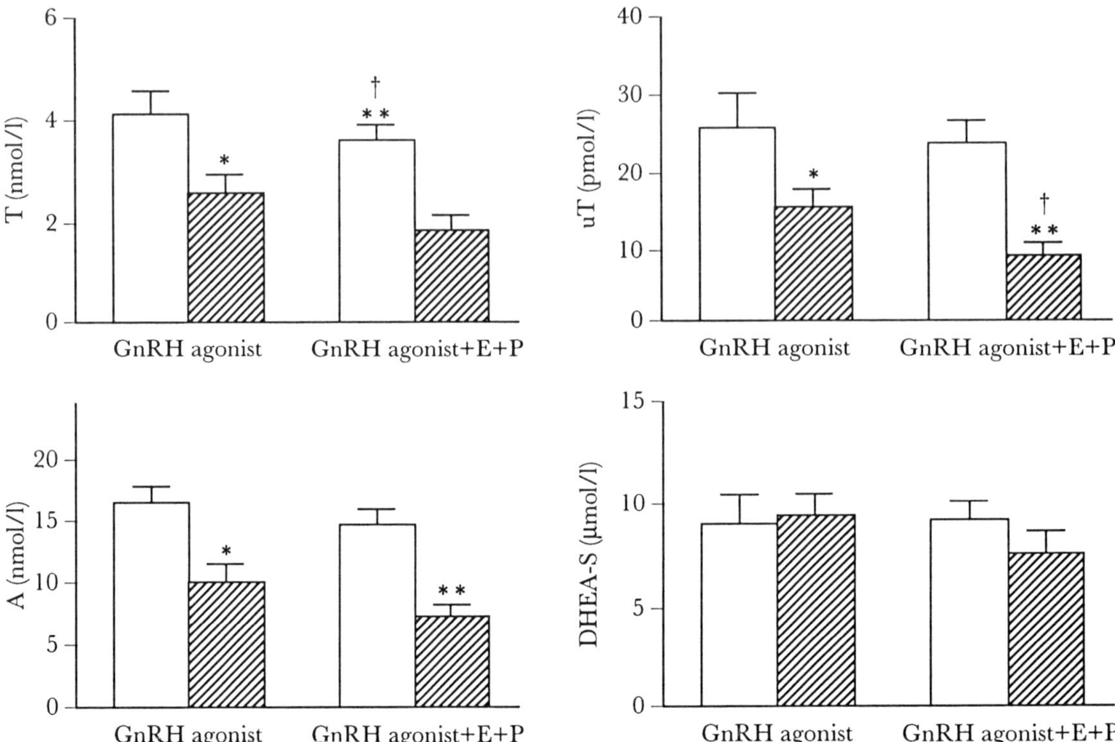

Figure 1 Effects of GnRH agonists alone and with hormonal replacement on serum androgen levels. A, androstenedione; E, estrogens; P, progestins; T, testosterone; uT, unbound testosterone; □, basal; ▨, 6 months

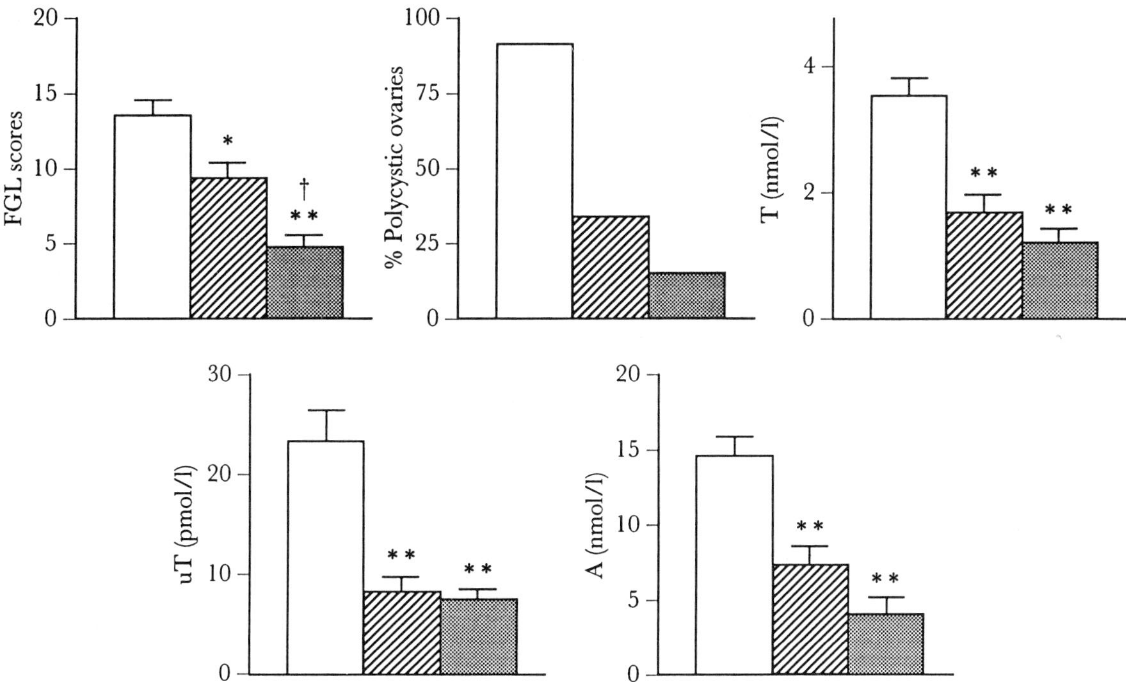

Figure 2 Effects of long-term GnRH agonists plus add-back steroid supplementation. A, androstenedione; FGL, Ferriman–Gallwey–Lorenzo; T, testosterone; uT, unbound testosterone; □, basal; ▨, 6 months; ▦, 1 year

decreased by about 55–70% after 6 months. Only one research group[11] reported disappointing results with very small decreases in hirsutism (10–15%), total testosterone (22%) and unbound testosterone (33%). In this report estradiol valerate (2 mg) was used as the estrogen supplement.

Table 1 Changes (percentages) in symptoms, lipids, high-density lipoprotein-C (HDL-C) and osteocalcin in the two groups

	GnRH agonists	GnRH agonist + estrogen
Vasomotor symptoms	100	0
Regular menses	0	83
Irregular menses	0	17
Amenorrhea	100	0
Total cholesterol	+11	0
HDL-C	−6	+2
Triglycerides	+3	+1
Osteocalcin	+40*	−6

*$p < 0.05$, change from pretreatment

Perhaps differences in the patients studied explain these differences in results.

IS STEROID SUPPLEMENTATION USEFUL IN THE TREATMENT OF OVARIAN HYPERANDROGENISM?

In our experience[9], estrogen supplementation enhanced the effects of GnRH agonists on the endocrine and clinical manifestations of ovarian hyperandrogenism. Serum FSH was reduced only in patients treated with combination therapy and the decrease of serum androgens was larger in patients using estrogen supplementation. In these patients, a more marked decrease of hirsutism was also observed. Other groups[11,13] have reported slightly different results. However, as already observed, the data of Tiitinnen and associates[11] are quite different from all others present in the literature and probably suggest that the GnRH agonist was not particularly effective in their patients. Another group[13] has recently reported results that are very similar to ours. Using oral

Table 2 Effect (percentages) of different models of estrogen supplementation on GnRH agonist therapy for ovarian hyperandrogenism

Estrogen	Reference number	Hirsutism improvement		Total testosterone	Free testosterone
		6 months	1 year		
Conjugated estrogens	9	−30	−55	−55	−52
Micronized estradiol	10	−23	—	−64	—
Estradiol valerate	11	−10	−15	−22	−33
Transdermal estradiol	12	−30	−50	−70	—
Oral contraceptives	13	−25	—	−70	−62
Oral contraceptives (with cyproterone acetate)	14	−26	—	−57	−76

contraceptives as the steroid supplement, Elkind-Hirsch and colleagues observed significant decreases in FSH and a larger reduction of serum androgens in patients treated with the combination therapy. However, they did not observe differences in the improvement of hirsutism in the two groups after 6 months of therapy. On the other hand, the reduction in the Ferriman–Gallwey–Lorenzo scores was very small after 6 months and true changes that may have occurred might have been difficult to detect.

We suggest that perhaps the more important advantage of using steroid supplementation is not the possible enhancement of the GnRH agonists but the possibility of prolonging the duration of GnRH agonist action and also the minimizing of side effects. With the use of GnRH agonists alone, treatment should not exceed 6 months, because of concerns of loss in bone mass[6]. It has been suggested that pituitary–ovarian suppression for longer than 6 months results in a loss of bone mass, which does not get replaced[6]. On the other hand, the clinical improvement of hirsutism is slow with any therapy and no results are generally seen before 3–4 months and then the effects progressively increase[1]. In our experience, in most patients, treatments of 1 year or more are generally necessary to get normal scores in the Ferriman–Gallwey–Lorenzo index. Accordingly, our patients treated with the GnRH agonists (both alone and with estrogen supplementation) experienced a slow reduction of hirsutism with significant decreases in Ferriman–Gallwey–Lorenzo scores only after 6 months. Normalization of the clinical

presentation was observed only in patients who were taking the combination therapy for 1 year[9]. A slow return from the possible peripheral (skin) effects of the androgens probably explains this phenomenon[16]. Serum levels of 3α-androstanediol-glucuronide, a peripheral androgen metabolite, decreased slowly and its reduction paralleled the decrease of hirsutism.

WHAT IS THE BEST REGIMEN FOR STEROID SUPPLEMENTATION?

As we have already observed, there are no substantial differences in endocrine and clinical results obtained, with the use of different regimens of steroid supplementation of GnRH agonist therapy for ovarian hyperandrogenism. All methods of steroid supplementation minimize the side effects of GnRH agonists. Normal menses are generally maintained and bleeding abnormalities (menometrorrhagia or oligomenorrhea) may easily be corrected by modifying the estrogen or progestin dose. There is an improvement in vasomotor symptoms and no changes in lipids. However, some concern has been expressed about using low doses of estrogens in premenopausal women treated with GnRH agonists. In fact, while 0.625 mg of conjugated estrogens or a correspondent dose of transdermal estradiol are sufficient to prevent bone loss in postmenopausal women[17], at least one study has shown that younger women require higher estrogen doses (1.25 mg of conjugated estrogens)[18].

In a recent study[12], using transdermal estradiol at a dose of 100 µg twice weekly as steroid supplementation of GnRH agonist therapy of young women with ovarian hyperandrogenism, a trend towards a progressive reduction of bone mass was observed in spite of the absence of changes in biochemical bone markers. In our initial report, we used low doses of conjugated estrogens and did not observe changes in osteocalcin. Recently, assessing bone mass by vertebral densitometry, we found a small but not significant reduction in bone mass. Although more data are needed and small variations of bone mass may not be clinically relevant in hyperandrogenic women who already have increased bone mass[19], we prefer to use higher doses of estrogens (1.25 mg of conjugated estrogens or oral contraceptives containing 35 µg of ethinylestradiol) and utilize the lower doses only when there are side effects or some contra-indication to the higher dose.

Another interesting option is the use of a contraceptive containing antiandrogens such as Diane (Schering, Berlin), which contains 2 mg of cyproterone acetate and may give some clinical advantage in terms of a more marked reduction of hirsutism. However, our data and those from the literature[14] do not show any further potentiation of the effect obtained by other methods of steroid supplementation.

HOW DOES GnRH AGONIST WITH ESTROGENS PLUS PROGESTINS COMPARE WITH OTHER CONVENTIONAL TREATMENTS OF OVARIAN HYPERANDROGENISM?

The data we have reviewed show that the combined administration of estrogens plus progestins with GnRH agonists is a safe and effective treatment of ovarian hyperandrogenism. However, to establish the place of this therapy in clinical practice, it is very important to compare this approach with other conventional treatments of ovarian hyperandrogenism. No published data are available. We have recently compared the effects of GnRH agonists and add-back therapy with cyproterone acetate, an antiandrogen widely used in Europe[18]. Sixty hirsute women affected by

ovarian hyperandrogenism were randomized to treatment with cyproterone acetate 2 mg (with 35 µg of ethinylestradiol) for 21 days, cyproterone acetate 50 mg (with ethinylestradiol 50 µg) in a reverse sequential regimen and GnRH agonists plus low doses of conjugated estrogens (0.625 mg). As shown in Figure 3, hirsutism decreased

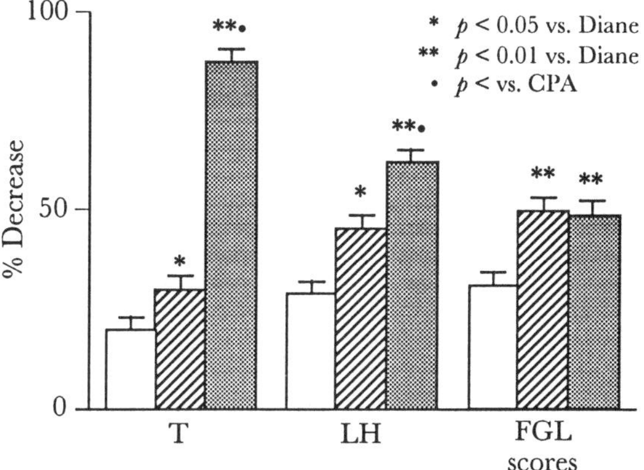

Figure 3 Comparisons of decreases in luteinizing hormone (LH), testosterone (T) and hirsutism (measured by Ferriman–Gallwey–Lorenzo [FGL] scores) in three groups of women with polycystic ovaries treated by Diane, high-dose cyproterone acetate (CPA) or GnRH agonists for 1 year. □, Diane; ▨, CPA; ▦, GnRH agonists

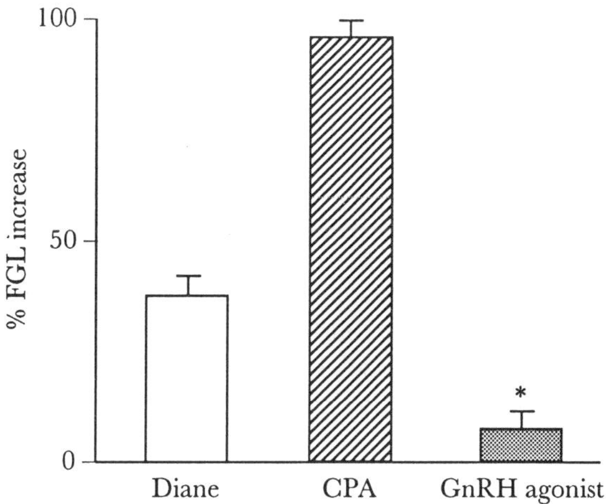

Figure 4 Percentage increase in hirsutism (measured by Ferriman–Gallwey–Lorenzo [FGL] scores) 6 months after withdrawal of different therapies. CPA, cyproterone acetate

significantly in all groups but GnRH agonists and cyproterone acetate at high doses were found to be more effective than cyproterone acetate at low doses (Diane). No differences in clinical results were observed when comparing GnRH agonists plus estrogens plus progestins with cyproterone acetate at high doses. Of some interest was the finding that GnRH agonists with add-back therapy resulted in a longer remission of hirsutism compared with cyproterone acetate. In fact, in spite of the rapid return of serum androgens to pretreatment values, hirsutism scores increased slowly and were still lower than pretreatment values after 1 year of therapy[20] (Figure 4). Similar behavior of Ferriman–Gallwey–Lorenzo scores after withdrawal of estrogens and GnRH agonists has been reported in a few patients by other authors[12]. These data suggest that combined administration of estrogens plus progestins with GnRH agonists is actually the best treatment to date for hirsutism due to ovarian hyperandrogenism. However, the higher costs of this treatment may prevent an exclusive endorsement of this form of treatment.

References

1. Lobo, R. A. (1995). Hirsutism, alopecia and acne. Beckler, K. L. (ed.) *Principles and Practice of Endocrinology and Metabolism*, 2nd edn, pp. 924–40. (Philadelphia: Lippincott)
2. Chang, F. J., Laufer, L. R., Meldrum, D. R., De Fazio, J., Lu, J. K. H., Vale, W. V., Rivier, J. E. and Judd, H. L. (1983). Steroid secretion in polycystic ovarian disease after ovarian suppression by a long acting gonadotropin releasing hormone agonist. *J. Clin. Endocrinol. Metab.*, **56**, 897–904
3. Andreyko, J. L., Monroe, S. E. and Jaffe, R. B. (1986). Treatment of hirsutism with a gonadotropin releasing hormone agonist (nafarelin). *J. Clin. Endocrinol. Metab.*, **63**, 854–9
4. Steingold, K., Ziegler, D. D., Cedars, M., Meldrum, D. R., Lu, J. K. and Judd, H. L. (1987). Clinical and hormonal effects of chronic gonadotropin releasing hormone agonist treatment in polycystic ovarian disease. *J. Clin. Endocrinol. Metab.*, **65**, 773–8
5. Corenblum, B. and Baylis, B. M. (1990). Medical therapy for the syndrome of familial virilization, insulin resistance and acanthosis inigricans. *Fertil. Steril.*, **53**, 421–5
6. Matta, W. H., Shaw, R. W., Hesp, R. and Evans, R. (1988). Reversible trabecular bone density loss following induced hypo-oestrogenism with the GnRH analogue buserelin in premenopausal women. *Clin. Endocrinol. (Oxf)*, **29**, 45–51
7. De Fazio, J., Meldrum, D. R., Laufer, L., Vale, W. V., Rivier, J. E. and Lu, J. K. H. (1983). Induction of hot flashes in menopausal women treated with a long acting GnRH-agonist. *J. Clin. Endocrinol. Metab.*, **56**, 445–8
8. Johansen, J. S., Riis, B. I., Hassager, C., Moen, M., Jacobson, J. and Christiansen, C. (1988). The effect of a gonadotropin releasing hormone agonist analog (nafarelin) on bone metabolism. *J. Clin. Endocrinol. Metab.*, **67**, 701-6
9. Carmina, E., Janni, A. and Lobo, R. A. (1994). Physiological estrogen replacement may enhance the effectiveness of the gonadotropin releasing hormone agonist in the treatment of hirsutism. *J. Clin. Endocrinol. Metab.*, **78**, 126–30
10. Morcos, R. N., Abdul-Malak, M.E., Shikora, E. *et al.* (1994). Treatment of hirsutism with a gonadotropin releasing hormone agonist and estrogen replacement therapy. *Fertil. Steril.*, **61**, 427–31
11. Tiitinnen, A., Seinberg, N., Steuman, U. and Ylikorkala, O. (1994). Estrogen replacement does not potentiate gonadotropin releasing hormone agonist induced androgen suppression in treatment of hirsutism. *J. Clin. Endocrinol. Metab.*, **79**, 447–51
12. Lemay, A. and Faure, N. (1994). Sequential estrogen–progestin addiction to gonadotropin releasing hormone agonist suppression for the chronic treatment of ovarian hyperandrogenism: a pilot study. *J. Clin. Endocrinol. Metab.*, **79**, 1716–22
13. Elkind-Hirsch, K. E., Anania, C., Mack, M. and Malina, K. R. (1995). Combination gonadotropin releasing hormone agonist and oral contraceptive therapy improves treatment of hirsute women with ovarian hyperandrogenism. *Fertil. Steril.*, **63**, 970–8
14. Rittmaster, R. (1988). Differential suppression of testosterone and estradiol in hirsute women with the superactive gonadotropin releasing hormone leuprolide. *J. Clin. Endocrinol. Metab.*, **67**, 651–5

15. Falsetti, L. and Pasinetti, E. (1994). Treatment of moderate and severe hirsutism by gonadotropin releasing hormone agonists in women with polycystic ovary syndrome and idiopathic hirsutism. *Fertil. Steril.*, **61**, 817–22

16. Carmina, E., Stanczyk, F. Z., Gentzschein, E. and Lobo, R. A. (1995). Time dependent changes in serum 3α-androstanediol glucuronide correlate with hirsutism scores after ovarian suppression. *Gynecol. Endocrinol.*, **9**, 215–20

17. Lindsay, R., Hart, D.M. and Clark, D.M. (1984). The minimum effective dose of estrogen for prevention of post-menopausal bone loss. *Obstet. Gynecol.*, **63**, 759–63

18. Sugimoto, A. K., Hodsman, A. B. and Nisker, J. A. (1993). Long term gonadotropin releasing hormone agonist with standard postmenopausal estrogen replacement failed to prevent vertebral bone loss in premenopausal women. *Fertil. Steril.* **60**, 672–4

19. Carmina, E. and Lobo, R. A. (1995). GnRH-agonist therapy for hirsutism is as effective as high dose cyproterone acetate but results in a longer remission. *Fertil. Steril.*, Suppl. (*Abstracts of the 41st Meeting of Reproductive Medicine*, Seattle, October 7–12 1995), abstr. 0.084

20. Di Carlo, C., Shoham, Z., MacDougall, J., Patel, A., Hall, M. L. and Jacob, H. S. (1992). Polycystic ovaries as a relative protective factor for bone mineral loss in young women with amenorrhea. *Fertil. Steril.*, **57**, 314–19

Section 5

Cancer

15

Combined androgen blockade with GnRH analogs and flutamide at all stages of prostate cancer

L. Cusan, J.-L. Gomez, P. Diamond, B. Candas and F. Labrie

INTRODUCTION

The best known and unanimously recognized characteristic of prostate cancer is its high sensitivity to androgen deprivation. In fact, among all hormone-sensitive cancers, prostate cancer is the one showing the best response to endocrine therapy. Accordingly, for more than 50 years[1], the exclusive treatment of advanced metastatic disease has been androgen deprivation. The two most relevant questions concerning endocrine therapy are thus:

(1) What is the best endocrine therapy; and

(2) When to start treatment?

It should already be mentioned that the results of recent clinical trials indicate that there are good reasons to believe that hormone therapy, in addition to remaining the first-line treatment of advanced disease, could well become part of any treatment of localized disease; endocrine therapy would therefore be the single therapy or part of therapy of any patient treated for prostate cancer.

ADRENAL ANDROGENS

Although castration (through orchiectomy or chemically by luteinizing hormone-releasing hormone (LHRH) agonists causes a 95% reduction in serum testosterone concentration, a much smaller effect is seen on the intraprostatic concentration of dehydrotestosterone (DHT), which is the only meaningful parameter of androgenic action in the prostatic tissue. In fact, after elimination of testicular androgens by medical or surgical castration, the intraprostatic concentration of DHT remains at approximately 40% of that measured in intact 65-year-old men (Figure 1A). As another measure of the importance of adrenal androgens in adult men, the serum levels of the main metabolites of androgens 5α-androstane-3α, 17β-diol (3α-diol), androsterone (ADT) and their glucuronidated derivatives are only reduced by 50–70%[2,3] following castration, thus reflecting the high level of adrenal precursor steroids converted into DHT in castrated men (Figure 1B). Contrary to the previous erroneous belief that the testes are responsible for 95% of total androgen production in men, as suggested by simple measurement of circulating serum testosterone, it is now well demonstrated that the prostatic tissue efficiently transforms the inactive adrenal steroid precursors dehydroepiandrosterone sulfate (DHEA-S), DHEA and androstenedione (Δ^4-dione) into the active androgen DHT.

PROSTATIC ANDROGENS

To stimulate prostatic growth, the adrenal steroid precursors DHEA-S and DHEA must be taken up by the prostatic tissue and be locally metabolized into active androgens. As illustrated in Figure 2, the formation of the active androgen DHT from DHEA involves three enzymatic activities: 3β-hydroxysteroid dehydrogenase/Δ^5-Δ^4 isomerase (3β-HSD), 17β-hydroxysteroid dehydrogenase (17β-HSD) and 5α-reductase. Alternatively, DHEA can be transformed into androst-5-ene-3β,17β-diol (Δ^5-diol) by 17β-HSD, whereas 3β-HSD catalyzes the conversion of the latter into testosterone.

The structure of two 3β-HSD, three 17β-HSD and two 5α-reductase human genes has been

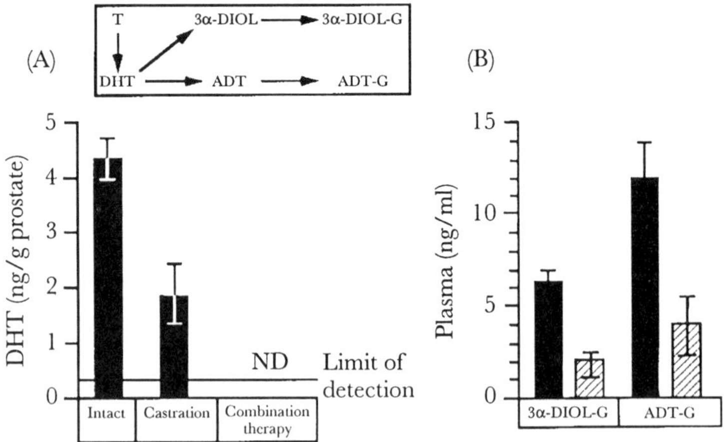

Figure 1 (A): effect of orchiectomy and combination therapy (addition of flutamide to orchiectomy or treatment with a luteinizing hormone releasing hormone superagonist) on the concentration of dihydrotestosterone (DHT) in human prostatic cancer tissue. Note that orchiectomy has only a partial inhibitory effect (approximately 60% reduction), whereas flutamide decreases intraprostatic DHT to undetectable levels. The lower limit of sensitivity of DHT measurement is 0.2 ng DHT/g tissue. About 40% of DHT is left in the prostatic cancer after castration, thus illustrating the need to block such a high level of androgens of adrenal origin left free to stimulate growth of prostate cancer after castration. (B): effect of castration on serum levels of the main metabolites of DHT, namely androsterone (ADT) and androstane-3α,17β-diol (3α-diol) and their respective glucoronated derivatives. ND, not detectable; ■, intact; ▨, castrated

elucidated[4]. The expression of genes specific for each of these enzymatic activities has been demonstrated in the human prostate, thus providing the explanation for the high level of DHT formation from DHEA in this tissue[4]. This new field of endocrinology has been called intracrinology[5]. This area of great promise for future therapeutic developments relates to the formation of active steroids in peripheral (intracrine) tissues from inactive precursors. These steroids act directly in the cells where their synthesis took place without being released in the extracellular compartment. These intracrine tissues, such as the human prostate, can thus control the synthesis and inactivation of androgens according to the local needs[5].

COMBINATION THERAPY IN STAGE D₂ PROSTATE CANCER

A first-line therapy?

Based on the knowledge that both the testes and the adrenals contribute about equally to androgen formation in men, combination therapy was developed to block simultaneously testicular and adrenal androgens at start of therapy in advanced prostate cancer[6] (Figure 2). The benefits of combination therapy first described in 1982 have been confirmed by four large-scale, double-blind and placebo-controlled randomized studies[7–10] (Table 1). In fact, these pivotal studies have confirmed and demonstrated the important advantages of combination therapy using a pure anti-androgen on all the objective and subjective parameters measured. Of particular importance is the observation that the simple addition of flutamide added, on average, 7.3[8] and 15.1[9] months of life while the use of an analog of flutamide, namely Anandron, added 5.4[7] and 7.3[10] months of life, respectively (Table 1). Studies that have not shown a benefit of combination therapy have had methodological problems such as too small a number of patients, inclusion of other than stage D₂ patients and no double-blind or placebo control[11,12].

In three of the combination therapy studies[6,9,10], the anti-androgen was added to the control arm at the time of progression, this addition leading to little or no significant benefit. Such results clearly

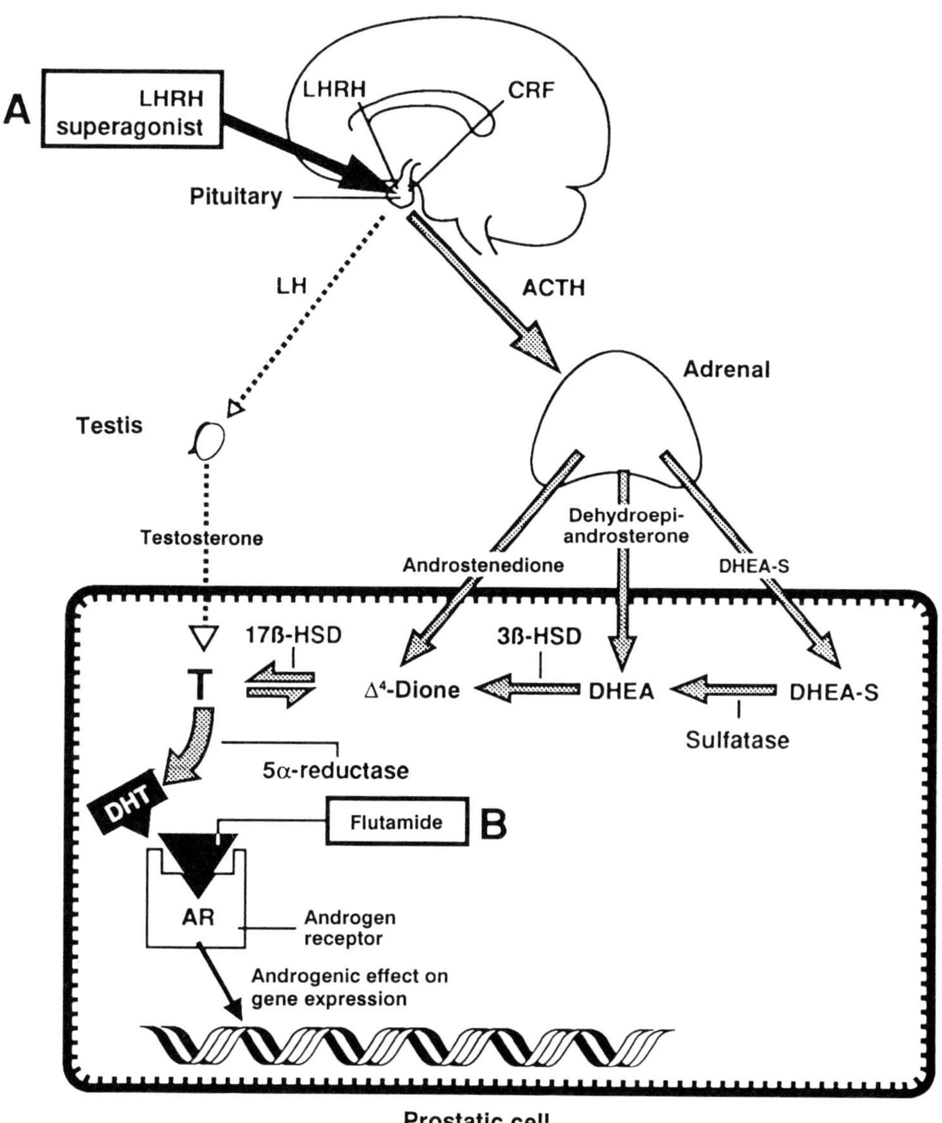

Figure 2 Schematic representation of the effect of combination therapy with a LHRH superagonist and a pure anti-androgen (flutamide) on prostrate cancer growth and of the biosynthetic steps involved in the formation of the active androgen dihydrostestosterone (DHT) from testicular testosterone as well as from the adrenal precursors dehydroepiandrosterone (DHEA), DHEA-sulfate (DHEAS-S) and androstenedione (Δ^4-dione) in human prostatic tissue. 17β-HSB = 17β-hydroxysteroid dehydrogenase; 3β-HSD = 3β-hydroxysteroid dehydrogenase/Δ^5-Δ^4-isomerase. The testis secretes testosterone (T) which is transformed into the more potent androgen dihydrotestosterone (DHT) by 5α-reductase in the prostate. Instead of secreting T or DHT directly, the adrenal secretes very large amounts of DHEA and DHEA-S which are transported in the blood to the prostate and other peripheral tissues. These inactive precursors are then transformed locally into the active androgens T and DHT. The genes encoding DHEA sulfatase, 3β-HSD, 17β-HSD and 5α-reductase are all expressed in the prostatic cells, thus providing 40% of the total DHT in this tissue. The anti-androgen blocks the access of DHT to the androgen receptor, thus greatly reducing the influence of androgens on genetic expression and prostate cancer cell growth, while testicular testosterone secretion is completely blocked by the LHRH superagonist or surgical castration (orchiectomy). CRF, corticotropin releasing factor; ACTH, adrenocorticotropic hormone

Table 1 Combination therapy with a pure anti-androgen and castration in double-blind, randomized, placebo-controlled and prospectives studies of stage D_2 disease

Study	Number of patients	Best response	No response	Pain improve-ment	PSA or PAP normal-zation	Duration of response (months)	Death due to cancer (months)	Death from all causes (months)
Béland et al.[7]*	194	46% vs. 20% $p < 0.01$	20% vs. 38% $p < 0.01$	$p < 0.05$	$p < 0.05$	Positive trend		24.3 vs. 18.9 (5.4) $p < 0.05$
National Cancer Institute (Crawford et al.[8]†)	602	$p < 0.05$		$p < 0.05$	$p < 0.05$	16.9 vs. 13.8 (3.1) $p < 0.05$		36.5 vs. 28.3 (7.3) $p < 0.05$
Janknegt et al.[10]*‡	423	41% vs. 24% $p < 0.01$	22% vs. 36% $p < 0.02$	$p < 0.05$	$p < 0.05$	19.0 vs. 14.9 (4.1) $p < 0.006$	37.1 vs. 29.8 (7.3)	27.3 vs. 24.2 (4.1)
European Organization for Research and Treatment of Cancer (Denis et al.[9]‡)	327			$p < 0.05$	$p < 0.05$	30.7 vs. 19.6 (11.1) $p < 0.008$	43.9 vs. 29.9 (15.1) $p < 0.007$	34.4 vs. 27.1 (7.3) $p < 0.02$

*Nilutamide and orchiectomy versus orchiectomy as control; †flutamide and luteinizing hormone-releasing hormone (LHRH) agonist versus LHRH agonist as control; ‡flutamide and LHRH agonist versus orchiectomy as control; NS, not significant; PAP, prostatic acid phosphatase; PSA, prostate-specific antigen

demonstrate the absolute need to use combination therapy at the start of treatment instead of at the time of relapse following failure of standard therapy.

The above-indicated observations argue extremely strongly against a two-step approach in the treatment of prostate cancer. It is thus clear that combination therapy should always be applied as first-line therapy because the same treatment loses most or all of its efficacy when used as second-line at the time of relapse following monotherapy. This approach of maximal androgen blockade at the start of therapy is supported by the well-known observation that patients relapsing after castration or treatment with estrogens, LHRH superagonists or an anti-androgen alone have a poor or no response to adrenalectomy, hypophysectomy or flutamide. Moreover, strongly supporting the harmful effect of exposure of prostate cancer cells to low androgen levels is the observation that low serum testosterone levels are associated with shorter survival following androgen deprivation[13]. Moreover, low pretreatment serum testosterone levels before the start of endocrine therapy are associated with a poor prognosis, this variable being even more important than the extent of bone metastases[13]. Such clinical data are well supported by the laboratory findings that low levels of androgens comparable to those found after castration in men induce the development of androgen-hypersensitive tumors that are resistant to antihormonal therapy[14]. In agreement with numerous previous studies, the European Organization for Research and Treatment of Cancer (EORTC) Trial 30 853 showed no difference between orchiectomy and orchiectomy associated with cyproterone acetate[15], thus demonstrating the absolute requirement to use a pure anti-androgen (flutamide or one of its analogs) in combination therapy instead of a mixed agonist–antagonist of androgen action such as cyproterone acetate.

Such dramatic and negative effects of partial blockade of androgens which leads to shorter survival[6–10] make unethical the use of any therapy having lower androgen-blocking capacity than the combination therapy using a pure anti-androgen in association with surgical or medical castration. In fact, it was judged unacceptable by the participants at the 1993 Geneva meeting on prostate cancer to treat men suffering from prostate cancer with any treatment exerting a blockade of androgens inferior to that achieved by combination therapy[16].

Greater response in 'minimal disease'?

An important observation made in all studies of stage D_2 prostate cancer patients who received the combination therapy as initial treatment is that prostate cancer is rapidly and extremely well controlled at the level of the prostate. Moreover, when progression of the disease occurs after an initial response, reappearance of the cancer takes place in the bones in approximately 98% of cases while progression at the level of the prostate is rare (2% of cases). These findings indicate clearly that combination therapy is most efficient in blocking cancer growth at the level of the prostate, while the main problem of hormonal treatment derives from tumors which have migrated and developed outside the prostatic area, usually in the bones. Such data strongly suggest that major efforts should be directed towards earlier treatment of the disease by combination therapy.

In order to further investigate the impact of early versus late treatment of metastatic prostate cancer, we have stratified our cohort of stage D_2 prostate cancer patients according to the number of bone lesions. As illustrated in Figure 3, the median survival is not yet reached at 8 years in the group of patients having 1–5 bone metastases, while survival is dramatically reduced to 3.56 years when the number of bone lesions increases to 6–10, thus representing a difference of more than 4.4 years of life. For the patients having 11–40 bone lesions, the calculated median survival was 2.36 years while it was reduced to 1.76 years

for those having disseminated disease or a superscan at the start of the same treatment.

Thus it is clear from the present data that the addition of a relatively small number of bone lesions has a major negative impact on survival. In fact, it can be seen in Figure 3 that when the number of bone metastases is larger than five, further increase in the number of metastases has less and less influence on the duration of survival under combination therapy, thus clearly demonstrating the major importance of not delaying treatment when the diagnosis of metastatic prostate cancer is made.

In agreement with these data, Crawford *et al.*[8] have reported that the patients who present with minimal disease display a much better response to combination therapy. In fact, recent analysis of the Intergroup National Cancer Institute (NCI) study has shown an advantage of 19.5 months of survival for the patients with minimal disease who received the combination of leuprolide and flutamide compared with those treated with leuprolide and placebo, while the median overall survival advantage calculated for the whole group of patients was only 7.3 months following combination therapy. Similarly, in the EORTC

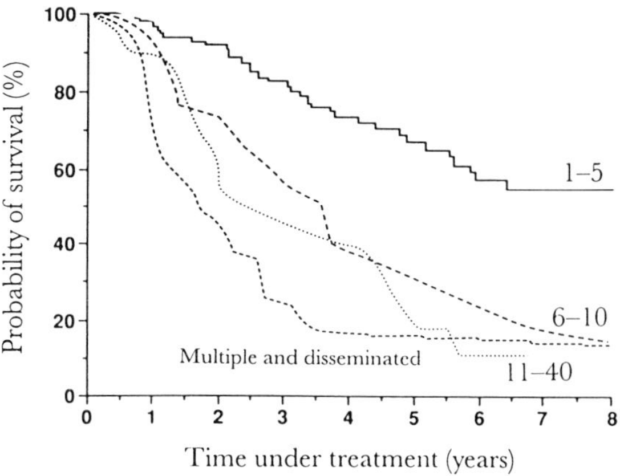

Figure 3 Probability of survival according to the number of bone metastases in previously untreated stage D_2 cancer prostate cancer patients who received combination therapy with flutamide and the luteinizing hormone-releasing hormone (LHRH) agonist [D-Trp[6], des-Gly-NH$_2$[10]]-LHRH ethylamide. Median survival: ——, 8 years (105 points); – – –, 3.56 years (45 points); ······, 2.36 years (50 points); ----, 1.76 (61 points)

30 853 trial, combination therapy with goserelin and flutamide in patients with a good (performance status 0–2, modest prostate-specific antigen [PSA], elevation and T category < 4) or intermediate prognosis led to a markedly improved disease-free survival as well as overall survival, compared with the total group of patients[9].

DIAGNOSIS OF LOCALIZED DISEASE

Since it is well recognized that the only opportunity for a significant reduction in prostate cancer deaths is treatment of localized disease before the appearance of metastases it is surprising that screening and early treatment remain controversial, despite the convincing evidence accumulated during the recent years clearly supporting early diagnosis and treatment. Much progress has, in fact, been made by several groups on the rational use of prostate-specific antigen and transrectal ultrasonography of the prostate for earlier diagnosis of prostate cancer while more efficient and well-tolerated curative therapies have been developed[17–29]. A highly efficient, easily applied, and low cost strategy for the detection of localized prostate cancer is now available[26].

Screening controversy

The controversy over screening results largely from the publication of few but much publicized reports on the potential value of deferred treatment for localized prostate cancer in men older than 70 years. The limited conclusions thus obtained have been erroneously extended to prostate cancer in general. In fact, all these reports are from uncontrolled studies which simply describe data collected from various series of selected patients. These case report studies were erroneously used as representatives of the standard evolution of untreated patients while, on the contrary, almost all of these patients were treated at first sign of progression[30–38]. Thus, somewhat surprisingly, the possibility of deferred treatment in a selected group of men older than 70 years has been used as an argument against screening. These data at best suggest that some selected patients having a life expectancy of less than 10 years can choose deferred treatment, despite an important risk of

dying from prostate cancer and a very high risk of suffering from metastatic disease within 10 years despite treatment at time of progression[34,38]. Those who used these data to argue against screening also missed the fundamental fact that in order to have the possibility of choosing deferred treatment, screening must be performed in order to detect prostate cancer at an early stage. In the absence of screening, most men will continue to be diagnosed at an advanced stage and will continue to die from prostate cancer at the same rate. In analogy with breast cancer, prostate cancer cannot be cured once it has escaped the primary organ. It is fundamental to recognize that the principal approach to efficient treatment should thus be early diagnosis and definitive therapy for patients who live long enough to benefit from it.

Efficiency of screening for prostate cancer

In order to avoid the well known and serious difficulties of treating prostate cancer discovered at a metastatic stage and to assess the potential benefits of diagnosis and treatment of the disease at a localized stage, we started, in 1989, the first prospective screening program in a randomly selected population of 60 000 men aged between 45 and 80 years in the Québec City area using serum PSA (prostate-specific antigen), DRE (digital rectal examination) and TRUS (transrectal ultrasonography) as independent screening tests in the first 1002 men[23], followed by an extension of the study to 7350 first-visit men[26]. Since these men have now been followed with annual PSA and DRE for up to 6 years, for a total of 14 554 follow up visits, it is of particular interest to analyze the results of these follow-up visits and be in a position to answer the following fundamental question: what is the efficiency of screening to detect prostate cancer at a localized and curable stage?

Since a major concern about screening is a potential increase in the number of cancers detected, it is important to see (Table 2) that only 117 cancers were found at 14 554 follow-up visits for an incidence of 0.8%, compared with a prevalence of 4.0% (322 cancers in 8029 men) at first visit. The percentage of men found having prostate cancer at follow-up visits is thus 5.0 times

Table 2 Correlation between serum prostate-specific antigen (PSA) levels and the presence of detectable prostate cancer in 45- to 80-year-old men at 8029 first visits and 14 554 follow-up visits. Transrectal ultrasonography was performed only when serum PSA was above 3.0 ng/ml and/or DRE (digital rectal examination) was positive

Serum PSA (ng/ml)	1st visit				Follow-up visits			
	Men		Prostate cancer		Visits		Prostate cancer	
	n	%	n	%	n	%	n	%
> 30	48	0.6	39	81.0	16	0.1	4	25.0
10.1–30	191	2.4	85	45.0	170	1.2	25	14.7
7.1–10	177	2.2	50	28.0	309	2.1	25	8.1
5.1–7.0	294	3.7	50	17.0	550	3.8	23	4.2
4.1–5.0	255	3.2	27	11.0	493	3.4	19	3.9
3.1–4.0	473	5.9	27	5.7	891	6.1	17	1.9
2.1–3.0	860	10.7	22	2.6	1544	10.6	3	0.2
1.1–2.0	2472	30.8	11	0.4	3969	27.3	—	0.0
0–1.0	3259	40.6	11	0.3	6612	45.4	1	< 0.1
All	8029	100.0	322	4.0	14 554	100.0	117	0.80

Table 3 Clinical stages of prostate cancers diagnosed at first and follow-up visits. The number of men examined at first visit is 8029 while 6343, 4939, 2524, 558, 187 and 3 men were examined at 1st, 2nd, 3rd, 4th and 5th follow-up visits

Stage	First visit		Follow-up visits					Total	
			1	2	3	4	5		
A_2			—	1	—	—	—	1	(0.9%)
B_0	9	(3.0%)	5	8	3	1	—	17	(15.0%)
B_1	109	(36.5%)	22	15	13	2	2	54	(47.8%)
B_2	94	(31.4%)	9	7	7	2	—	25	(22.1%)
C_1	26	(8.7%)	5	2	2	1	—	10	(8.8%)
C_2	35	(11.7%)	2	3	—	—	—	5	(4.4%)
D_0	2	(0.7%)	—	—	—	—	—	0	
D_1	6	(2.0%)	—	—	—	—	—	0	
D_2	18	(6.0%)	1	—	—	—	—	1	(0.9%)
Not available	23		2	1	1	—	—	4	
Total	322		46	37	26	6	2	117	

Adjusted chi-square test: frequency distribution of stages A + B + C and D at first visit versus follow-up visits, significantly different, $p < 0.05$

lower than at first visit. It is important to mention that of the 117 prostate cancers diagnosed at follow-up visits, 114 were PSA positive and only three (2.6%) were missed by PSA and found by DRE, thus demonstrating the unique importance of serum PSA to detect prostate cancer, especially at annual follow-up screening visits. For comparison, at first visit, 86.3% of cancers were PSA positive and 13.7% were found by DRE in the presence of normal PSA.

The most important finding, however, is that only one out of 117 (0.9%) cancers diagnosed at follow-up visits was metastatic compared with 8.7% at first visit (Table 3). The only stage D_2

prostate cancer was diagnosed at the first follow up visit and was most probably missed at first visit. Stage C_2 prostate cancers, on the other hand, decreased from 11.7% at first visit to only 4.4% at follow ups. Stages B_0 increased from 3.0% at first visit to 15% at follow-up visits while stage B_1 disease increased from 36.5% to 47.8% and stage B_2 cancers, on the other hand, decreased from 31.4% to 22.1%.

The present study clearly demonstrates that screening with PSA can, in practical terms, eliminate the diagnosis of advanced or incurable prostate cancer. If every man simply follows the recommendations of the American Cancer Society, namely annual screening starting at the age of 50 years, the proportion of localized or potentially curable disease can be increased from approximately 40% in the absence of screening[39,40] to close to 100%. In fact, in the present study, the proportion of stage D metastatic cancers at follow-up visits is only 0.9%, while 99.1% of patients are diagnosed at a localized stage and are thus candidates for curative therapy. In fact, if one starts screening at the age of 50 years, all subsequent visits should be equivalent to the follow-up visits of the present study, thus permitting diagnosis of prostate cancer at a localized stage in nearly all men.

It is also important to indicate that the present study confirms that screening does not detect an important proportion of small cancers[26,41]. It is known that one-third of men older than 50 years have incidental prostate cancer found at autopsy while, on the other hand, only 10% of men develop clinical prostate cancer during their lifetime[42]. This apparent paradox has generated widespread arguments against screening by extrapolating that screening would automatically detect these small and still insignificant cancers which are found at autopsy or following transurethral resection of the prostate for treatment of benign prostatic hyperplasia, thus potentially leading to unnecessary and even harmful treatment. The facts, however, are quite different: the available screening techniques, namely PSA, DRE, and TRUS cannot detect such small autopsy cancers in the absence of random biopsies[21,23,26]. Screening performed as described above is usually not sufficiently sensitive to detect cancers having a

diameter smaller than 0.75 cm: of the 49 cancers diagnosed in our study, who were subsequently randomized to radical prostatectomy alone and could thus be measured with precision in the surgical specimen, only two (4.1%) had a volume smaller than 0.3 ml or a diameter smaller than 0.75 cm. Using PSA and DRE followed by TRUS, only 7% of detected cancers have been found to be microfocal and low in grade (for a review[25]). A strong argument supporting these findings is provided by the observation that 75% of men who developed prostate cancer with an elevated PSA died from this cancer[43].

DOWNSTAGING OF LOCALIZED DISEASE BY COMBINATION THERAPY

Unfortunately, not all men who are thought to have organ-confined prostate cancer at diagnosis are found to have organ confined disease at surgery. In fact, in 50–60% of cases the pathological analysis of the specimen obtained at radical prostatectomy shows that the cancer is more advanced than originally predicted at diagnosis[44–50]. Since the prognosis of stage C or D_1 prostate cancer is poor, the risk that 50% or more of prostate cancers expected to be localized at diagnosis are found to be not curable at surgery can easily explain the lack of enthusiasm for radical prostatectomy and the controversies surrounding the diagnosis and treatment of early stage prostate cancer.

A possible means of improving the proportion of patients with organ-confined disease and cancer negative margins at surgery was suggested clearly by the observation that patients treated by combination therapy using a pure anti-androgen associated with medical or surgical castration for metastatic disease show a much more rapid and marked regression of their cancer in the prostatic area compared with distant metastatic disease[6,51,52]. Moreover, it is well recognized that when recurrence of the disease occurs, progression of the cancer at the level of the prostate is a rare event while, instead, the bones are the usual site of progression. Since prostate cancer localized into the prostatic area is so highly sensitive to androgen deprivation, it is logical to use

Table 4 Effect of 3-month neoadjuvant combination therapy with the anti-androgen flutamide and a luteinizing hormone-releasing hormone agonist on positive margins at radical prostatectomy in stages B and C prostate cancer

Group	Negative margins	Positive margins	Total
Control	47 (66.2%)	24 (33.8%)	71
Combination therapy	83 (92.2%)	7 (7.8%)	90
Total			161

Chi-square test: $p < 0.001$

combination therapy to downstage prostate cancer in men diagnosed as having localized prostate cancer before performing radical surgical prostatectomy.

Following an encouraging preliminary trial[18] we have conducted a prospective and randomized clinical trial in order to assess precisely the potential advantages of neoadjuvant combination therapy with the pure anti-androgen flutamide and an LHRH agonist administered for 3 months before radical prostatectomy compared with surgery alone[25].

As shown in Table 4, the incidence of cancer-positive surgical margins was reduced highly significantly to only 7.8% (seven of 90) in the group of patients who received an LHRH superagonist and flutamide for 3 months before radical prostatectomy compared with 33.8% (24 of 71) in the group of men who had no endocrine therapy before radical prostatectomy (chi-square test, $p < 0.001$). Figure 4 shows that the decrease in cancer-positive surgical margins is of major amplitude at all stages of the disease except at stage B_0 and C_1. In fact, while cancer-positive margins were found in the surgical specimens in 25.5% of stage B_1, 58.8% of stage B_2 and 80% of stage C_2 control patients, the incidence of positive margins decreased to 2.3% in stage B_1, 10.8% in stage B_2, and 14.3% in stage C_2 patients who received combination therapy for 3 months before surgery.

It is then of particular interest to examine the final staging at histopathological examination of the specimen obtained at surgery compared with clinical staging at diagnosis and to determine the effect of combination therapy at each stage of the disease. Upstaging is particularly striking at stages B_1 and B_2 in the control untreated group. In fact, of 39 cancers originally classified as B_1, 21 showed a more advanced stage at surgery, including five with C_1 and 10 with C_2 disease (Table 5). Similarly, of 17 cancers originally classified as B_2 disease in the control group, three became C_1, eight became C_2 and two became D_1 disease. On the other hand, it can also be seen in Table 5 that downstaging following neoadjuvant combination therapy was frequent at all stages of the disease: in the patients originally classified as having B_1 disease, 14 of 43 (32.5%) tumors originally classified as having a mean diameter of 1.0 to 1.5 cm decreased to < 1.0 cm while no cancer was found in six patients after thorough examinations of additional histological sections. Downstaging was seen in 13 of 29 (44.8%) of patients originally classified as having stage B_2 disease. Although the number of patients is small, the downstaging effect was particularly important in patients originally classified as having C_1 disease

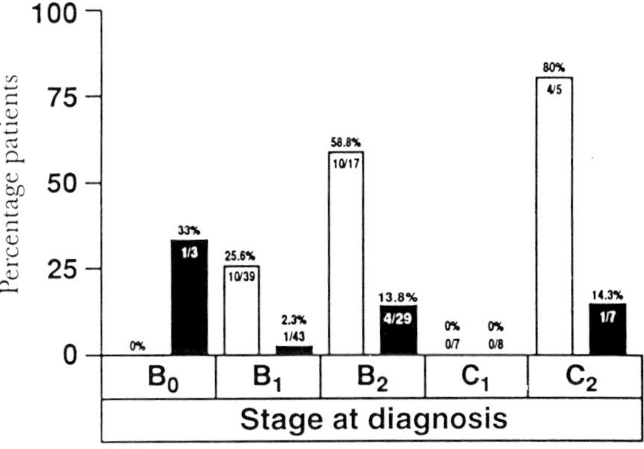

Figure 4 Effect of 3-month neoadjuvant combination therapy with flutamide and a luteinizing hormone-releasing hormone agonist on cancer-positive surgical margins at radical prostatectomy according to the clinical stage at diagnosis. Data are expressed as percentage of patients in each group. The number within the bars indicates the number of patients having cancer-positive margins in each group. □, control; ■, combination therapy

Table 5 Effect of 3-month neoadjuvant combination therapy with flutamide and leuprolide acetate on the final histopathological stage at surgery compared with the initial clinical stage at diagnosis

Original		Final histopathological stage at surgery						
Stage	No.	NC	B_0	B_1	B_2	C_1	C_2	D_1
A. Control, untreated:								
B_0	3	0	1	0	1	1	0	0
B_1	39	0	7	11	6	5	10	0
B_2	17	0	0	3	1	3	8	2
C_1	7	0	1	1	2	3	0	0
C_2	5	0	0	0	1	0	1	3
B. 3-month neoadjuvant combination therapy:								
B_0	3	0	1	0	1	1	0	0
B_1	43	6	14	11	7	3	2	0
B_2	29	0	2	11	6	5	3	2
C_1	8	0	2	1	3	1	1	0
C_2	7	0	1	2	2	1	0	1

NC, no cancer

at diagnosis where six of eight (75.0%) had downstaging, and in patients originally classified at diagnosis as stage C_2 where six of seven cancers (85.7%) were downstaged following neoadjuvant combination therapy.

The essential objective of treatment of early stage prostate cancer is complete removal or elimination of cancer tissue. Although the long-term effects of androgen deprivation achieved by neoadjuvant combination therapy on survival remain to be assessed by long-term follow up of the patients, the present data show that androgen deprivation induces prostate cancer cell death or apoptosis at a relatively high rate in the prostate area, under the influence of combination therapy: such cancer cell death leads to a relatively rapid downstaging of the disease. After only 3 months of neoadjuvant combination therapy with flutamide and an LHRH agonist, cancer-positive surgical margins decreased from 33.8% to only 7.8% while organ-confined disease increased from 49.3% to 77.8%.

Because the aim of neoadjuvant therapy is to cause a maximal reduction in prostatic androgen levels to induce maximal atrophy, apoptosis and death of prostate cancer cells, combination therapy using a pure anti-androgen[6,23,51] in association with a LHRH superagonist is the most logical approach. The use of a LHRH superagonist alone, an anti-androgen alone, or an inhibitor of androgen formation alone is not recommended because partial blockade of androgens is likely to induce the development of tumors resistant to androgen blockade[5,53,54]. This would be a major concern to patients having incomplete removal of the cancer or positive margins at surgery.

Although the effects of the present approach on survival remain to be determined by long-term follow up, it is reasonable to expect that patients with localized disease at final histopathological staging following radical prostatectomy should have a life expectancy not unlike that of men of similar age with no prostate cancer[55,56]. It remains to be seen, however, if cancer cell death or apoptosis induced by combination therapy in the prostatic area as clearly demonstrated in the present study occurs to the same extent at distant micrometastatic sites. The answer to this important question will also be provided by long-term follow up of these patients.

Previous studies have shown that combination endocrine therapy decreases the total volume of the prostate and of the cancer[18,27,53,57–62]. The present data show, in the first randomized study, that neoadjuvant combination therapy leads not only to downsizing of the prostate and tumor but also to a true downstaging of prostate cancer. Lee *et al.*[27] have also clearly demonstrated that prostate cancer cell death is induced by combination therapy in the prostatic area.

References

1. Huggins, C. and Hodges, C. V. (1941). Studies of prostatic cancer. I. Effect of castration, estrogen and androgen injections on serum phosphatases in metastatic carcinoma of the prostate. *Cancer Res.*, **1**, 293–307
2. Moghissi, E., Ablan, F. and Horton, R. (1984). Origin of plasma androstanediol glucuronide in men. *J. Clin. Endocrinol. Metab.*, **59**, 417–21
3. Bélanger, A., Brochu, M. and Cliche, J. (1986). Levels of plasma steroid glucuronides in intact and castrated men with prostatic cancer. *J. Clin. Endocrinol. Metab.*, **62**, 812–15
4. Labrie, F., Simard, J., Luu-The, V., Pelletier, G., Belghmi, K. and Bélanger, A. (1994). Structure, regulation and role of 3β-hydroxysteroid dehydrogenase, 17β-hydroxysteroid dehydrogenase and aromatase enzymes in formation of sex steroids in classical and peripheral intracrine tissues. In Sheppard, M. C. and Stewart, P. M. (eds.) *Hormone, Enzymes and Receptors,* pp. 451–74.(London: Baillière's Clinical Endocrinology and Metabolism, Baillière Tindall)
5. Labrie, F. (1991). Intracrinology. *Mol. Cell. Endocrinol.*, **78**, C113–18
6. Labrie, F., Dupont, A. and Bélanger, A. (1985). Complete androgen blockade for the treatment of prostate cancer. In de Vita, V. T., Hellman, S. and Rosenberg, S. A. (eds.) *Important Advances in Oncology*, pp. 193–217. (Philadelphia: Lippincot)
7. Béland, G., Elhilali, M., Fradet, Y., Laroche, B., Ramsey, E. W., Trachtenberg, J., Venner, P. M. and Tewari, H. D. (1988). Total androgen blockade versus castration in metastatic cancer of the prostate. In Motta, M. and Serio, M. (eds.) *Hormonal Therapy of Prostatic Diseases: Basic and Clinical Aspects,* pp. 302–11. (Bussum: Medicom)
8. Crawford, D., Eisenberger, M. A., McLeod, D. G., Spaulding, J. T., Benson, R., Dorr, F. A., Blumenstein, D. A., Davis, M. A. and Goodman, P. J. (1989). A controlled trial of leuprolide with and without flutamide in prostatic carcinoma. *N. Engl. J. Med.*, **321**, 419–24
9. Denis, L., Carneiro de Moura, J. L., Bono, A., Sylvester, R., Wheeton, R., Newling, D. and Pauno, M. D. (1993). Goserelin acetate and flutamide vs bilateral orchiectomy: a phase III EORTC trial (30853). *Urology*, **42**, 119–29
10. Janknegt, R. A., Abbou, C. C., Bartoletti, R., Bernstein-Hahn, L., Bracken, B., Brisset, J. M., Silva, F. C. d., Knonagel, H. and Venner, P. (1993). Orchiectomy and anandron (Nilutamide) or placebo as treatment of metastatic prostatic cancer in a multinational double-blind randomized trial. *J. Urology*, **149**, 77–83
11. Iversen, P., Christensen, M. G., Friis, E., Hornbol, P., Hvidt, V., Iversen, H. G., Klarskov, P., Krarup, T., Lund, F., Mogensen, P., Pedersen, T., Rasmussen, F., Rose, C., Skaarup, P. and Wolf, H. (1990). A phase III trial of zoladex and flutamide versus orchiectomy in the treatment of patients with advanced carcinoma of the prostate. *Cancer*, **66**, 1058–66
12. Lunglmayr, G. (1990). A multicenter trial comparing the luteinizing hormone releasing hormone analog Zoladex, with Zoladex plus flutamide in the treatment of advanced prostate cancer. The International Prostate Cancer Study Group. *Eur. Urol.*, **18** (Suppl. 3), 28–9
13. Soloway, M. S., Ishikawa, S., Zwang, R. V. d. and Todd, B. (1989). Prognostic factors in patients with advanced prostate cancer. *Urology*, **33**, 53–6
14. Labrie, F., Veilleux, R. and Fournier, A. (1988). Low androgen levels induce the development of androgen-hypersensitive cells clones in Shionogi mouse mammary carcinoma cells in culture. *J. Natl. Cancer Inst.*, **80**, 1138–47
15. Robinson, R. G., Spicer, J. A., Preston, D. F., Wegst, A. V. and Martin, N. L. (1994). Treatment of metastatic bone pain with strontium-89. *Int. J. Rad. Appl. Instrum.*, **14**, 219–22
16. Labrie, F. (1993). GnRH agonists in prostate cancer. In *The State of the Art*, pp. 103–21. (New York: Parthenon)
17. Lee, F., Torp-Pedersen, S. T., Siders, D., Littrup,

P. J. and McLeary, R. D. (1989). Transrectal ultrasound in the diagnosis and staging of prostatic carcinoma. *Radiology*, **170**, 609–15

18. Monfette, G., Dupont, A. and Labrie, F. (1989). Temporary combination therapy with flutamide and Tryptex as adjuvant to radical prostatectomy for the treatment of early stage prostate cancer. In Labrie, F., Lee, F. and Dupont, A. (eds.) *Early Stage Prostate Cancer: Diagnosis and Choice of Therapy*, pp. 41–51. (New York: Excerpta Medica)

19. Cooner, W. H., Mosley, B. R., Jr, C. L. R., Beard, J. H., Pond, H. S., Terry, W. J., Igel, T. C. and Kidd, D. D. (1990). Prostate cancer detection in a clinical urological practice by ultrasonography, digital rectal examination and prostate-specific antigen. *Urology*, **143**, 1146–54

20. Whitmore, W. (1990). Natural history of low-stage prostatic cancer and the impact of early detection. *Urol. Clin. North Am.*, **17**, 689–97

21. Catalona, W. J., Smith, D. S., Ratliff, T. L., Dodds, K. M., Coplen, D. E., Yuan, J. J., Petros, J. A. and Andriole, G. L. (1991). Measurement of prostate-specific antigen in serum as a screening test for prostate cancer. *N. Engl. J. Med.*, **324**, 1156–61

22. Oesterling, J. E. (1991). Prostate specific antigen: a critical assessment of the most useful tumor marker for adenocarcinoma of the prostate. *J. Urol.*, **145**, 907–23

23. Labrie, F., Dupont, A., Suburu, R., Cusan, L., Tremblay, M., Gomez, J. L. and Emond, J. Serum prostatic specific antigen (PSA) as prescreening test for prostate cancer. *J. Urol.*, **147**, 846–52

24. Lee, F., Littrup, P. J., Loft-Christensen, L. B. S. K., McHugh, T. A., Siders, D. B., Mitchell, A. E. and Newby, J. E. (1992). Predicted prostate specific antigen results using transrectal ultrasound gland volume. *Cancer*, **70** (Suppl.), 211–20

25. Labrie, F., Dupont, A., Cusan, L., Gomez, J. L., Diamond, P., Koutsilieris, M., Suburu, R., Fradet, Y., Lemay, M., Têtu, B., Emond, J., and Candas, B. (1993). Downstaging of localized prostate cancer by neoadjuvant therapy with flutamide and lupron: the first controlled and randomized trial. *Clin. Invest. Med.*, **16**, 511–21

26. Labrie, F., Dupont, A., Suburu, R., Cusan, L., Gomez, J. L., Koutsilieris, M., Diamond, P., Emond, J., Lemay, M. and Têtu, B. (1993). Optimized strategy for detection of early stage, curable prostate cancer: role of prescreening with prostatic-specific antigen. *Clin. Invest. Med.*, **16**, 426–41

27. Lee, F., Siders, D. B., Newby, J. E., McHugh, T. A. and Solomon, M. H. (1993). The role of transrectal ultrasound-guided staging biopsy and androgen ablation therapy prior to radical prostatectomy. *Clin. Invest. Med.*, **16**, 458–70

28. Littrup, P. J., Goodman, A. C. and Mettlin, C. J. (1993). The benefit and cost of prostate cancer early detection. The Investivators of the American Cancer Society–National Prostate Cancer Project. *CA Cancer J. Clin.*, **43**, 143–9

29. Mettlin, C. (1993). Early detection of prostate cancer following repeated examinations by multiple modalities: results of the American Cancer Society National Prostate Cancer Detection Project. *Clin. Invest. Med.*, **16**, 440–7

30. Larsson, A. and Norlen, B. J. (1985). Five-year follow up of patients with localized prostatic carcinoma initially referred for expectant treatment. *Scand. J. Urol. Nephrol.*, **19**, 30

31. Moskovitz, B., Nitecki, S. and Richter-Levin, D. (1987). Cancer of the prostate: is there a need for aggressive treatment? *Urol. Int.*, **42**, 49–52

32. Goodman, C. M., Busuttil, A. and Chisholm, G. D. (1988). Age, and size and grade of tumour predict prognosis in incidentally diagnosed carcinoma of the prostate. *Br. J. Urol.*, **62**, 576–80

33. Orestano, F. (1991). Problems of wait-and-see policy in incidental carcinoma of the prostate. In Altwein, F. and Schneider, W. (eds.) *Incidental Carcinoma of the Prostate*, pp. 162–6. (Berlin-Heidelberg: Springer Verlag)

34. Whitmore Jr, W. F., Warner, J. A. and Thompson, I. M. (1991). Expectant management of localized prostatic cancer. *Cancer*, **67**, 1091–6

35. Adolfsson, J., Carstensen, J. and Lowhagen, T. (1992). Deferred treatment in clinically localized prostatic carcinoma. *Br. J. Urol.*, **69**, 183–7

36. Johansson, J. E., Adami, H. O., Andersson, S. O., Bergstrom, R., Holmberg, L. and Krusemo, U. B. (1992). High 10-year survival rate in patients with early, untreated prostatic cancer. *J. Am. Med. Assoc.*, **267**, 2191–6

37. Jones, G. W. (1992). Prospective, conservative management of localized prostate cancer. *Cancer*, **70**, 307–10

38. Chodak, G. W., Thisted, R. A., Gerber, G. S., Johansson, J.-E., Adolfsson, J., Jones, G. W., Chisholm, G. D., Moskovitz, B., Livne, P. M. and Warner, J. (1994). Results of conservative management of clinically localized prostate cancer. *N. Engl. J. Med.*, **330**, 242–8

39. Murphy, G. P., Natarajan, N. and Pontes, J. E. (1982). The national survey of prostate cancer in the United States by the American College of Surgeons. *J. Urol.*, **127**, 928–34

40. Schmidt, J. D., Mettlin, C. J., Natarajan, N., Peace, B. B., Beart Jr, R. W., Wincheste, D. P. and Murphy, G. P. (1986). Trends in patterns of care for prostatic cancer, 1974–1983: results of surveys by the American College of Surgeons. *J. Urol.*, **136**, 416–21

41. Catalona, W. J. (1994). Management of cancer of the prostate. *N. Engl. J. Med.*, **331**, 996–1004

42. Epstein, J. I., Walsh, P. C., Carmichael, M. and Brendler, C. B. (1994). Pathologic and clinical findings to predict tumor extent of nonpalpable (stage Tlc) prostate cancer. *J. Am. Med. Assoc.*, **271**, 368–74

43. Gann, P. H., Hennekens, C. H. and Stampfer, M. J. (1995). A prospective evaluation of plasma prostate-specific antigen for detection of prostatic cancer. *J. Am. Med. Assoc.*, **273**, 289–94

44. Boxer, R. J., Kaufman, J. J. and Goodwin, W. E. (1977). Radical prostatectomy for carcinoma of the prostate: 1951–1976. A review of 329 patients. *J. Urol.*, **117**, 208–13

45. Veenema, R. J., Gursel, E. O. and Lattimer, J. K. (1977). Radical retropubic prostatectomy for cancer: a 20-year experience. *J. Urol.*, **117**, 330–1

46. Catalona, W. J. and Stein, A. J. (1982). Staging errors in clinically localized prostatic cancer. *J. Urol.*, **127**, 452–6

47. Elder, J. S., Jewett, H. J. and Walsh, P. C. (1982). Radical perineal prostatectomy for clinical stage B2 carcinoma of the prostate. *J. Urol.*, **127**, 704–6

48. Lange, P. H. and Narayan, P. (1983). Understaging and undergrading of prostate cancer. Argument for postoperative radiation as adjuvant therapy. *Urology*, **21**, 113–18

49. Gibbons, R. P., Correa Jr, R. J., Brannen, G. E. and Weissman, R. M. (1989). Total prostatectomy for clinically localized prostate cancer: long-term results. *J. Urol.*, **141**, 564–6

50. Brawer, M. K. and Lange, P. H. (1990). Adjuvant therapy after radical prostatectomy. *Probl. Urol.*, **4**, 461–72

51. Labrie, F., Dupont, A., Bélanger, A., Cusan, L., Lacourcière, Y., Monfette, G., Laberge, J. G., Emond, J., Fazekas, A. T. A., Raynaud, J. P. and Husson, J. M. (1982). New hormonal therapy in prostatic carcinoma: combined treatment with an LHRH agonist and an antiandrogen. *J. Clin. Invest. Med.*, **5**, 267–75

52. Labrie, F., Bélanger, A., Dupont, A., Luu-The, V., Simard, J. and Labrie, C. (1993). Science behind total androgen blockade: from gene to combination therapy. *Clin. Invest. Med.*, **16**, 487–504

53. Labrie, F. and Veilleux, R. (1988). Maintenance of androgen responsiveness by glucocorticoids in Shionogi mammary carcinoma cells in culture. *J. Natl. Cancer Inst.*, **80**, 966–70

54. Labrie, F., Bélanger, A., Simard, J., Labrie, C. and Dupont, A. (1993). Combination therapy for prostate cancer: endocrine and biological basis of its choice as new standard first line therapy. *Cancer*, **71**, 1059–67

55. Walsh, P. C. and Jewett, H. J. (1980). Radical surgery for prostatic cancer. *Cancer*, **45**, 1906–11

56. Brendler, C. B. and Walsh, P. C. (1992). The role of radical prostatectomy in the treatment of prostate cancer. *CA Cancer. J. Clin.*, **42**, 212–22

57. Solomon, M. H. (1990). Radical prostatectomy following androgen blockade. In Lee, F. and McLeary, R. L. (eds.) *5th International Symposium on Transrectal Ultrasound in the Diagnosis and Management of Prostate Cancer*, Chicago

58. Labrie, F. (1991). Endocrine therapy for prostate cancer. Endocrinol. *Metab. Clin. North Am.*, **20**, 845–72

59. Andros, E. A., Danesghari, F. and Crawford, E. D. (1993). Neoadjuvant hormonal therapy in stage C carcinoma of the prostate. *Clin. Invest. Med.*, **16**, 510–15

60. Fair, W. F., Aprikian, A. G., Cohen, D., Sogani, P. and Reuter, V. (1993). Use of neoadjuvant androgen deprivation therapy in clinical localized prostate cancer. *Clin. Invest. Med.*, **16**, 516–22

61. Schulman, C. C. and Sassine, A. N. (1993). Neoadjuvant hormonal deprivation before radical prostatectomy. *Clin. Invest. Med.*, **16**, 523–31

62. Solomon, M. H., McHugh, T. A., Dorr, R. P., Lee, F. and Siders, D. B. (1993). Hormone ablation therapy as neoadjuvant treatment to radical prostatectomy. *Clin. Invest. Med.*, **16**, 532–8

Treatment of patients with advanced prostate cancer with LHRH antagonist Cetrorelix

16

D. Gonzàlez-Bàrcena, A. V. Schally, A. M. Comaru-Schally, A. Cortez-Morales, M. Vadillo-Buenfil and A. Molina-Ayala

INTRODUCTION

In 1971 isolation, structural determination and synthesis of the luteinizing hormone (LH) and follicle stimulating hormone (FSH) from porcine hypothalami were achieved by Schally *et al.*[1]. Subsequently, attempts were made to replace or delete different amino acids within the parent molecule in order to obtain analogs with higher receptor-binding affinities. To date more than 3000 analogs of luteinizing hormone-releasing hormone (LHRH) have been developed. Long-term chronic administration of potent long-acting LHRH agonistic analogs leads to pituitary desensitization and inhibition of sex steroid levels. Clinical applications of agonistic analogs of LHRH are expanding steadily. They are used for treatment of precocious puberty, endometriosis, uterine leiomyomas and hormone-dependent malignant neoplasms, especially those of prostate, breast and ovary[2–9].

Early antagonistic analogs of LHRH had a relatively low potency, but in the first clinical study with the antagonist D-Phe[2], D-Trp[3], D-Phe[6]-LHRH it was demonstrated that a single injection of a large dose (90 mg) can suppress gonadotropin levels and the response to exogenous LHRH[10].

Insertion of D-arginine in position 6 of LHRH antagonists increased the inhibitory activity, with [Ac-D-(4Cl)-Phe1[2], D-Trp[3], D-Arg[6], D-Ala[10]]-LHRH being active at doses of 1–3 µg in rats[2]. However, antagonists with D-Arg or related basic residues in position 6 induce histamine liberation resulting in transient edema and other anaphylactoid reactions[11]. The side effects of this class of antagonists delayed their clinical use in humans.

Among the new generation of LHRH antagonists, '(Ac-D-Nal (2)[1], D-Phe(4Cl)[2], (D-Pal (3)[3], D-Cit[6], D-Ala[10])-LHRH' (Cetrorelix, SB-75) was shown to be one of the most powerful analogs, free of allergenic effects and extremely active in small doses[12]. Since 1988, the authors have been carrying out various clinical studies with the antagonist Cetrorelix in normal men, climacteric women and patients with gonadal dysgenesis[13], benign prostatic hyperplasia and advanced prostate cancer[14,15]. In view of the authors encouraging results, they decided to use the LHRH analog SB-75 (Cetrorelix) to treat a group of patients with advanced prostate carcinoma.

PATIENTS AND METHODS

Thirty-six prostatic cancer patients at stage D2 volunteered for this study.

Group I

Sixteen patients with a mean age of 71.3 ± 1.86 years (range 55–84 years) received 0.5 mg twice a day subcutaneously. Initially three were treated for only 6 weeks in order to evaluate the safety of the analog. Thereafter these 16 patients received the SB-75 Cetrorelix for up to 37 months (mean 18.25 months).

Group II

Twenty patients with mean age of 70.2 ± 1.7 years (range 53–84 years) initially received a higher

Table 1 Clinical profiles and laboratory data of the patients with prostatic adenocarcinoma before treatment with the LHRH antagonist SB-75 (Cetrorelix)

	Age (years)	PSA (0–4 ng/ml)*	Serum free testosterone (41.6–138 pmol/l)*	Tumor differentiation (Gleason)	Months of Cetrorelix administration
Group I	71.31±1.86 (55–84)**	441.55±102 (37.9–1438.7)**	50.47±5.14 (17.33–80.5)**	5.71±0.36 (4–9)**	18.25±3.04 (3–37)**
Group II	70.2±1.7 (53–84)**	1159.78±381.75 (4.0–5577)**	56.04±5.97 (30.5–105.9)**	6.75±0.58 (2–10)**	13.35±1.3 (0.5–21)**

*Normal values; ** range ; PSA, prostate-specific antigen

dose of SB-75 (Cetrorelix), 5 mg twice a day subcutaneously for the first 2 days and thereafter 0.800 mg twice a day subcutaneously for up to 21 months (mean 13.3 ± 1.3 months, range 0.5–21 months). All patients required high doses of potent analgesics for severe bone pain and also had elevated levels of the serum prostate-specific antigen (PSA). Six were paraplegic and one had paraparesis due to spinal cord invasion of metastatic prostatic cancer. The antagonistic analog (SB-75, Cetrorelix) was synthesized and provided by ASTA Medica, Frankfurt, Germany. For injection, the analog was dissolved in a 5% mannitol solution and was then sterilized in an autoclave for 15 min at 18 p.s.i. and 120°C. For the injection, each dose was diluted to 1 ml.

The patients were admitted to the endocrinology department of the Hospital de Especialidades, Centro Médico La Raza del Instituto Mexicano del Seguro Social in Mexico. Informed consent was obtained from all patients after the therapeutic options available had been explained. The study was approved by the Hospital Ethics and Scientific Research Committee (protocol 92-690-753).

RESULTS

Table 1 shows the clinical profiles and laboratory data of both groups of patients with prostatic cancer before administration of the LHRH antagonist Cetrorelix. Before therapy all patients had elevated levels of prostate-specific antigen (PSA) and normal serum values of free testosterone.

Group I

During treatment 13 of the 16 patients showed a clinical remission of prostate cancer, one remained stable and two did not respond. Three patients in remission died due to serious coexisting illness (disseminated tuberculosis at 6 months, pneumonia at 4 months and myocardial infarction at 15 months). Five patients relapsed during the treatment, three at about 8 months and two at 13 and 17 months, respectively. At the relapse time four patients received ketoconazole (in mean doses of 600 mg per day orally) in addition to Cetrorelix. Three patients showed additional remission. In one patient who maintained nearly normal serum-free testosterone levels the dose of Cetrorelix was increased to 5 mg twice a day for 48 hours, followed by 0.8 mg twice a day subcutaneously, and he subsequently showed new remission.

Four patients who were in remission abandoned the therapy for non-medical reasons, two at 3 months, and two at 13 and 29 months, respectively.

Group II

Eighteen of 20 patients showed clinical remission; one remained stable, one did not respond and died of cancer at 10 months. One patient who was in remission died from diabetic ketoacidosis after 16 months of therapy. One patient who was in remission decided to discontinue the therapy because of a decrease of the erectile function and libido. During the Cetrorelix therapy four of the 18 patients who were on remission relapsed at 5,

Table 2 Inhibition of serum free testosterone* and PSA** levels in prostatic cancer patients after administration of LHRH antagonist SB-75 (Cetrorelix)

		Days			Months					
	Basal	*0.5*	*3*	*5*	*1*	*2*	*3*	*4*	*5*	*6*
Free testosterone:										
group I	58.24	10.02	6.25	2.54	6.81	3.71	5.61	6.17	5.12	1.18
group II	54.09	10.50	7.85	3.84	5.16	9.17	1.53	0.72	1.03	2.86
Prostate-specific antigen:										
group I	461.2				112	94	185	230	303	239
group II	1184.1				453	399	169	68	19	55

*Normal 41.6–138 pmol/l; **normal 0–4 ng/ml

8, 16 and 17 months, respectively. Two received additional therapy; two patients received a double dose of Cetrorelix, one showed additional remission and one partial remission.

Other findings

Seven patients (three in group I and four in group II) had spinal cord invasion of metastatic prostatic cancer; of these, six were paraplegic due to metastatic lesions in the thoracic vertebrae and one had paraparesis because of metastatic compression at L4 and S1 levels. After therapy the neurological symptoms regressed in all the patients. Five patients were able to walk with a cane and one had shown 60% improvement of the neurological injury.

In the 31 patients who showed remission after the first week of treatment with Cetrorelix, a significant decrease in bone pain and reversal of the signs of prostatism were observed. In spite of the individual variations, PSA levels fell gradually in both groups.

Before initiation of therapy both groups I and II had serum levels of free testosterone within normal limits. After the first dose of Cetrorelix free testosterone fell. The percentage of inhibition at 12 hours was about 80% for both groups. During chronic therapy, the majority of patients maintained persistent testosterone inhibition (Table 2). Two patients in group I and three in group II maintained subnormal values of free testosterone.

DISCUSSION

Development of modern antagonists such as Cetrorelix (SB-75)[12,16–18], Detirelix[3,19,20], Nal-Glu antagonist[21–24], antide[25,26] and Ganirelix[27] has made possible a variety of clinical studies. Among these antagonists, Cetrorelix (SB-75) was shown to be one of the most powerful analogs, free of allergenic side effects and extremely active in small doses. SB-75 can be administered safely to human beings by intravenous, intramuscular and subcutaneous routes for prolonged periods of time[13]. While repeated administration of LHRH agonists is required to inhibit LH and FSH and reduce the levels of sex steroids, similar effects can be obtained with a single administration of LHRH antagonists.

Regression of experimental prostatic carcinoma after administration of agonistic analogs of LHRH was first reported by Redding and Schally in 1981[4]. During the past decade thousands of patients with prostatic cancer have been treated with LHRH agonists. Acceptance of these analogs is excellent and in a survey of patients who were offered a choice between orchidectomy and LHRH agonists the analogs were selected as primary treatment more than 70% of the time[28].

During the first few days of administration of LHRH agonists, plasma testosterone rises because of increased LH release from the pituitary. This initial rise in testosterone may be responsible for elevation of prostatic acid phosphatase and increase in bone pain[29,30]. The flare-up of disease, which is usually transient, may occur during the first 2 weeks of treatment until receptor down-regulation takes place. The worsening of clinical symptoms occurs in about 10% of patients and the expanding tumor may cause spinal compression or cauda equina damage, with irreversible neurological loss (paraplegia). Severe fatal reactions have been observed in occasional patients[31]. In such patients, LHRH agonists cannot be used as single drugs because of the possibility of flare-up caused by the transient stimulation of LH, FSH and sex steroid release, which occur during the first few days of administration. The authors' results show that the initial and chronic administration of LHRH antagonist SB-75 (Cetrorelix) is an effective therapy for the management of advanced prostate cancer. The use of SB-75 avoids the initial release of sex steroids that is produced by LHRH agonists as well as the adverse effects of estrogen therapy and the psychological impact of surgical castration. Patients who did not respond in spite of persistent inhibition of serum testosterone during the administration of the SB-75 had androgen-insensitive prostate cancer.

ACKNOWLEDGEMENTS

We are grateful to ASTA Medica (Frankfurt, Germany) for supplying the antagonist LHRH analog SB-75 (Cetrorelix). It is a pleasure to acknowledge useful discussions and valuable advice from Professor J. Engel, Dr K. Burk and Dr Th. Reissmann from ASTA Medica.

References

1. Schally, A. V., Nair, R. M. G., Redding, T. W. and Arimura, A. (1971). Isolation of the luteinizing hormone and follicle-stimulating hormone releasing hormone from porcine hypothalami. *J. Biol. Chem.*, **246**, 7230–6

2. Schally, A. (1989). The use of LH-RH analogs in gynecology and tumor therapy. In Belfort, P., Pinotti, J.A. and Eskes, T. K. A. B. (eds.) *Advances in Gynecology and Obstetrics. General Gynecology*, Vol. 6, pp. 3–20. (Carnforth, UK: Parthenon Publishing)

3. Vickery, B.H. (1986). Comparison of the potential for therapeutic utilities with gonadotropin-releasing hormone agonists and antagonists. *Endocr. Rev.*, **7**, 115–24

4. Redding, T. W. and Schally, A. V. (1981). Inhibition of prostate tumor growth in two rats models by chronic administration of D-Trp-6-LH-RH. *Proc. Natl. Acad. Sci. USA*, **78**, 6509–12

5. Parmar, H., Lightman, S. L., Allen, L., Phillips, R. H., Edwards, L. and Schally, A. V. (1985). Randomized controlled study of orchidectomy versus long-acting D-Trp-6-LH-RH microcapsules in advanced prostatic carcinoma. *Lancet*, **ii**, 1202–5

6. Zorn, J. R., Tanger, C. H., Roger, M., Grenier, J., Comaru-Schally, A. M. and Schally, A. V. (1986). Therapeutic hypogonadism induced by a delayed-release preparation of microcapsules of D-Trp-6-luteinizing hormone-releasing hormone: a preliminary study in eight women with endometriosis. *Int. J. Fertil.*, **31**, 11–27

7. George, M., Lhomme, C., Lefort, J., Gras, C., Comaru-Schally, A. M. and Schally, A. V. (1989). Long term use of an LH-RH agonist in the management of uterine leiomyomas. A study of 17 cases. *Int. J. Fertil.*, **34**, 19–24

8. Parmar, H., Nicoll, J., Stockdale, A., Cassoni, F., Phillips, R. H., Lightman, S. and Schally, A. V. (1977). Advanced ovarian carcinoma. Response to the agonist D-Trp-6-LH-LH. *Cancer Treat. Rep.*, **69**, 1341

9. Dutta, A. S. (1988). LH-RH antagonists. *Drugs Future*, **13**, 761–87

10. Gonzalez-Barcena, D., Kastin, A. J., Coy, D. H., Nikolics, K. and Schally, A. V. (1977). Suppression of gonadotropin release in man by inhibitory analogue of luteinizing hormone-releasing hormone. *Lancet*, **2**, 997–8

11. Schmidt, F., Sundaram, K., Thau, R. B. and Bardin, C. W. (1984). (Ac-D-Dal (2), 4FD-Phe, D-Trp, D-Arg)-LH-RH, a potent antagonist of LHRH, produces transient edema and behavioral changes in rats. *Contraception*, **29**, 283–9

12. Reissmann, Th., Engel, J., Kutscher, B., Bernd, M., Hilgard, P., Peukert, M., Szelenyi, I., Reichert, S., Gonzalez-Barcena, D., Nieschiang, E., Comaru-Schally, A. M. and Schally, A. V. (1994). Cetrorelix. *Drugs Future*, **19**, 228–37

13. Gonzàlez-Bàrcena, D., Vadillo-Buenfil, M., Garcia Procel, E., Guerra-Arguero, L., Cardenas Cornejo, I., Comaru-Schally, A. M. and Schally, A. V.

(1994). Inhibition of luteinizing hormone, follicle-stimulating hormone and sex-steroid levels in men and women with a potent antagonist analog of luteinizing hormone-releasing hormone, Cetrorelix (SB-75). *Eur. J. Endocrinol.*, **131**, 286–92

14. Gonzàlez-Bàrcena, D., Vadillo-Buenfil, M., Gomez-Orta, F., Fuentes-Garcia, M., Cardenas Cornejo, I., Graef Sanchez, A., Comaru-Schally, A. M. and Schally, A. V. (1994). Responses to the antagonistic analog of LH-RH (SB-75, Cetrorelix) in patients with benign prostatic hyperplasia and prostatic cancer. *Prostate*, **24**, 84–92

15. Gonzàlez-Bàrcena, D., Vadillo-Buenfil, M., Cortez-Morales, A., Fuentes-Garcia, M., Cardenas-Cornejo, I., Comaru-Schally, A. M. and Schally, A. V. (1995). Luteinizing hormone-releasing hormone antagonist Cetrorelix as primary single therapy in patients with advanced prostatic cancer and paraplegia due to metastatic invasion of spinal cord. *Urology*, **45**, 275–81

16. Bajusz, S., Kovacs, M., Gazdag, M., Bokser, L., Karashima, T., Csernus, V. J., Janaky, T., Guoth, J. and Schally, A. V. (1986). Highly potent antagonists of luteinizing hormone-releasing hormone free of edematogenic effects. *Proc. Natl. Acad. Sci. USA*, **85**, 1637–41

17. Bajusz, S., Csernus, V. J., Janaky, T., Bokser, L., Fekete, M. and Schally, A. V. (1988). New antagonist of LHRH. II Inhibition and potentiation of LHRH by closely related analogues. *Int. J. Pept. Protein Res.*, **32**, 425–35

18. Schally, A. V., Srkalovic, G., Szende, B., Redding, T. W., Korkut, E., Szepeshazi, K., Bokser, L., Pinski, J., Groot, K., Serfozo, P., Comaru-Schally, A. M., Bajusz, S., Gonzalez-Barcena, D., Reissmann, T., Hilgard, P. and Engel, J. (1990). New antagonistic analogues of LH-RH: experimental oncological and clinical studies. Advances in the study of GnRH analogues. The basic science of GnRH analogues. In Lunenfeld, D. (ed.) *Proceedings of the International Symposium on GnRH Analogues*, November 1990, Geneva, Switzerland, Vol. 2, pp. 25–35. (Carnforth, UK: Parthenon Publishing Group)

19. Andreyko, J. L., Monroe, S. E., Marshall, L. A., Fluker, M. R., Neremberg, C. A. and Jaffe, R. B. (1992). Concordant suppression of serum immunoreactive luteinizing hormone (LH), follicle stimulating hormone, alpha subunit, bioactive LH, and testosterone in postmenopausal women by a potent gonadotropin releasing hormone antagonist (Detirelix). *J. Clin. Endocrinol. Metab.*, **74**, 399–405

20. Pavlou, S. N., Wakefield, G. B., Island, S. P., Hoffman, P. G., LePage, M. E., Chang, R. L., Nerenger, C. A. and Kovaks, W. J. (1987). Suppression of pituitary–gonadal function by a potent new luteinizing hormone-releasing hormone antagonist in men. *J. Clin. Endocrinol. Metab.*, **64**, 931–6

21. Pavlou, S. N., Wakefield, G. B., Schleschter, N. L., Linder, J., Souza, K. H., Kamilaris, T. C., Konidaris, S., Rivier, J. F., Vale, W. W. and Toglia, M. (1989). Mode of suppression of pituitary and gonadal function after acute or prolonged administration of luteinizing hormone-releasing hormone antagonist in normal men. *J. Clin. Endocrinol. Metab.*, **68**, 446–54

22. Jockenhovel, F., Bhasin, S., Steiner, B. S., Rivier, J. E., Vale, W. W. and Swerdloff, R. S. (1988). Hormonal effects of single gonadotropin-releasing hormone antagonist doses in men. *J. Clin. Endocrinol. Metab.*, **66**, 1065–70

23. Leal, J. A., Williams, R. F., Danforth, D. R., Gordon, K. and Hodgen, G. D. (1988). Prolonged duration of gonadotropin inhibition by a third generation GnRH antagonist. *J. Clin. Endocrinol. Metab.*, **67**, 1325–7

24. Matikainen, T., Ding, Y. Q., Vergara, M., Huhtaniemi, I., Couzinet, B. and Schaison, G. (1992). Differing responses of plasma bioactive and immunoreactive follicle-stimulating hormone and luteinizing hormone to gonadotropin-releasing hormone antagonist and agonist treatments in postmenopausal women. *J. Clin. Endocrinol. Metab.*, **75**, 820–5

25. Bagatell, C. J., Conn, P. M. and Bremner, W. J. (1993). Single-dose administration of gonadotropin-releasing hormone antagonist, Nal-Lys (antide) to healthy men. *Fertil. Steril.*, **60**, 680–5

26. Behre, H. M., Klein, B., Steinmeyer, E., McGregor, G. P., Voigt, K. and Nieschlag, E. (1992). Effective suppression of luteinizing hormone and testosterone by single doses of the new gonadotropin-releasing hormone antagonist Cetrorelix (SB-75) in normal men. *J. Clin. Endocrinol. Metab.*, **75**, 393–8

27. Rabinovici, J., Rothman, P., Monroe, S. E., Neremberg, C. and Jaffe, B. (1992). Endocrine effects and pharmacokinetic characteristics of a potent new gonadotropin-releasing hormone antagonist (Ganirelix) with minimal histamine-releasing properties: studies in postmenopausal women. *J. Clin. Endocrinol. Metab.*, **75**, 1220–5

28. Crawford, D. E. (1990). Hormonal therapy of

prostatic carcinoma. Defining the challenge. *Cancer*, **66** (Suppl.), 1035–8

29. Labrie, F., Dupont, A., Belanger, A. and Lachance, R. (1987). Flutamide eliminates the risk of disease flare in prostatic cancer patients treated with a luteinizing hormone-releasing hormone agonist. *J. Urol.*, **138**, 804–6

30. Kuhn, J. M., Billebaud, T., Navratil, H., Moulonguet, A., Fiet, J., Grise, P., Louis, J. F., Costa, P., Husson, J. M., Dahan, R., Bertagna, C. and Edelstein, R. (1984). Prevention of the transient adverse effects of a gonadotropin-releasing hormone analogue (buserelin) in metastatic carcinoma by administration of an antiandrogen (nilutamide). *N. Engl. J. Med.*, **321**, 413–18

31. Kahan, A., Delrieu, F., Amor, B., Chiche, B. and Steg, A. (1984). Disease flare induced by D-Trp[6] LHRH analogue in patients with metastatic prostatic cancer. *Lancet*, **i**, 971–2

17

GnRH agonists in premenopausal breast cancer

A. Manni

INTRODUCTION

It is now well established that approximately one-third of human breast cancers depend upon estrogen for continued growth. While in postmenopausal women estrogen derive primarily from peripheral aromatization of adrenal androgen precursors, in premenopausal subjects estrogens are primarily of ovarian origin. Therefore, ovariectomy has been the standard endocrine therapy of hormone responsive premenopausal breast cancer since 1896, when Beatson first reported objective tumor regressions in some premenopausal patients who had undergone castration[1].

Since ovariectomy requires surgery and is irreversible, medical means of suppressing ovarian estrogen production have been pursued actively. The introduction of potent non-steroidal anti-estrogens (e.g. tamoxifen) raised the possibility of achieving a medical castration by inhibiting estrogen action at the target tissue level[2]. Tamoxifen has indeed been found to exert an anti-tumor effect in premenopausal patients which is comparable to that of ovariectomy[3,4]. It is of concern, however, that this treatment markedly stimulates estrogen production by the ovaries and is unable to completely suppress menses in the majority of patients[5]. Furthermore, ovariectomy performed at the time of disease progression in patients taking tamoxifen has been shown to induce palliation in a significant number of patients[6,7]. Thus, tamoxifen does not appear to be able to induce a complete medical castration and its use in this group of patients should probably be restricted to research clinical trials. Inhibition of estrogen biosynthesis with the aromatase inhibitor aminoglutethimide has also been found to be unable to induce a medical castration[8], presumably as a result of the compensatory increase in gonadotropin secretion overriding the enzymatic block. The introduction of potent gonadotropin releasing hormone (GnRH) analogs offers the best possibility of achieving a complete medical ovariectomy. The chronic administration of these compounds has been shown to induce a paradoxic suppression of pituitary gonadotropin secretion mediated by both GnRH receptor down-regulation and postreceptor events[9,10]. The development of effective depot preparations which require only one injection a month has greatly increased the feasibility of GnRH analog therapy in premenopausal patients with breast cancer[11]. Consistent suppression of ovarian function has only been observed with parenteral injections of the analogs. Chronic intranasal therapy has been found to induce an incomplete suppression of ovarian function in most patients[12], probably as a result of the poor absorption of these compounds through this route (approximately 2%).

In this chapter the endocrine and anti-tumor effects of GnRH analog therapy in pre-menopausal women with advanced breast cancer are reviewed briefly. In addition, recent data on the potential merit of combined GnRH analogs and anti-estrogen therapy are summarized and discussed.

GnRH ANALOG MONOTHERAPY

Endocrine effects

Figure 1 illustrates the author and his colleagues' data for daily subcutaneous leuprolide administration which have now been confirmed by other investigators using a variety of GnRH analogs[13]. Similar results have also been obtained with once-monthly depot injections. As can be

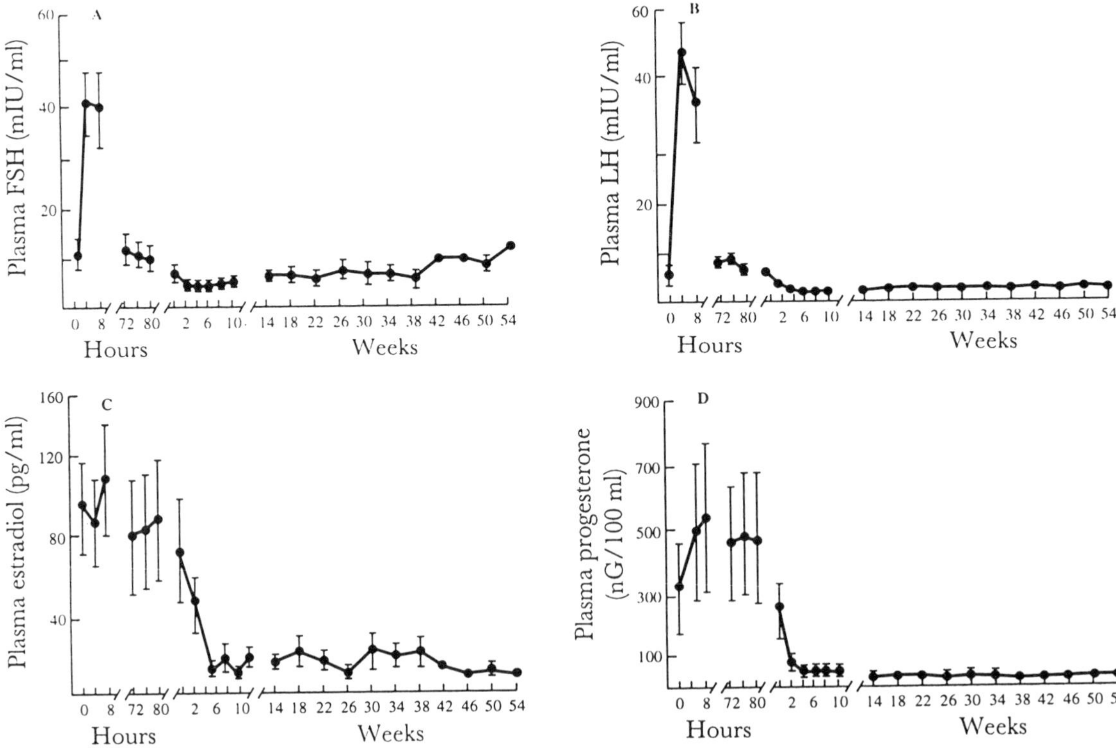

Figure 1   Plasma FSH, LH, estradiol and progesterone levels in premenopausal patients with advanced breast cancer treated chronically with leuprolide. Modified from Santen, R. J., Manni, A. and Harvey, H. (1986). Gonadotropin releasing hormone (GnRH) analogs for the treatment of breast and prostatic carcinoma. *Breast Cancer Res. Treat. J.*, **7**, 129–45[14]. Reproduced with permission of Kluwer Academic Publiahers

seen, both plasma luteinizing hormone (LH) and follicle stimulating hormone (FSH) rose transiently during the initial 4 days of therapy before falling to suppressed levels. Estradiol levels varied markedly during the first week of treatment but fell to postmenopausal levels after 4 weeks and remained at these concentrations thereafter. The lack of a consistent early rise (hormonal flare) in estradiol differed from the uniform increase in testosterone observed in men with prostate cancer during the same time period[14]. It is conceivable that the variability of initial estradiol responses observed in our patients may have reflected the fact that they began treatment at variable times during their menstrual cycle. As expected, plasma progesterone fell to castrate levels within a similar time frame (Figure 1). Plasma estrone and estrone sulfate also fell to levels measured routinely in postmenopausal women with breast cancer. No consistent changes were observed in the serum

levels of androstenedione, prolactin and cortisol during leuprolide administration. Taken collectively, these data demonstrate that a selective inhibition of ovarian function without significant alterations in adrenal secretion results from GnRH analog administration. Complete suppression of ovarian activity resulting in amenorrhea has been observed in all patients chronically treated with GnRH analogs by the author's team and other investigators[11,13].

Clinical results

Several clinical trials of GnRH analogs for treatment of premenopausal women with breast cancer have now been published. A summary of these various studies reported by the author and his colleagues in a recent review[15] revealed a 41% objective response rate in 238 unselected patients and 51% in 126 women with estrogen-receptor

Table 1 Clinical efficacy of goserelin plus tamoxifen versus goserelin alone in 318 premenopausal patients with advanced breast cancer*

	Randomized treatment		
	Goserelin alone ($n = 159$)	*Goserelin plus tamoxifen* ($n = 159$)	p *value*
Objective response (CR + PR), *n* (%)	50 (31)	60(38)	0.24
complete response	8 (5)	12 (8)	
partial response	42 (26)	48 (30)	
No change, *n* (%)	51 (32)	42 (26)	
Progression, *n* (%)	49 (31)	47 (30)	
Median duration of response, weeks (range)	59 (12–216)	88 (8–196)	
Median time to first progression, weeks (range)	23 (0–216)	28 (0–196)	0.03
Median survival, weeks (range)	127 (0–303)	140 (0–298)	0.25

*From Jonat, W., Kaufmann, M., Blamey, R. W. *et al.* (1995). A randomised study to compare the effect of the luteinizing hormone releasing hormone (LHRH) analogue goserelin with or without tamoxifen in pre- and perimenopausal patients with advanced breast cancer. *Eur. J. Cancer*, **31A**, 137–42[19]. Reproduced with permission of Elsevier Science Ltd. CR, complete response; PR, partial response

positive tumors. Subsequent trials have shown similar results. Median durations of response have been reported between 10–16 months. Overall, the results of therapy with GnRH analogs are similar to those expected from ovariectomy.

Toxicity

A remarkable lack of significant clinical toxicity with these compounds has been a consistent finding[15]. As expected, hot flushes are the most common side effect as a result of cessation of ovarian function. A few patients have experienced mild, local discomfort at the injection site. In contrast to the situation in prostate cancer, the phenomenon of 'tumor flare' has not been well documented with this form of hormonal therapy in premenopausal patients with breast cancer. This probably results from the lack of a consistent early rise in estradiol discussed earlier in the chapter (Figure 1).

COMBINATION THERAPY WITH GnRH ANALOGS AND ANTI-ESTROGENS

The rationale for this combined approach would be to obtain a complete blockade of estrogen action. The administration of anti-estrogens could in fact potentiate the anti-tumor effect of these compounds by blocking the action at the tumor site of the residual postmenopausal levels of estrogens observed during chronic therapy with GnRH analogs. Furthermore, co-administration of anti-estrogens may prevent the flare phenomenon, observed on rare occasions in some patients. It may shorten the time required for tumor regression to occur since it takes several weeks for the GnRH analogs to optimally suppress ovarian steroidogenesis. An initial concern with this approach was the observation by Klijn and De Jong[16] that the addition of tamoxifen to goserelin treatment caused reappearance of progesterone secretion in some patients as a result of the stimulatory effect of tamoxifen on the pituitary–gonadal axis. It is probable, however, that this finding was due to the intranasal administration of goserelin, which is ineffective in suppressing pituitary gonadotropin secretion due to poor absorption. Subsequent studies using parenteral GnRH analog administration have failed to confirm this finding. Walker *et al.*[17] observed that the combination of the anti-estrogen tamoxifen (40 mg daily) and goserelin (3.6 mg depot every 4 weeks) resulted in a more effective suppression

Table 2 Clinical efficacy of goserelin plus tamoxifen versus goserelin alone in the subgroup of 115 patients with skeletal metastasis only*

	Randomized treatment		
	Goserelin (n = 62)	Goserelin plus tamoxifen (n = 53)	p value
Objective response (CR + PR), n (%)	15 (24)	23 (43)	0.03
Median duration of response, weeks (range)	60 (15–159)	111 (11–193)	
Median time to progression, weeks (range)	24 (4–159)	70 (4–193)	0.005
Number of deaths, n (%)	35 (56)	18 (34)	
Median survival, weeks (range)	124 (5–238)	221 (4–236)	0.009

From Jonat, W., Kaufman, M., Blamey, R. W. *et al.* (1995). A randomised study to compare the effect of luteinizing hormone releasing hormone (LHRH) analogue goserelin with or without tamoxifen in pre- and perimenopausal patients with advanced breast cancer. *Eur. J. Cancer*, **31A**, 137–42[19]. Reproduced with permission of Elsevier Science Ltd. CR, complete response; PR, partial response

of circulating concentrations of FSH and a further small, but significant, decline in serum estradiol levels than observed with goserelin alone.

A multicenter study by the Italian Trials in Medical Oncology (ITMO) Group tested the endocrine and clinical effects of monthly subcutaneous injections of goserelin (3.6 mg) in association with tamoxifen (20 mg daily) as first-line therapy in 64 premenopausal patients with advanced disease[18]. An overall response rate of 41% was observed with a median time to response and a median response duration of 4 and 13 months, respectively. Serum estrogen levels were reduced into the postmenopausal range in association with marked suppression of LH and FSH. The authors concluded that although the clinical results were not better than expected with GnRH analog therapy alone, the concurrent use of goserelin and tamoxifen proved to be a feasible approach in the management of premenopausal advanced breast cancer which needed to be tested in a randomized, controlled, clinical trial. The results of such a study involving 318 pre- and perimenopausal patients with advanced breast cancer has recently been reported by Jonat *et al.*[19]. The patients were randomized to receive goserelin (3.6 mg subcutaneously every 28 days) or the combination of goserelin plus tamoxifen (40 mg once daily). As can be seen in Table 1, the clinical efficacy of the two regimens was quite similar with the exception of a modest but significant prolongation in median time to first progression observed with the combination treatment. It is of interest that, when the analysis was restricted to the 115 patients with skeletal metastasis only, statistically significant differences in objective response rate, time to disease progression and overall survival in favor of the combination therapy were observed (Table 2). As discussed by the authors, this finding needs to be prospectively confirmed before any firm conclusions can be reached. Both treatments were equally well tolerated with hot flushes being the most common side effect.

References

1. Beatson, G. T. (1896). On the treatment of inoperable cases in carcinoma of the mamma: suggestion for new method of treatment with illustrative cases. *Lancet*, **ii**, 104–7

2. Manni, A., Trujillo, J. E., Marshall, J. S., Brodkey, J. and Pearson, O. H. (1979). Antihormone treatment of stage IV breast cancer. *Cancer*, **43**, 444–50

3. Ingle, J. N., Krook, J. E., Green, S. J., Kubista, T. P., Everson, K. L., Ahmann, D. L., Chang, M. N., Bisel, H. F., Windschitl, H. E. and Twito, D. L. (1986). Randomized trial of bilateral oophorectomy versus tamoxifen in premenopausal women with metastatic breast cancer. *J. Clin. Oncol.*, **4**, 178

4. Buchanan, R. B., Blamey, R. W., Durrant, K. R., Howell, A., Paterson, A. G., Preece, P. E., Smith, D. C., Williams, C. J. and Wilson, R. G. (1986). A randomized comparison of tamoxifen with oophorectomy in premenopausal patients with advanced breast cancer. *J. Clin. Oncol.*, **4**, 1326

5. Manni, A. and Pearson, O. H. (1980). Antiestrogen-induced remissions in premenopausal women with stage IV breast cancer: effects on ovarian function. *Cancer Treat. Rep.*, 64, 779–85

6. Sawka, C. A., Pritchard, K. I., Paterson, A. H. G., Sutherland, D. J. A., Thomson, D. B., Shelley, W. E., Myers, R. E., Mobbs, B. G., Malkin, A. and Meakin, J. W. (1986). Role and mechanism of action of tamoxifen in premenopausal women with metastatic breast carcinoma. *Cancer Res.*, **46**, 3152–6

7. Hoogstraten, B., Fletcher, W. S., Gad-el-Mawla, N., Maloney, T., Altman, S. J., Vaughn, C. B. and Foulkes, M. A. (1982). Tamoxifen and oophorectomy in the treatment of recurrent breast cancer. *Cancer Res.*, **42**, 4788–91

8. Santen, R. J., Samojlik, E. and Wells, S. A. (1980). Resistance of the ovary to blockade of aromatization with aminoglutethimide. *J. Clin. Endocrinol. Metab.*, **51**, 473–7

9. Conn, P. M. (1986). The molecular basis of gonadotropin releasing hormone action. *Endocr. Rev.*, **7**, 3–10

10. Jinnah, H. A. and Conn, P. M. (1986). GnRH action at the pituitary: basic research and clinical applications. *Endocr. Rev.*, **7**, 11

11. Kaufmann, M., Jonat, W., Kleeberg, U., Eirmann, W., Janicke, F., Hilfrich, J., Kreienberg, R., Albrecht, M., Weitzel, H. K., Schmid, H., Strunz, P., Schachner-Wunschmann, E., Bastert, G. and Maass, H. and the German Zoladex Trial Group (1989). Gosrelin, a depot gonadotropin releasing hormone agonist in the treatment of premenopausal patients with metastatic breast cancer. *J. Clin. Oncol.*, **7**, 1113–19

12. Klijn, J. G. M. and De Jong, F. H. (1982). Treatment with a luteinizing hormone-releasing hormone analogue (Buserelin) in premenopausal patients with metastatic breast cancer. *Lancet*, **ii**, 1213

13. Harvey, H. A., Lipton, A., Max, D. T., Pearlman, H. G., Diaz-Perches, R. and de la Garza, J. (1985). Medical castration produced by the GnRH analogue leuprolide to treat metastatic breast cancer. *J. Clin. Oncol.*, **3**, 1068

14. Santen, R. J., Manni, A. and Harvey, H. (1986). Gonadotropin releasing hormone (GnRH) analogs for the treatment of breast and prostatic carcinoma. *Breast Cancer Res. Treat.*, **7**, 129–45

15. Santen, R. J., Manni, A., Harvey, H. and Redmond, C. (1990). Endocrine treatment of breast cancer in women. *Endocr. Rev.*, **11**, 1–45

16. Klijn, J. G. M. and De Jong, F. H. (1984). Long term treatment with the LH-RH agonist Buserelin (Hoe 66) for metastatic breast cancer in single and combined drug regimens. In Labrie, F., Belanger, A. and Dupont, A. (eds.) *LH-RH and its Analogues*, pp. 425–37. (Dordrecht: Elsevier)

17. Walker, K. J., Walker, R. F., Turkes, A., Robertson, J. F. R., Blamey, R. W., Griffiths, K. and Nicholson, R. I. (1989). Endocrine effects of combination antioestrogen and LH-RH agonist therapy in premenopausal patients with advanced breast cancer. *Eur. J. Cancer Clin. Oncol.*, **25**, 651–4

18. Buzzoni, R., Biganzoli, L., Bajetta, E., Celio, L., Fornasiero, A., Mariana, L., Zilembo, N., Di Bartolomeo, M., Di Leo, A., Arcangeli, G., Aitini, E., Farina, G., Schieppati, G., Galluzzo, D. and Martinetti, A. (1995). Combination goserelin and tamoxifen therapy in premenopausal advanced breast cancer: a multicentre study by the ITMO group. *Br. J. Cancer*, **71**, 1111–14

19. Jonat, W., Kaufmann, M., Blamey, R. W., Howell, A., Collins, J. P., Coates, A., Eiermann, W., Jänicke, F., Njordenskold, B., Forbes, J. F. and Kolvenbag, G. J. C. M. (1995). A randomised study to compare the effect of the luteinising hormone releasing hormone (LHRH) analogue goserelin with or without tamoxifen in pre- and perimenopausal patients with advanced breast cancer. *Eur. J. Cancer*, **31A**, 137–42

Treatment of postmenopausal breast cancer

18

K. H. Baumann and L. Kiesel

INTRODUCTION

Breast cancer is the most common malignant disease among women. One in nine women will develop breast cancer during her lifetime[1]. Endocrine factors, among others, particularly estrogens, are known to be involved in breast cancer development and progression. Research efforts have been focused on understanding the hormonal regulatory pathways and their mediators. Gonadotropin-releasing hormone (GnRH) analogs have become a center of interest because:

(1) They have a regulatory influence on the pituitary–gonadal axis; and

(2) Data has accumulated indicating direct effects on target tissues other than the pituitary.

HORMONAL REGULATION OF BREAST CANCER

In 1896 Beatson[2] established the inhibitory effect on human breast cancer progression that occurred when the ovaries were surgically removed. Ovariectomy led to a remarkably better course of the malignant disease compared with women whose ovaries were still intact. Since then the role of hormones, especially of estrogen on human breast cancer development and progression, has been investigated widely (for a review see[3,4]). Estrogen is known to regulate a series of factors closely related to cell proliferation (for a review see[5]). Consequently, the use of estrogen antagonists in the treatment of estrogen receptor (ER)-positive breast tumors in postmenopausal women has emerged as a powerful strategy in breast cancer therapy[6,7]. Similarly, premenopausal breast cancer patients gain benefits by down-regulation of ovarian steroid synthesis due to chronic GnRH analog treatment[7–12].

It is disappointing, however, that not all ER-positive breast tumors are sensitive to anti-estrogen therapy or estrogen reduction by GnRH analogs. Even more alarming is the fact that initially anti-estrogen sensitive tumors may become resistant to anti-estrogen therapy[5]. Combined, both groups comprise approximately 30% of all ER-positive breast tumors[13]. The biological basis of estrogen-induced cancer proliferation and progression and the steps towards the development of estrogen independency are multifactorial[5,14]. Formerly estrogen-dependent processes become autonomous. Pathways are activated which circumvent the requirement for estrogen and mutations of the estrogen receptor gene are also well known[15–17]. Biological and molecular diversity of the tumor cell population also contributes to the failure of anti-cancer treatment regimens[18]. Anti-estrogen therapy and/or down-regulation of estrogen synthesis targets and down-regulates only estrogen-dependent steps; other mechanisms do not approach the anti-estrogenic concept.

Development towards estrogen independence and anti-estrogen resistance calls for additional therapeutic strategies in human breast cancer. Based on experimental data which will be outlined later, GnRH analogs have proved to be powerful anti-proliferative agents with very few side effects in animals[19–21]. Two mechanisms are responsible for GnRH analog action on chronic application:

(1) Suppression of the hypophyseal gonadotropin synthesis and secretion followed by down-regulation of ovarian steroid hormone production[22].

(2) Direct antiproliferative effects on breast tumor cells have been demonstrated experimentally[23,24].

Table 1 Reported clinical effects of GnRH analogs on postmenopausal breast cancer patients

GnRH agonist	Patients objective	Response	Reference
Clinical trials:			
goserelin	6	0	31
buserelin	18	0	32
leuprorelin	40	7.5	33
triptorelin	15	20	34
goserelin	10	20	35
goserelin	6	0	36
buserelin	14	14	37
goserelin	28	11	38
leuprorelin	15	0	39
buserelin	26	0	40
buserelin	3	0	41
leuprorelin	15	0	42
goserelin	52	7.5	43
Case reports:			
triptorelin	2	100	44
goserelin	1	100	45

Case reports and clinical trials now provide more insight into the potency of GnRH analogs as therapeutic in postmenopausal breast cancer patients. In the main, experimentally observed attenuation of tumor growth has not been confirmed clinically.

GnRH ANALOGS IN POST-MENOPAUSAL BREAST CANCER PATIENTS: CLINICAL TRIALS

Experimental results of tumor growth inhibition and the detection of GnRH receptors in human breast cancer tissues[25–27] here favored the idea of the direct anti-tumor effects of GnRH analogs in breast cancer patients. However, only minor evidence exists for direct anti-proliferative effects of GnRH analogs on postmenopausal breast tumors[28,29]. A number of clinical studies (for a review see[30]) provide contradictory results on the effectiveness of GnRH analog therapy in postmenopausal breast cancer patients (Table 1[31–45]). All studies, however, included only a small number of postmenopausal patients.

Clinical trials have been contradictory to *in vitro* and *in vivo* observations on the effectiveness of GnRH analogs; in most cases a therapeutic beneficial effect on postmenopausal breast cancer patients has not been discussed and the objective response to GnRH analog treatment has been short-lived. The successful treatment reported by Schwartz *et al.*[44] was achieved by using a very large dosage of a GnRH agonist; other investigations have used dosages as low as 1/100 to 1/1000 of this amount. Some observations that might partly explain the lack of beneficial activity of treatment with GnRH analogs are:

(1) The patients had advanced breast cancer and most of them were pretreated.

(2) GnRH analog concentrations sufficient to exert direct anti-proliferative effects as determined experimentally were possibly not achieved in the tumor target tissues.

(3) The studies did not investigate the breast tumors for the presence of specific GnRH binding sites; thus no relation can be drawn between therapeutic efficiency and GnRH receptor status.

Consequently, it is clear that GnRH analogs in the adjuvant therapy of advanced and pretreated breast cancers are of only modest potency. It must be kept in mind that selection for highly

Table 2 Characterization (affinity constants [K_A] and maximal binding capacities [B_{max}]) of GnRH analogs binding to human breast cancer tissues and MCF-7 human breast cancer cells. The nucleotide sequence of the GnRH receptor in mammary cancer cells was recently characterized[56]

| | High affinity | | Low affinity | | |
Tissue/cell line	K_A (10^9 M^{-1})	B_{max} (nM)	K_A (10^6 M^{-1})	B_{max} (nM)	Reference
Human breast cancer	4.7	0.027	1.60	2.66	26
Human breast cancer	—	—	0.02	—	24
Human breast cancer	2.5	0.100	61.80	17.50	27
MCF-7	7.7	0.020	45.30	15.50	*
MCF-7	—	—	3.30	—	21

*Baumann and Kiesel, unpublished

malignant and therapy-resistant cancer cell clones might have occurred during previous treatments.

Nevertheless, the hypothesis that GnRH analogs exert direct anti-proliferative therapeutic effects in postmenopausal breast cancers cannot be excluded completely by the clinical trials performed so far. A trial with postmenopausal breast cancer patients having detectable levels of GnRH binding sites in cancer biopsies would therefore be an appropriate way to investigate the hypothesis further. The use of a radioreceptor assay for the detection of specific GnRH binding sites in human breast cancer cells is, however, controversial[25–27,46]. Combinations of GnRH receptor assays and/or immunohistochemistry and/or molecular biology (e.g. reverse transcription–polymerase chain reaction) offer different methods with which to determine GnRH receptor status. Data on experimental potency and bioavailability in humans of different GnRH analogs might also support a decision to identify the most promising peptide to target expressed and detected GnRH receptors in breast tissues.

EXPERIMENTAL BACKGROUND FOR DIRECT GnRH ANALOG ACTION ON BREAST CANCER CELLS

The concept of 'programmed cell death' has existed for more than two decades (for a review see[47,48]) and involves a set of specifically activated genes and their products which ultimately lead to cell death. Cancer can be seen as an imbalance between cell proliferation and cell death; it would be reasonable, therefore, to search for strategies increasing the number of cells undergoing apoptosis, thus shifting the equation towards equality or superiority of dying cells. Reduction of estrogen-dependent tumor masses by estrogen antagonists is partly a result of apoptosis and/or cell cycle arrest[49]. The question arises as to whether breast tumors are sensitive to apoptosis inducers other than anti-estrogens, which is important in the case of the progression to anti-estrogen resistance and originally estrogen-independent and/or ER-negative breast tumors. As has been shown by many investigators, GnRH analogs are capable of inducing apoptosis in sensitive target cells in different tumor models[20,50].

Direct anti-proliferative effects of GnRH analogs require specific GnRH binding sites on the targeted human breast cancer cells. GnRH analogs bind to specific receptors located on the cell surface membrane. The hypophyseal GnRH receptor has been cloned and biochemically characterized[51–53]. Using the biochemical approach several research groups have demonstrated the expression of GnRH receptor[25–27] and the induction of second messenger pathways in human breast cancer cells by GnRH analogs[54,55]. Approximately one-half the tested human breast cancer tissues express specific GnRH binding sites. Scatchard blot analysis has revealed high- and low-affinity binding sites for GnRH (Table 2). The number of receptors in breast cancer tissues is much less compared with that of the pituitary. The distribution of GnRH receptor content in breast cancer biopsies of 140

Table 3 GnRH analogs binding to human breast cancer samples. For methods and additional data refer to reference[27]

	Number (n)	Mean GnRH analog binding (fmoles/mg ± SEM)	Number of samples with GnRH analog binding ≥ 3 fmoles/mg (n(%))
All women	235	6.4 ± 0.53	121 (51.5)
Postmenopausal women	140	6.9 ± 0.7	42 (44.2)
Premenopausal women	95	5.6 ± 0.8	79 (56.4)

SEM, standard error of the mean

postmenopausal women is shown in Figure 1. Detection of GnRH receptors did not correlate in any direction (Figure 2) with the presence of steroid receptors[27,26]. The GnRH receptor content in human breast cancer biopsies was not significantly different between pre- and postmenopausal women (Table 3).

The presence of specific GnRH analog binding sites in human breast cancer tissues provides an important link between clinical use of GnRH analogs and the encouraging results obtained from *in vitro* and *in vivo* investigations demonstrating a dose-dependent growth inhibition of breast cancer cells by GnRH agonists and antagonists, most probably mediated by specific GnRH receptors in tumor cells. Both cell cycle arrest[57] and the induction of apoptosis[50,58] were described. A clearly disturbing feature in some experimental investigations is the high GnRH analog concentration necessary to achieve significant effects (>0.1 μM of GnRH analog). New GnRH analogs were developed which down-regulated tumor cell proliferation at lower concentrations[50,54,59]. Additionally, *in vivo* models underlined that sufficient amounts of GnRH analog reach the target tissues in mice[50,58]. If the newly synthesized GnRH analogs achieve serum levels sufficient for tumor inhibition at the experimental stage, the door might reopen for testing in GnRH receptor positive human breast cancers.

DRUG TARGETING, A CHANCE FOR GnRH ANALOGS?

In recent years the concept of drug targeting has expanded from laboratories into clinics. Specific

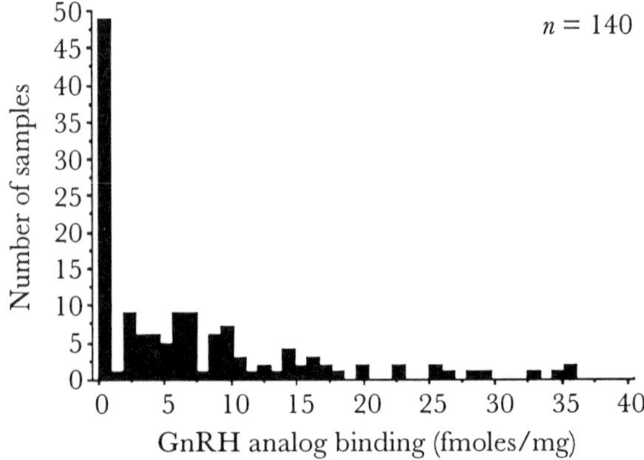

Figure 1 Distribution of gonadotropin releasing hormone (GnRH) analog binding content in breast cancer biopsies of postmenopausal women. For methods and analysis refer to reference[27]

antibodies or ligands which recognize their target counterparts on the surface of tumor cells are coupled with cytotoxic moieties, finally resulting in an accumulation of anti-cancer drugs in tumor cells. Thus, higher amounts of cytotoxic drugs reach the cells than would be possible by uncoupled direct application of cytotoxic agents. Furthermore, side effects of the toxic drugs might be diminished. The presence of GnRH receptors also offers an exciting possibility for drug targeting. Cytotoxic moieties are either coupled to GnRH analogs or alternatively, antibodies to the GnRH receptor may be used as carriers. In the former case, in animal studies, such drugs accumulated in targeted breast cancer tissues and increased the cytotoxic effect on tumor cells[60-62]. Experimental data using this approach has demonstrated the

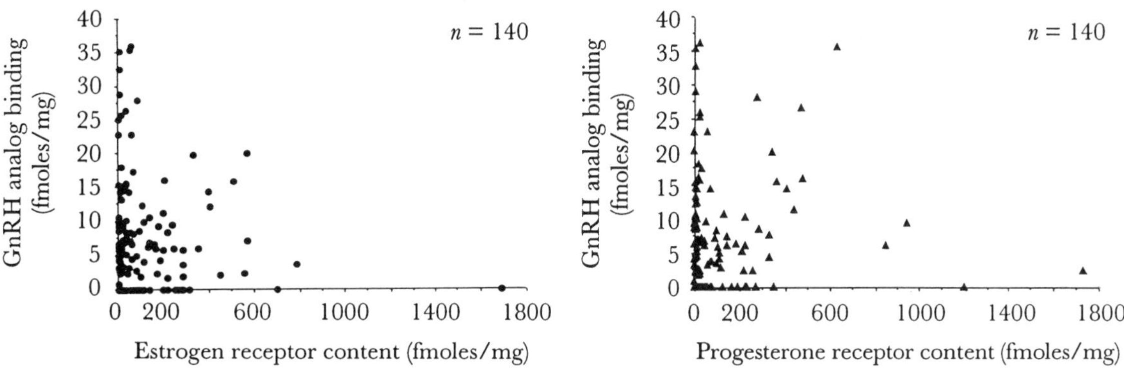

Figure 2 The gonadotropin-releasing hormone (GnRH) analog binding content in breast cancer biopsies of postmenopausal women is drawn against the estrogen-receptor (left) and progesterone receptor levels (right). For methods and analysis refer to reference[27]

increase in anti-tumor efficiency of the coupled drug[61,62]. Investigating cancer samples for the expression of GnRH receptor would enable selected use of these compounds.

Taken together, the use of GnRH analogs as an adjuvant therapy in postmenopausal breast cancer patients has suffered a major setback because of the lack of evidence of direct anti-cancer effects in patients, and application in a drug targeting regimen is not yet confirmed as a successful strategy in humans. Newly developed, more potent, GnRH analogs have not yet been tested for direct anti-cancer activity in humans.

BREAST CANCER PREVENTION WITH GnRH ANALOGS: ARTIFICIAL MENOPAUSE

One field remains open for GnRH analogs: the induction of artificial menopause by chronic GnRH analog application as a tumor preventive measure[63,64]. Estrogen is a potent tumor initiator and promotor in breast cancer development. The women most at risk from this type of cancer are those whose breast tissue has not undergone differentiation in the course of a completed pregnancy and those with a genetic risk for breast cancer. Thus, for breast cancer prevention, it is necessary to either induce terminal differentiation of the mammary epithelial cells or to reduce the tumorigenic effects of estrogens in women with (based on current knowledge) increased risk for

breast cancer. The systemic effect of GnRH analog therapy as a preventive strategy would consist mainly of estrogen reduction by reversible down-regulation of ovarian sex steroid synthesis. Combining GnRH analogs with low-dose hormone replacement therapy (HRT) would counteract side effects of the artificial postmenopausal state[65,66]. Low-dose HRT may not significantly abrogate the tumor-preventive measures[67–69]; long-term trials[70] have still to determine whether such a concept would lead to a reduction in breast cancer incidence, and also lack the side effects associated with estrogen depletion.

It also remains to be shown whether systemic GnRH analog and/or local GnRH-like peptides exert any direct preventive function for cancer. GnRH-like peptides have been detected in human benign and malignant breast tissues[71–73]; the role of these peptides is not yet known.

ELEVATED GONADOTROPIN LEVELS IN POSTMENOPAUSAL WOMEN

The role of increased gonadotropins in postmenopausal women and its relation to breast cancer has, so far, been poorly investigated. Thus, the down-regulation of gonadotropins[74–77] by chronic GnRH analog treatment and its significance for the treatment of breast cancer are even less well understood. Investigating the action of gonadotropins on breast epithelial cells may yield further information about additional direct or indirect mechanisms of GnRH action with respect to breast cancer development and progression in postmenopausal women.

CONCLUSION

Clinical data on the treatment of postmenopausal breast cancer patients with earlier generations of GnRH agonists mainly have not confirmed the growth inhibitory effects of GnRH analogs on human breast cancers shown previously in *in vitro* and *in vivo* studies. Nevertheless, the presence of GnRH receptors as well as GnRH-like peptides in breast cancer specimens still suggest a biological role for these molecules in breast cancer growth regulation. Additionally, the presence of GnRH receptors offers an opportunity for drug targeting using cytotoxic drugs coupled to GnRH analogs or receptor antibodies. The role of GnRH analogs as tumor preventive agents (with respect to primary and secondary prevention) in women at risk for developing breast cancer and any direct effects remain to be investigated.

References

1. Moore, D. H., Moore II, D. H. and Moore, C. T. (1983). Breast carcinoma etiological factors. *Adv. Cancer Res.*, **40**, 189–253
2. Beatson, G. T. (1896). On the treatment of inoperable cases of carcinoma of the mamma: suggestions for a new method of treatment with illustrative cases. *Lancet*, **ii**, 104–7
3. Rochefort, H. (1994). Hormonal regulations of breast cancers from cell lines to patients. *Presse Med.*, **23**, 1211–16
4. Clarke, R., Skaar, T., Baumann, K., Leonessa, F., James, M., Lippman, J., Thompson, E. W., Freter, C. and Brunner, N. (1994). Hormonal carcinogenesis in breast cancer: cellular and molecular studies of malignant progression. *Breast Cancer Res. Treat.*, **31**, 237–48
5. Clarke, R., Bruenner, N., Katzenellenbogen, B., Thompson, R., Norman, M., Koppi, C., Paik, S., Lippman, M. and Dickson, R. (1989). Progression from hormone dependent to hormone independent growth in MCF-7 human breast cancer cells. *Proc. Natl. Acad. Sci. USA*, **86**, 3649–53
6. Baum, M. (1990). The role of endocrine therapy in primary breast cancer. *J. Steroid. Biochem.*, **36**, 187–9
7. Manni, A. (1989). Endocrine therapy of metastatic breast cancer. *J. Endocrinol. Invest.*, **12**, 357–72
8. Miller, W. R. (1990). Endocrine treatment for breast cancers: biological rationale and current progress. *J. Steroid. Biochem. Mol. Biol.*, **37**, 467–80
9. Brambilla, C., Escobedo, A., Artioli, R., Lechuga, M. J. and Motta, M. (1992). Treatment of premenopausal advanced breast cancer with goserelin – a long-acting luteinizing hormone releasing hormone agonist. *Anticancer Drugs*, **3**, 3–8
10. Davidson, N. E. (1994). Ovarian ablation as treatment for young women with breast cancer. *Monogr. Natl. Cancer Inst.*, 1994, 95–9
11. Klijn, J. G. and de Jong, F. (1982). Treatment with a luteinising-hormone-releasing-hormone analogue (buserelin) in premenopausal patients with metastatic breast cancer. *Lancet*, **i**, 1213–6
12. Klijn, J. G. (1992). LH-RH agonists in the treatment of metastatic breast cancer: ten years' experience. *Recent Results Cancer Res.*, **124**, 75–90
13. Rose, C. and Mouridsen, H. T. (1989). Endocrine management of advanced breast cancer. *Horm. Res.*, **32** (Suppl. 1), 189–97
14. Clarke, R., Thompson, E., Leonessa, F., Lippman, J., McGarvey, M. and Bruenner, N. (1993). Hormone resistance, invasiveness and metastatic potential in human breast cancer. *Breast Cancer Res. Treat.*, **24**, 227–39
15. Castles, C. G., Fuqua, S. A., Klotz, D. M. and Hill, S. M. (1993). Expression of a constitutively active estrogen receptor variant in the estrogen receptor-negative BT-20 human breast cancer cell line. *Cancer Res.*, **53**, 5934–9
16. Fuqua, S. A. W., Allred, D. C. and Auchus, R. J. (1993). Expression of estrogen receptor variants. *J. Cell. Biochem. Suppl.*, **17G**, 194–7
17. Fuqua, S. A. W. (1994). Estrogen receptor mutagenesis and hormone resistance. *Cancer*, **74**, 1026–9
18. Dexter, D. L. and Calabresi, P. (1982). Intraneoplastic diversity. *Biochim. Biophys. Acta*, **695**, 97–112

19. DeSombre, E. R., Johnson, E. S. and White, W. F. (1976). Regression of rat mammary tumors effected by a gonadoliberin analog. *Cancer Res.*, **36**, 3830–3

20. Szende, B., Lapis, K., Redding, T. W., Srkalovic, G. and Schally, A. V. (1989). Growth inhibition of MXT mammary carcinoma by enhancing programmed cell death (apoptosis) with analogs of LHRH and somatostatin. *Breast Cancer Res. Treat.*, **14**, 307–14

21. Vincze, B., Palyi, I., Daubner, D., Kremmer, T., Szamel, I., Bodrogi, I., Sugar, J., Seprodi, J., Mezo, I., Teplan, I. and Echardt, S. (1991). Influence of luteinizing hormone-releasing hormone agonists on human mammary carcinoma cell lines and their xenografts. *J. Steroid. Biochem. Mol. Biol.*, **38**, 119-26

22. Rabin, M. N. and McNeil, L. W. (1980). Pituitary and gonadal desensitization after continuous luteinzing hormone-releasing hormone infusion in normal females. *J. Clin. Endocrinol. Metab.*, **51**, 873–6

23. Miller, W. R., Scott, W. N., Morris, R., Fraser, H. M. and Sharpe, R. M. (1985). Growth of human breast cancer cells inhibited by a luteinizing hormone-releasing hormone agonist. *Nature*, **313**, 231–3

24. Eidne, K. A., Flanagan, C. A., Harris, N. S. and Millar, R. P. (1987). Gonadotropin-releasing hormone (GnRH)-binding sites in human breast cancer cell lines and inhibitory effects of GnRH antagonists. *J. Clin. Endocrinol. Metab.*, **64**, 425–32

25. Eidne, K. A., Flanagan, C. A. and Millar, R. P. (1985). Gonadotropin-releasing hormone binding sites in human breast carcinoma. *Science*, **229**, 989–91

26. Fekete, M., Wittliff, J. and Schally, A. (1989). Characteristics and distribution of receptors for (D-TRP⁶)-luteinizing hormone-releasing hormone, somatostatin, epidermal growth factor, and sex steroids in 500 biopsy samples of human breast cancer. *J. Clin. Lab. Anal.*, **3**, 137–47

27. Baumann, K. H., Kiesel, L., Kaufmann, M., Bastert, G. and Runnebaum, B. (1993). Characterization of binding sites for a GnRH-agonist (buserelin) in human breast cancer biopsies and their distribution in relation to tumor parameters. *Breast Cancer Res. Treat.*, **25**, 37–46

28. Harris, A. L., Carmichael, J., Cantwell, B. M. and Dowsett, M. (1989). Zoladex: endocrine and therapeutic effects in post-menopausal breast cancer. *Br. J. Cancer*, **59**, 97–9

29. Nicholson, R. I. and Walker, K. J. (1989). GnRH agonists in breast and gynaecologic cancer treatment. *J. Steroid. Biochem.*, **33**, 801–4

30. Emons, G. and Schally, A. V. (1994). The use of luteinizing hormone releasing hormone agonists and antagonists in gynaecological cancers. *Hum. Reprod.*, **9**, 1364–79

31. Nicholson, R. I., Walker, K. J., Turkes, A., Dyas, J., Plowman, P. N., Williams, M. and Blamey, R. W. (1985). Endocrinological and clinical aspects of LHRH action (ICI 118630) in hormone dependent breast cancer. *J. Steroid. Biochem.*, **23**, 843–7

32. Waxman, J. H., Harland, S. J., Coombes, R. C., Wrigley, P. F. M., Malpas, J. S., Powles, T. and Lister, T. A. (1985). The treatment of postmenopausal women with advanced breast cancer with buserelin. *Cancer Chemother. Pharmacol.*, **15**, 171–3

33. Santen, R. J., Manni, A. and Harvey, H. (1986). Gonadotropin-releasing hormone (GnRH) analogs for the treatment of breast and prostatic carcinoma. *Breast Cancer Res. Treat.*, **7**, 129–45

34. Mathe, G., Keiling, R., Vovan, M. L., Gastiaburu, J., Prevot, G., Vannetzel, J. M. and Misset, J. L. (1986). Phase II trial of D-Trp-6-LHRH in advanced breast cancer. *Eur. J. Cancer Clin. Oncol.*, **22**, 723

35. Plowman, P. N., Nicholson, R. I. and Walker, K. J. (1986). Remission of postmenopausal breast cancer during treatment with the luteinising hormone releasing hormone agonist ICI 118630. *Br. J. Cancer*, **54**, 903–9

36. Wander, H. E., Kleeberg, U. R., Schachner-Wünschmann, E. and Nagel, G. A. (1987). A long-acting depot preparation of a synthetic GnRH agonist (Zoladex) in the treatment of pre- and postmenopausal advanced breast cancer. *J. Steroid. Biochem.*, **28** (Suppl.), 1049

37. Lissoni, P., Barni, S., Crispino, S., Cattaneo, G. and Tancini, G. (1988). Endocrine and clinical effects of an LHRH analogue in pretreated advanced breast cancer. *Tumori*, **74**, 303–8

38. Harris, A. L., Carmichael, J., Cantwell, B. M. and Dowsett, M. (1989). Zoladex: therapeutic effects in postmenopausal breast cancer. *Horm. Res.*, **1**, 213–6

39. Crighton, I. L., Dowsett, M., Lal, A. and Smith, I. E. (1989). Use of luteinizing hormone-releasing hormone agonist (leuprolin) in advanced postmenopausal breast cancer: clinical and endocrine effects. *Br. J. Cancer*, **60**, 644–8

40. Vici, P., Veltri, E., Carpano, S., Di, L. L. and Lopez, M. (1991). Buserelin therapy in

postmenopausal patients with advanced breast carcinoma. *Clin. Ter.*, **136**, 195–9

41. Höffken, K. (1992). LH-RH agonists in the treatment of premenopausal patients with advanced breast cancer. *Recent Results Cancer Res.*, **124**, 91–104

42. Dowsett, M., Jacobs, S., Aherne, J. and Smith, I. E. (1992). Clinical and endocrine effects of leuprorelin acetate in pre- and postmenopausal patients with advanced breast cancer. *Clin. Ther.*, **14** (Suppl. A), 97–103

43. Saphner, T., Troxel, A. B., Tormey, D. C., Neuberg, D., Robert, N. J., Pandya, K. J., Edmonson, J. H., Rosenbluth, R. J. and Abeloff, M. D. (1993). Phase II study of goserelin for patients with postmenopausal metastatic breast cancer. *J. Clin. Oncol.*, **11**, 1529–35

44. Schwartz, L., Guiochet, N. and Keiling, R. (1988). Two partial remissions induced by an LHRH analogue in two postmenopausal women with metastatic breast cancer. *Cancer*, **62**, 2498–500

45. Cassano, A., Astone, A., Garufi, C., Noviello, M. R., Pietrantonio, F. and Barone, C. (1989). A response in advanced post-menopausal breast cancer during treatment with the luteinising hormone releasing hormone agonist – Zoladex. *Cancer Lett.*, **48**, 123–4

46. Mullen, P., Bramley, T., Menzies, G. and Miller, B. (1993). Failure to detect gonadotrophin-releasing hormone receptors in human benign and malignant breast tissue and in MCF-7 and MDA-MB-231 cancer cells. *Eur. J. Cancer*, **29A**, 248–52

47. Kerr, J. F. R., Wyllie, A. H. and Currie, A. R. (1972). Apoptosis: a basic biological phenomenon with wide-ranging implications in tissue kinetics. *Br. J. Cancer*, **26**, 239–57

48. Schwartzman, R. and Cidlowski, J. (1993). Apoptosis: the biochemistry and molecular biology of programmed cell death. *Endocrine Rev.*, **14**, 133–51

49. Watanabe, Y., Sawada, N., Isomura, H., Satoh, H., Hirata, K. and Mori, M. (1995). Estrogen-depleted condition induces apoptosis of rat mammary cancer cells after entering the S-phase of the cell cycle. *Cell. Struct. Funct.*, **20**, 125–32

50. Reissmann, T., Hilgard, P., Harleman, J. H., Engel, J., Comaru, S. A. and Schally, A. V. (1992). Treatment of experimental DMBA induced mammary carcinoma with Cetrorelix (SB-75): a potent antagonist of luteinizing hormone-releasing hormone. *J. Cancer Res. Clin. Oncol.*, **118**, 44–9

51. Tsutsumi, M., Zhou, W., Millar, R. P., Mellon, P. L., Roberts, J. L., Flanagan, C. A., Dong, K., Gillo, B. and Sealfon, S. C. (1992). Cloning and functional expression of a mouse gonadotropin-releasing hormone receptor. *Mol. Endocrinol.*, **6**, 1163–9

52. Kakar, S. S., Musgrove, L. C., Devor, D. C., Sellers, J. C. and Neill, J. D. (1992). Cloning, sequencing, and expression of human gonadotropin-releasing hormone (GnRH) receptor. *Biochem. Biophys. Res. Commun.*, **189**, 289–95

53. Clayton, R. N. and Catt, K. J. (1980). Receptor-binding affinity of gonadotropin-releasing hormone analogs: analysis by radioligand-receptor assay. *Endocrinology*, **106**, 1154–9

54. Keri, G., Balogh, A., Horvath, A., Mezo, I., Vadasz, Z., Bokonyi, G., Bajor, T., Vantus, T., Teplan, I., Horvath, J., Csuka, O. and Nicholson, R. I. (1992). Novel antitumor peptide hormones and their effect on signal transduction. *J. Steroid. Biochem. Mol. Biol.*, **43**, 105–10

55. Lee, M. T., Liebow, C., Kamer, A. R. and Schally, A. V. (1991). Effects of epidermal growth factor and analogues of luteinizing hormone-releasing hormone and somatostatin on phosphorylation and dephosphorylation of tyrosine residues of specific protein substrates in various tumors. *Proc. Natl. Acad. Sci. USA*, **88**, 1656–60

56. Kakar, S. S., Grizzle, W. E. and Neill, J. D. (1994). The nucleotide sequences of human GnRH receptors in breast and ovarian tumors are identical with that found in pituitary. *Mol. Cell. Endocrinol.*, **106**, 145–9

57. Mullen, P., Scott, W. N. and Miller, W. R. (1991). Growth inhibition observed following administration of an LHRH agonist to a clonal variant of the MCF-7 breast cancer cell line is accompanied by an accumulation of cells in the G0/G1 phase of the cell cycle. *Br. J. Cancer*, **63**, 930–2

58. Szepeshazi, K., Milovanovic, S., Lapis, K., Groot, K. and Schally, A. V. (1992). Growth inhibition of estrogen independent MXT mouse mammary carcinomas in mice treated with an agonist or antagonist of LH-RH, an analog of somatostatin, or a combination. *Breast Cancer Res. Treat.*, **21**, 181–92

59. Nicholson, R. I. and Keri, G. (1992). Antitumour activity of folligen, a novel gonadotropin-releasing hormone analogue against DMBA-induced tumours in the rat. *Tumour Biol.*, **13**, 44–50

60. Janaky, T., Juhasz, A., Rekasi, Z., Serfozo, P., Pinski, J., Bokser, L., Srkalovic, G., Milovanovic, S., Redding, T. W., Halmos, G. (1992). Short-

chain analogs of luteinizing hormone-releasing hormone containing cytotoxic moieties. *Proc. Natl. Acad. Sci. USA*, **89**, 10203–7

61. Janaky, T., Juhasz, A., Bajusz, S., Csernus, V., Srkalovic, G., Bokser, L., Milovanovic, S., Redding, T. W., Rekasi, Z., Nagy, A. and Schally, A. V. (1992). Analogues of luteinizing hormone-releasing hormone containing cytotoxic groups. *Proc. Natl. Acad. Sci. USA*, **89**, 972–6

62. Milovanovic, S. R., Monje, E., Szepeshazi, K., Radulovic, S. and Schally, A. (1993). Effect of treatment with LHRH analogs containing cytotoxic radicals on the binding characteristics of receptors for luteinizing-hormone-releasing hormone in MXT mouse mammary carcinoma. *J. Cancer Res. Clin. Oncol.*, **119**, 273–8

63. Bernstein, L., Ross, R. K. and Henderson, B. E. (1992). Prospects for the primary prevention of breast cancer. *Am. J. Epidemiol.*, **135**, 142–52

64. Sismondi, P., Biglia, N., Giai, M. and Defabiani, E. (1994). GnRH analogs in benign breast disease and breast cancer chemoprevention. A challenge for the year 2000. *Eur. J. Gynaecol. Oncol.*, **15**, 108–14

65. Adashi, E. Y. (1994). Long-term gonadotrophin-releasing hormone agonist therapy: the evolving issue of steroidal 'add-back' paradigms. *Hum. Reprod.*, **9**, 1380–97

66. Pike, M. C. and Spicer, D. V. (1993). The chemoprevention of breast cancer by reducing sex steroid exposure – perspectives from epidemiology. *J. Cell. Biochem. Suppl.*, **17G**, 26–36

67. Bonnier, P., Romain, S., Giacalone, P. L., Laffargue, F., Martin, P. M. and Piana, L. (1995). Clinical and biologic prognostic factors in breast cancer diagnosed during postmenopausal hormone replacement therapy. *Obstet. Gynecol.*, **85**, 11–7

68. Grady, D., Rubin, S. M., Petitti, D. B., Fox, C. S., Black, D., Ettinger, B., Ernster, V. L. and Cummings, S. R. (1992). Hormone therapy to prevent disease and prolong life in postmenopausal women [see comments]. *Ann. Intern. Med.*, **117**, 1016–37

69. Spicer, D., Shoupe, D. and Pike, M. (1991). Gonadotropin-releasing hormone agonist plus add-back sex steroids to reduce risk of breast cancer (letter). *J. Natl. Cancer Inst.*, **83**, 1763

70. Spicer, D. V., Pike, M. C., Pike, A., Rude, R., Shoupe, D. and Richardson, J. (1993). Pilot trial of a gonadotropin hormone agonist with replacement hormones as a prototype contraceptive to prevent breast cancer. *Contraception*, **47**, 427–44

71. Seppälä, M. and Wahlström, T. (1980). Identification of luteinizing hormone-releasing factor and alpha subunit of glykoprotein hormones in ductal carcinoma of the mammary gland. *Int. J. Cancer*, **26**, 267–8

72. Harris, N., Dutlow, C., Eidne, K., Dong, K. W., Roberts, J. and Millar, R. (1991). Gonadotropin-releasing hormone gene expression in MDA-MB-231 and ZR-75-1 breast carcinoma cell lines. *Cancer Res.*, **51**, 2577–81

73. Ikeda, M., Taga, M., Sakakibara, H., Minaguchi, H. and Vonderhaar, B. K. (1995). Detection of messenger RNA for gonadotropin-releasing hormone (GnRH) but not for GnRH receptors in mouse mammary glands. *Biochem. Biophys. Res. Commun.*, 207, 800–6

74. Couzinet, B., Lahlou, N., Thomas, G., Thalabard, J. C., Bouchard, P., Roger, M. and Schaison, G. (1991). Effects of gonadotrophin releasing hormone antagonist and agonist on the pulsatile release of gonadotrophins and alpha-subunit in postmenopausal women. *Clin. Endocrinol. (Oxf.)*, **34**, 477–83

75. Kolp, L. A., Pavlou, S. N., Urban, R. J., Rivier, J. C., Vale, W. W. and Veldhuis, J. D. (1992). Abrogation by a potent gonadotropin-releasing hormone antagonist of the estrogen/progesterone-stimulated surge-like release of luteinizing hormone and follicle-stimulating hormone in postmenopausal women. *J. Clin. Endocrinol. Metab.*, **75**, 993–7

76. Matikainen, T., Ding, Y. Q., Vergara, M., Huhtaniemi, I., Couzinet, B. and Schaison, G. (1992). Differing responses of plasma bioactive and immunoreactive follicle-stimulating hormone and luteinizing hormone to gonadotropin-releasing hormone antagonist and agonist treatments in postmenopausal women. *J. Clin. Endocrinol. Metab.*, **75**, 820–5

77. Oppenheim, D. S., Bikkal, H., Crowley, W. J. and Klibanski, A. (1992). Effects of chronic GnRH analogue administration on gonadotrophin and alpha-subunit secretion in postmenopausal women. *Clin. Endocrinol. (Oxf.)*, **36**, 559–64

Comparison of a GnRH analog and an anti-estrogen for the treatment of advanced or progressive ovarian cancer

W. Jäger and E. Beck

INTRODUCTION

Several animal experiments and epidemiological observations suggest that gonadotropins may be involved in the etiology and growth of ovarian cancer[1-3]. The two most important epidemiological observations which tend to support this hypothesis are the reduced incidence of ovarian cancer in patients using oral contraceptives over several years and the increased incidence of ovarian cancer in postmenopausal patients. The last observation deserves further consideration, since all ovarian cancer patients become hypergonadotropic after surgery (removal of the ovaries) and according to that hypothesis high gonadotropin levels could stimulate remaining cancer cells to further growth.

With the development of gonatropin releasing hormone (GnRH) analogs the reversible blockade of pituitary gonadotropin release became feasible and the effect of a reduction of the gonadotropins on the course of ovarian cancer could be evaluated. Because of some favorable effects observed in initial clinical studies, the Bavarian Oncology Study Group (BOSG) decided to begin a randomized trial in 1989 to evaluate the role of GnRH analogs for the treatment of ovarian cancer[4-7]. As all the members of the BOSG considered hormonal therapies as palliative treatment the study was not performed in patients with primary disease but only in patients with progressive ovarian cancer, in whom all other treatment modalities were exhausted ('last-line' therapy). To test the hypothesis that a reduction of gonadotropins leads to reduced growth, survival time was the main outcome variable. Treatment for the control arm tamoxifen was chosen because all participating clinicians had gained experience with the substance in breast cancer patients. It did not have severe side effects and did not reduce gonadotropin levels.

PATIENTS AND METHODS

Between May 1989 and May 1991, 73 patients with (far) advanced ovarian cancer were randomly assigned by four university departments of gynecology to receive the GnRH analog or the anti-estrogen.

Patients were considered eligible for the study when progression of ovarian cancer was diagnosed and all established treatment modalities (e.g. repeated surgery or different chemotherapies) were exhausted. The diagnosis of progressive ovarian cancer was made by each clinic according to its follow-up program after surgery and primary treatment (growing tumors by clinical examination, computerized axial tomography [CAT] scan, ultrasound, increasing cancer antigen [CA]-125 levels by more than 100% within 4 weeks). The informed written consent of patients was obtained. Randomization was performed centrally by telephone using a block randomization and the center as a strata variable.

Treatment began immediately after randomization. Patients received either 30 mg/day tamoxifen (Nolvadex®, ICI Pharma, Plankstadt, Germany) (at that time the usual dosage in Germany for treatment of metastatic breast cancer), or an intramuscular injection of 3.2 mg triptorelin (Decapeptyl®, Ferring GmbH, Kiel, Germany) at 28-day intervals.

Menopausal status at the time of primary surgery was defined by the date of the last menstrual period as documented in the records. The histological results were obtained from hospital records at the time of primary treatment. Hormone-receptor measurements had not been performed routinely at primary surgery so these data were not available for most patients. Of the patients, 77% had serous ovarian cancer, 53% histological grade II and 40% grade III disease; 87% of the patients had primary stage III or IV ovarian cancer.

After randomization the follow-up examinations were repeated every 3 months. It was generally agreed by the investigators that a precise documentation of response would not be possible in those patients with massive tumor spread; therefore, the efficacy of the two treatment arms was evaluated only on the survival time after randomization.

The initial plan was to enter 174 patients in order to detect an increase in 1-year survival time from 30% to approximately 47% (relative risk 1.6) with a power of 80%. Due to initial negative impressions and the availability of other treatment modalities most clinics lost interest and the number of patients entering the study diminished continuously. As a result an unplanned interim analysis was carried out and the inclusion of patients was stopped. Fifty-eight patients died before the end of the study. The median observation time was 8 months.

Survival time was calculated from the date of randomization until death or the date last seen. Estimations of survival probabilities were performed according to the Kaplan–Meier method[8]; p-values for treatment comparisons and for the investigation of prognostic factors were based on the log rank-test.

RESULTS

All relevant clinical parameters were nearly equally distributed between the two groups. Before the start of treatment most patients had elevated luteinizing hormone (LH) and follicle stimulating hormone (FSH) levels with estradiol levels in the postmenopausal range. In all patients assigned to the GnRH analog arm, LH and FSH serum levels were suppressed immediately after initiation of therapy, while in the tamoxifen group only a slight but not significant reduction of the gonadotropin levels appeared. No drug-induced severe toxicity or side effects were observed.

The median survival after randomization was 6 months. No significant difference in survival after randomization was observed between the two groups either in pre- or in postmenopausal patients (Figures 1 and 2). However, the survival rates of premenopausal patients were significantly better than those of postmenopausal patients. The estimate of the relative risk for tamoxifen versus triptorelin was 0.96 with 95% confidence intervals 0.57–1.63.

No clinical remission was observed and CA-125 levels usually increased. In only three patients, no obvious progression with stable CA-125 levels was diagnosed for periods of 26, 27 and 36 months. Two of these patients received tamoxifen and one patient triptorelin. In the univariate analysis a tendency (although not significant) for longer survival was detected in patients whose interval between primary surgery and inclusion in this study was greater than 18 months.

DISCUSSION

The results of our study demonstrated that the reduction of gonadotropins did not improve the course of progressive ovarian cancer. The survival times of patients treated with triptorelin were in the same range as the survival times of patients treated with tamoxifen.

The median survival time for both treatment arms was only 6 months. These results differed from previously published data, which gave a more optimistic impression[4–7].

In a retrospective analysis of our own previous study the stabilization of disease was observed mainly in patients who had a long interval between primary disease and recurrence. These patients seem to have a generally longer survival time, although the reasons are not known.

The main disadvantage of the study was that the calculated number of patients could not be included within the scheduled time interval. This was based on the fact that most patients died within a few months after randomization, so that the clinicians considered the treatment to be insufficient and enrolled the patients in

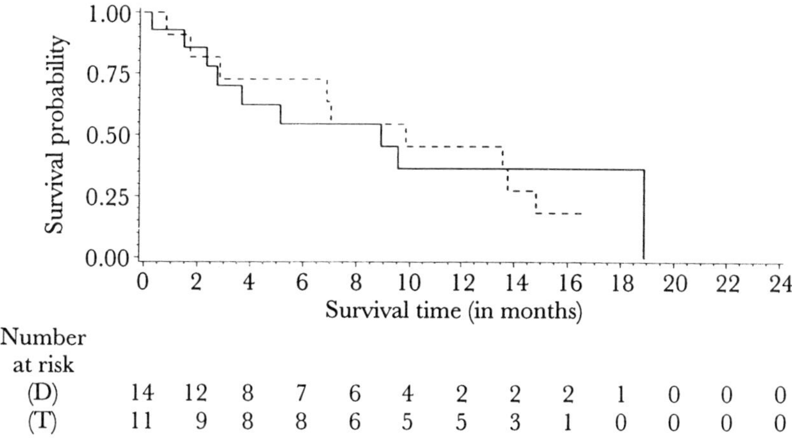

Figure 1 Kaplan–Meier estimation of the survival time after randomization for premenopausal patients. ——, Decapeptyl (D); - - -, tamoxifen (T)

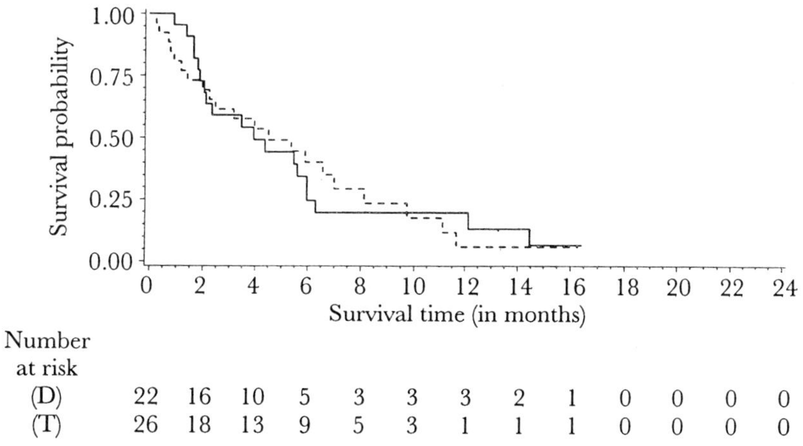

Figure 2 Kaplan–Meier estimation of the survival time after randomization for postmenopausal patients. ——, Decapeptyl (D); - - -, tamoxifen (T)

forthcoming new treatment studies using taxol. Although there were only 73 patients, the results of the unplanned interim analysis with an estimated risk of 0.96 for the treatment effect was seen as sufficient evidence to stop the trial. We must admit that even for a strong effect (relative risk 1.6) the power was only approximately 45%, but nevertheless the comparison between tamoxifen and triptorelin in 73 patients is one of the first studies in ovarian cancer to randomize between two hormone therapies.

It was difficult to compare the data of our study with the results of other treatment studies in advanced or recurrent ovarian cancer, based on two facts:

(1) There are relatively few published studies on hormone therapies in ovarian cancer, most of which have to be considered as case reports; and

(2) Most studies (including chemotherapy studies) are not randomized, have remissions or progressions as outcome variable and do not report survival times.

With few exceptions evaluable studies arrive at a median survival time of 9 months after initiation of the 'second-line' therapy. Compared to the median survival time of 6 months obtained in our study, it seems probable that none of the currently available treatments offer profound benefits for progressive ovarian cancer. Even the results obtained by taxol treatment do not seem to differ substantially from those obtained with other chemotherapeutic substances or with the survival times observed during tamoxifen or GnRH analog treatment[9]. If, therefore, a patient with progressive ovarian cancer is considered for palliative treatment, hormone therapies may be preferred since at least they do not subject the patient to heavy side effects. Based on the results of our study there is no difference if the patient receives tamoxifen or a GnRH analog

References

1. Cramer, D. W. (1990). Epidemiology aspects of early menopause and ovarian cancer. *Ann. N.Y. Acad. Sci.*, **592**, 363–75
2. Biskind, M. S. and Biskind, G. S. (1944). Development of tumors in the rat ovary after transplantation into the spleen. *Proc. Soc. Exp. Biol. Med.*, **55**, 176–9
3. Wimalasena, J., Dostal, R. and Meehan, D. (1992). Gonadotrophins, estradiol, and growth factors regulate epithelial ovarian cancer cell growth. *Gynecol. Oncol.*, **46**, 345–50
4. Parmar, H., Rustin, G., Lightman, S. L., Phillips, R. H., Hanham, I. W. and Schally, A.V. (1988). Reponse to D-Trp-6-luteinizing hormone releasing hormone (Decapeptyl) microcapsules in advanced ovarian cancer. *Br. Med. J.*, **269**, 1229.
5. Jäger, W., Wildt, L. and Lang, N. (1989). Some observations on the effect of a GnRH analog in ovarian cancer. *Eur. J. Obstet. Gynecol. Reprod. Biol.*, **32**, 137–48
6. Bruckner, H. W. and Motwani, B. T. (1989). Treatment of advanced refractory ovarian carcinoma with a gonadotrophin-releasing hormone analogue. *Am J. Obstet. Gynecol.*, **161**, 1216–18
7. Kullander, S., Rausing, A. and Schally, A. V. (1987). LHRH agonist treatment in ovarian cancer. In Klijn, J. G. M. (ed.) *Hormonal Manipulation of Cancer: Peptides, Growth Factors, and NEW (Anti)Steroidal Agents*, pp. 353–5. (New York: Raven Press)
8. Kaplan, E. L., and Meier, D. (1958). Nonparametric estimation from incomplete observations. *J. Am. Stat. Assoc.*, **53**, 471–81
9. Kohn, E. C., Sarosy, G., Bicher, A., Link, C., Christian, M., Steinberg, S. M., Rothenberg, M., Adamo, D. O., Davis, P., Ognibene, F. P., Cunnion, R. E. and Reed, E. (1994). Dose-intense taxol: high response rate in patients with platinum-resistant recurrent ovarian cancer. *J. Natl. Cancer Inst.*, **86**, 18–24

Treatment of ovarian cancer with LHRH antagonists

20

G. Emons, O. Ortmann, G. Irmer, V. Müller, K.-D. Schulz and A. V. Schally

INTRODUCTION

Epithelial ovarian cancer is the most common cause of death from gynecological malignancies in the western world[1]. Despite efforts aimed at early detection, most cases are diagnosed only at advanced stage. Cytoreductive surgery in combination with platinum-based chemotherapy has produced a substantial clinical improvement in these patients, yielding high response rates (up to 80%) and increased short- and medium-term survival[1–5]. Although this strategy may increase long-term survival in some favorable subgroups[6], the overall effects on survival have been poor[1,4]. Most patients, even in one-third of women in whom second look operations show complete pathological remissions, eventually relapse and ultimately die of chemoresistant disease[1,3–5]. The advent of new chemotherapeutic agents such as the taxanes raises some hopes that this situation may gradually improve, but even the new cytotoxic drugs will probably not solve the basic problem of chemoresistance development[7–9]. Chemotherapy regimens used in ovarian cancer patients have relevant acute toxicity. In addition, long-term sequelae such as secondary leukemia or myelodysplasia have to be considered[10–12]. Endocrine therapies, based on anti-estrogens, progestagens, their combinations, androgens and anti-androgens, have demonstrated no or only marginal efficacy in this disease (for a review see[1,13–16]).

With the isolation, determination of structure of luteinizing hormone-releasing hormone (LHRH) and the development of agonistic and antagonistic analogs[17], this class of peptides has attracted the attention of oncologists involved in the development of new endocrine therapies for epithelial ovarian cancer[14,18]. This interest in the use of LHRH analogs in epithelial ovarian cancer is based on two putative mechanisms of action:

(1) The suppression of endogenous gonadotropins which might be a mitogenic stimulus for ovarian cancer; and

(2) The direct anti-tumor effects of LHRH analogs, which could be mediated through specific receptors found in these tumors (for a review see[14–18]).

So far these investigations have been performed mainly with agonistic analogs of LHRH, since potent LHRH antagonists free of edematogenic side effects have only recently become available[17,18].

SUPPRESSION OF ENDOGENOUS GONADOTROPINS BY LHRH AGONISTS IN WOMEN WITH OVARIAN CANCER

Based on epidemiological and experimental data, it has been suggested that the growth of epithelial ovarian cancer may be stimulated by gonadotropins (for a review see[14–18]). Agonists of LHRH, which induce a suppression of endogenous gonadotropins, reduced the growth of xenografted human epithelial ovarian cancers in nude mice[19,20]. In 1985, Parmar and colleagues[21] reported on a patient with advanced epithelial ovarian cancer who had relapsed after surgery, chemo- and radiotherapy and who was then treated with the LHRH agonist triptorelin. Concomitant with the suppression of gonadotropins was a marked shrinkage of the tumor mass, lasting for 12 months[21]. A subsequent series of phase II trials by several groups has shown that treatment with LHRH agonists of patients with refractory advanced ovarian cancer led to objective remissions in 12% (21 of the 171 patients who could be evaluated) and stable disease in 19% (32 of 171 patients). Duration of the response varied between 26 and 98 weeks[22–30] (for a review see[14–16]).

These findings have been evaluated recently in a double-blind controlled clinical trial by investigators in Finland, Sweden, Israel and Germany. One hundred and thirty-five patients in whom advanced ovarian cancer (FIGO stage III or IV) had been diagnosed for the first time were included in the study. After surgical treatment and staging, the patients were randomized to receive either a long-acting preparation of the LHRH agonist triptorelin (Decapeptyl-Depot®, Ferring, Kiel, Germany) or placebo. For ethical reasons all patients received a first-line chemotherapy based on cisplatin or carboplatin and, if necessary, also salvage chemotherapies. Triptorelin or placebo were administered for 4 years or until death[31,32]. Although LHRH agonist treatment consistently suppressed luteinizing hormone (LH)- and follicle stimulating hormone (FSH)-serum levels, no significant effects on progression free and overall survival were observed in comparison to the placebo group (Emons *et al.* for the Decapeptyl–Ovarian Cancer Group, in preparation).

Erickson *et al.*[33] recently reported on a phase II trial of cyclophosphamide, cisplatin and the LHRH agonist leuprolide acetate after the debulking of stage III or IV epithelial ovarian cancers in 33 patients. They found that FSH levels were consistently suppressed by LHRH agonist treatment, but the efficacy of chemotherapy was not improved when comparisons were made with historical controls. The results of these trials suggest that the suppression of endogenous gonadotropins by conventional doses of LHRH agonists has no relevant beneficial effects in patients with advanced epithelial ovarian cancer who receive standard surgical cytoreduction and cytotoxic chemo-therapy.

Thus the approach to suppress endogenous gonadotropins by LHRH agonists has, so far, demonstrated only marginal activity in phase I/II trials on ovarian cancer patients in the salvage situation. The response rates of 12% objective remissions and 19% of disease stabilizations still must be substantiated in controlled trials.

DIRECT ANTI-TUMOR EFFECTS OF LHRH AGONISTS IN OVARIAN CANCER

Receptors for LHRH

In 1989, specific binding sites for LHRH were demonstrated by our group in 80% of ovarian cancer biopsies tested ($n = 32$)[34,35]. These binding sites were of the low affinity/high capacity type ($K_a = 1.4 \times 10^5$ M^{-1}; $B_{max} = 209 \pm 69$ pmol/mg membrane protein with a molecular weight of 63.3 kDa)[34,35]. Using an improved radioreceptor assay, we were recently able to demonstrate two classes of LHRH binding sites in the human ovarian cancer cell lines EFO-21 and EFO-27, one with a high affinity ($K_{d1} = 1.5$ or 1.7 nM) and the other with a low affinity ($K_{d2} = 7.5$ or 4.3 μM)[36]. Similar high affinity LHRH binding sites were detected in epithelial ovarian cancer biopsies[37]. In addition, the expression of messenger ribonucleic acid (mRNA) for the LHRH receptor identical to that for human pituitary LHRH receptor[38] was demonstrated in these ovarian cancer cell lines and six of eight biopsy samples[37]. Using different techniques, Imai *et al.*[39] demonstrated high affinity LHRH binding sites (K_d in the nM range) and expression of LHRH receptor mRNA in the human epithelial ovarian cancer cell lines MCAS, SK-OV3 and Ca OV-3, as well as in 21 of 23 primary epithelial ovarian cancers. Yano *et al.*[40] reported a specific high affinity LHRH binding site ($K_d = 1.4$ nM) in the human epithelial ovarian cancer cell line OV-1063. Receptor internalization assay showed that the ligand–receptor complex was internalized at 37°C, indicating the presence of biologically active LHRH receptors on these ovarian cancer cells[40]. Kakar *et al.*[41] recently demonstrated by nucleotide sequencing of the LHRH receptor complementary (c)DNA from a malignant ovarian tumor that it was identical to that of the human pituitary LHRH receptor. In contrast to the findings discussed above, Peterson *et al.*[42] were not able to detect specific LHRH receptors in ovarian cancer cell lines BG-1, OVCAR-3 and two primary epithelial ovarian tumors. Connor *et al.*[43] found no specific LHRH binding in the epithelial ovarian cancer cell lines OVCAR-3, 222, 2774 and three clones of the A 2780 line. Thus it could be concluded that a large proportion, but not all, of the established epithelial ovarian cancer cell lines express LHRH receptors. However, our findings[37] as well as those of Imai *et al.*[39], which are based on the detection of both high affinity LHRH binding sites as well as mRNA for the human pituitary receptor, indicate that the vast majority of primary epithelial ovarian cancers expresses receptors for LHRH.

LHRH-immunoactivity and bioactivity as well as the expression of mRNA for LHRH was detected by Ohno *et al.*[44] in three primary epithelial ovarian cancers and the cell line SK-OV 3. Utilizing a distinct LHRH antibody and a LHRH bioassay and different polymerase chain reaction primers than Ohno *et al.*[44], our group demonstrated the presence of LHRH immunoactivity and bioactivity as well as the mRNA for LHRH in the epithelial ovarian cancer cell lines EFO-21, EFO-27 and in eight of eight primary ovarian cancers[37].

Inhibition of growth of ovarian cancer cell lines

First studies on the *in vitro* effects of the LHRH agonist buserelin on ovarian cancer cell lines (OVCNOVA, OV-166, and OV-1255) by Slotman *et al.*[45] showed only minor, but statistically significant antiproliferative effects. Thompson *et al.*[46] found a dose-dependent inhibition of the *in vitro* proliferation of the ovarian cancer cell line 2774 induced by high concentrations (1 μM, 100 μM) of the LHRH agonist leuprolide.

We demonstrated recently, that the *in vitro* proliferation of the human ovarian cancer cell lines EFO-21 and EFO-27 was time- and dose-dependently inhibited by the LHRH agonist [D-Trp^6] LHRH (triptorelin)[36]. In both cell lines a significant reduction of cell number (to 86–87.5% of controls) was observed even at a 1 nM concentration of the analog. This effect became maximal at 10 μM triptorelin, the cell number being reduced to 65.5–68% of controls[36]. As both cell lines have high affinity binding sites for triptorelin (K_d 1.4–1.7 nM)[36] and express the mRNA for the human pituitary LHRH receptor[37], we suggested that the effects of triptorelin might be mediated through these LHRH receptors. Yano *et al.*[40] could demonstrate a similar dose-dependent inhibition of growth of human epithelial ovarian cancer cell line OV-1063 by triptorelin in the range of 10 nM to 10 μM. As mentioned above,

the OV-1063 cell line also expresses biologically active LHRH receptors[40]. Connor *et al.*[43] evaluated possible direct anti-tumor effects of the LHRH agonists buserelin and leuprolide in the ovarian cancer cell lines OVCAR-3, 222, 2774 and three subclones of A 2780. They observed a statistically significant reduction (16% at maximum) of cell growth in the OVCAR-3 and the A 2780-parent cell line with buserelin, but no dose-related response pattern was seen[43]. Leuprolide produced significant dose-dependent inhibition of growth in all six cell lines, but only when its concentration was raised to 100 μM[43]. As mentioned, the authors failed to detect specific LHRH binding sites in these six cell lines when using ^{125}I-labeled buserelin as radioligand[43]. The reason for the discrepancy between the findings of Yano *et al.*[40] and our own[36] on one hand and those of Connor *et al.*[43] on the other are apparent. The EFO-21, EFO-27 and OV-1063 cell lines express LHRH receptors with a K_d in the range of 1.4–1.7 nM[36,37,40] and their proliferation is significantly inhibited by triptorelin concentrations in the nanomolar range[36,40]. The cell lines tested by Connor *et al.*[43] and also by Peterson *et al.*[42] expressed no high affinity LHRH binding and hence their proliferation was inconsistently inhibited by buserelin and reduced by leuprolide only at 100 μM concentrations[43]. It is also possible that the specific LHRH agonist used as radioligand for the measurement of binding sites and for assessment of direct anti-proliferative effects might have contributed to these discrepancies. The work of Imai *et al.*[39], Yano *et al.*[40] and our own[36,37] provides reasonable evidence that the ovarian cancer cell lines EFO-21, EFO-27, MCAS, SK-OV3, CaOV-3 and OV-1063 express LHRH-receptors. As shown by Imai *et al.*[39] and our group[37], the vast majority of primary ovarian cancers similarly contains LHRH receptors. Ohno *et al.*[44] and our group[37] have also demonstrated that the cell lines SK-OV3, EFO-21 and EFO-27, as well as almost all primary ovarian cancers studied so far, express LHRH. Thus, it seems reasonable to speculate that most epithelial ovarian cancers have a local regulatory system based on the expression of LHRH and its receptor which might be a target for direct anti-tumor effects of LHRH analogs. The data on direct anti-proliferative effects of triptorelin on the ovarian cancer cell lines EFO-21, EFO-27 and OV-1063, which express LHRH receptors, support this concept. Future work using primary cultures of epithelial ovarian cancers should clarify the issue of whether the LHRH receptors found in the majority of biopsy samples obtained at surgery[37,39] mediate direct anti-tumor effects of LHRH agonists. However, concentrations of LHRH agonists necessary to induce direct anti-tumor activity *in vitro* probably cannot be achieved in the human *in vivo* by the administration of usual doses of LHRH agonists (for detailed discussion see Emons and Schally[14]). The development of new LHRH analogs such as those containing cytotoxic radicals (see Schally *et al.*, this volume) or of potent LHRH antagonists might permit a better exploitation of direct anti-tumor effects in the treatment of ovarian cancer.

DIRECT ANTI-TUMOR EFFECTS OF LHRH ANTAGONISTS IN OVARIAN CANCER

Recently, potent LHRH antagonists such as Cetrorelix, which are free of edematogenic and anaphylactic side effects, have become available for preclinical and clinical testing (for a review see Schally[17], Schally *et al.*[18], Emons and Schally[14]). While there already exists considerable clinical experience with LHRH antagonists in the treatment of prostatic cancer (for a review see González-Bàrcena, this volume) or in ovulation induction (for a review see Bouchard, this volume), only preclinical work has been performed so far on the use of these new compounds in ovarian cancer.

Our group demonstrated that the LHRH antagonists SB-75 (Cetrorelix) and Hoe-013 (Ramorelix) displaced ^{125}I-labeled triptorelin from plasma membranes of EFO-21 and EFO-27 human ovarian cancer cells in a way similar to unlabeled triptorelin[36]. The proliferation of the EFO-21 cell line was dose-dependently inhibited by Cetrorelix and Ramorelix with an efficacy similar to the agonist triptorelin. In the EFO-27 line, however, both LHRH antagonists had no anti-proliferative effects[36]. Interestingly, Cetrorelix partly antagonized the anti-proliferative effects of triptorelin in a dose-dependent way in the EFO-27 line[36]. Yano *et al.*[40] reported that the

growth of human epithelial ovarian cancer cell line OV-1063 was dose-dependently inhibited by Cetrorelix (10 nM to 10 μM) and that this inhibition was greater than that obtained with the agonist triptorelin. ^{125}I-labeled triptorelin could be displaced equally well by unlabeled triptorelin and Cetrorelix, suggesting that both analogs were bound to the same receptor on OV-1063 cells[40].

Connor *et al.*[43] observed no effect of the LHRH antagonist antide on the proliferation of the six ovarian cancer cell lines tested by them (see above), which presumably had no LHRH receptors[43]. Manetta *et al.*[47] failed to detect direct anti-proliferative *in vitro* effects of the LHRH antagonist Cetrorelix in the ovarian cancer cell lines UCI 101, UCI 107, PA-1, OVCAR-3, UCLA 222 and the three subclones of A2780 in concentrations ranging from 1 nM to 100 μM. No data on LHRH receptor expression in these cell lines were given[47].

Thus, so far clear direct anti-proliferative activity of LHRH antagonists on ovarian cancer cells has been demonstrated only in the EFO-21[36] and OV-1063[40] cell lines, which are both known to express LHRH receptors[36,41]. However, the results obtained in the EFO-27 cell line, which has been shown to have LHRH receptors and in which the LHRH agonist triptorelin has clear anti-proliferative activity[36], suggests that the mechanism of action of LHRH analogs in ovarian cancer is not uniform but that individual response patterns exist in different ovarian cancer cell lines[36].

It may be more rewarding to test direct anti-tumor effects of LHRH analogs in primary cell cultures from biopsy specimens obtained at surgery, which could be more related to the *in vivo* situation than the use of established ovarian cancer cell lines which might have lost important characteristics of the original tumor.

In this context it is noteworthy that, in the endometrial cancer cell lines HEC-1A and Ishikawa, we could also demonstrate the expression of high affinity LHRH binding sites as well as of LHRH and its mRNA[48,49]. In our hands the proliferation of these cell lines was equally well inhibited in a time- and dose-dependent fashion by both the LHRH agonist triptorelin and the LHRH antagonist Cetrorelix[48]. These direct actions were probably mediated through the high affinity LHRH binding sites[48]. As the majority of endometrial cancers express specific LHRH binding sites[50,51], the use of LHRH agonists and antagonists in this malignant disease deserves further attention.

Only few data are available on the effects of LHRH antagonists on the growth of human ovarian cancers heterotransplanted into the nude mouse. Manetta *et al.*[47] reported on a significant growth inhibition of xenografts of UCI 107 ovarian cancer by Cetrorelix[47]. As they had not observed a direct effect of Cetrorelix on the proliferation of this cell line *in vitro*, they concluded that this finding might be a result of inhibition of the pituitary–gonadal axis and gonadotropin secretion by Cetrorelix[47].

Yano and colleagues[52] compared the effects of chronic administration of the LHRH agonist triptorelin and of the antagonist Cetrorelix on growth of OV-1063 human epithelial ovarian cancer xenografts in nude mice[52]. Both treatments reduced uterine and ovarian weights and serum LH levels, indicating that a comparable suppression of pituitary–gonadal axis was obtained with either analog. Tumor growth, however, was significantly inhibited only by the LHRH antagonist Cetrorelix and not by the agonist triptorelin, a finding indicating that direct anti-tumor effects of Cetrorelix and not the suppression of pituitary–gonadal axis was the relevant mechanism of action[52]. In addition, it could be shown that chronic treatment with Cetrorelix greatly reduced the concentrations of receptors for epidermal growth factor (EGF) and insulin-like growth factor-I (IGF-I)[52], as well as the levels of mRNA for EGF receptors[53], in the tumors, phenomena that might be related to tumor growth inhibition. If these results could be extended to additional ovarian cancer cell lines, this may indicate that for the inhibition of proliferation of ovarian cancer *in vivo*, LHRH antagonists would be superior to agonistic analogs.

CONCLUSIONS

Some epidemiological and experimental data suggest that the suppression of gonadotropins by LHRH analogs may be useful for the treatment of epithelial ovarian cancer, but the available clinical data show that the therapeutical impact of such a strategy is marginal at best. A considerable body of evidence has been accumulated during the past few years, indicating that the majority of epithelial ovarian cancers expresses LHRH and its receptor. Work performed in ovarian cancer cell lines which express LHRH and its receptor has clearly shown that this putative local regulatory system based on LHRH could be used *in vitro* as a site of attack for both LHRH agonists and LHRH antagonists, inducing growth inhibition. Much work remains to be done before all the processes involved in this local system and the exact mechanism of action of LHRH analogs on this system can be understood. In addition, the problems of conflicting results obtained in different ovarian cancer cell lines have to be reconciled. Even after solving these problems, it is doubtful that conventional LHRH agonists at the doses used today can be effective for the exploitation of direct anti-tumor effects mediated through LHRH receptors in epithelial ovarian cancer. It should be noted that most LHRH agonists used in clinical trials and practice today have been designed to exert maximal activity at the pituitary level. Direct effects on ovarian cancer and other extrapituitary sites may be only a side-action of these analogs. Potent LHRH antagonists free of side effects are now available and must be thoroughly investigated, since they could prove superior to the agonists in the treatment of ovarian cancer. Experimental work on LHRH antagonists in ovarian cancer is in progress and phase I/phase II clinical trials are in preparation.

ACKNOWLEDGEMENT

Experimental work was supported by the Deutsche Forschungs-gemeinschaft (SFB-215, B10, Graduiertenkolleg 'Zell- und Tumor-biologie'), Ferring Arzneimittel GmbH, Kiel, Germany, and the P. E. Kempkes and A. and U. Kulemann Foundations, Marburg, Germany.

References

1. Ozols, R. F., Rubin, S. C., Dembo, A. J. and Robboy, S. (1992). Epithelial ovarian cancer. In Hoskins, W. J., Perez, S. A. and Young, R. C. (eds.) *Principles and Practice of Gynecologic Oncology*, pp. 731–81. (Philadelphia: Lippincott)

2. Hoskins, W. J. (1994). Epithelial ovarian carcinoma: principles of primary surgery. *Gynecol. Oncol.*, **55**, 591–6

3. Stewart, L. A. for the Advanced Ovarian Cancer Trialist Group (1991). Chemotherapy in advanced ovarian cancer: an overview of randomized clinical trials. *Br. Med. J.*, **303**, 884–93

4. Christian, M. C. and Trimble, E. L. (1994). Salvage chemotherapy for epithelial ovarian carcinoma. *Gynecol. Oncol.*, **55**, S143–50

5. National Institutes of Health Consensus Development Conference Statement (1994). Ovarian cancer: screening, treatment and follow-up. *Gynecol. Oncol.*, **55**, S4–14

6. Neijt, J. (1994). Advances in the chemotherapy of gynecologic cancer. *Curr. Opin. Oncol.*, **6**, 531–8

7. ten Bokkel Huinink, W. W., Eisenhauer, E. and Swenerton, K. for the Canadian–European Taxol Cooperative Trial Group (1993). Preliminary evaluation of a multicenter randomized comparative study of TAXOL (paclitaxel) dose and infusion length in platinum treated ovarian cancer. *Cancer Treat. Rev.*, **19** (Suppl. C), 79–86

8. Trimble, E. L., Adams, J. D., Vena, P., Hawkins, M. J., Friedman, M. A., Fisherman, J. S., Christian, M. C., Canetta, R., Onetto, N., Hayn, R. and Arbuck, S. G. (1993). Paclitaxel for platinum-refractory ovarian cancer: results from the first 1,000 patients registered to National Cancer Institute treatment referral center 9103. *J. Clin. Oncol.*, **11**, 2405–10

9. McGuire, W. P., Hoskins, W. J., Brady, M. F., Kucera, P. E., Partridge, E. E., Look, K. Y. and Davidson, M. for the Gynecologic Oncology Group (1995). Taxol and cisplatin (TP) improves outcome in advanced ovarian cancer as compared to cytoxan and cisplatin (CP). *31st Annual Meeting, American Society of Clinical Oncology*, May, Los Angeles, abstr. 771

10. Kaldor, J. M., Day, N. E., Petterson, F., Clarke, E. A., Pedersen, D., Mehnert, W., Bell, J., Host, H., Prior, P., Karjalainen, S., Neal, F., Koch, M., Band, P., Choi, W., Kirn, V. P., Arslan, A., Zaren, B., Belch, A. R., Storm, H., Kittelmann, B., Fraser, P. and Stovall, M. (1990). Leukemia following chemotherapy for ovarian cancer. *N. Engl. J. Med.*, **322**, 1–6

11. Cheruku, R., Hussain, M., Tyrkus, M. and Edelstein, M. (1993). Myelodysplastic syndrome after cis-platin therapy. *Cancer*, **72**, 213–18

12. Colon-Otero, G., Malkasian, G. P. and Edmonson, J. H. (1993). Secondary myelodysplasia and acute leukemia following carboplatin-containing chemotherapy for ovarian cancer. *J. Natl. Cancer Inst.*, **85**, 1858–60

13. Rao, B. R. and Slotman, B. J. (1991). Endocrine factors in common epithelial ovarian cancer. *Endocr. Rev.*, **12**, 14–26

14. Emons, G. and Schally, A. V. (1994). The use of luteinizing hormone releasing hormone agonists and antagonists in gynecological cancers. *Hum. Reprod.*, **9**, 1364–79

15. Emons, G. and Schulz, K.-D. (1995). New developments in the hormonal treatment of endometrial and ovarian cancer. In Jonat, W. and Kaufmann, M. (eds.) *Hormone Dependent Tumors, Basic Research and Clinical Studies*, in press. (Basel: Karger)

16. Emons, G. and Schulz, K.-D. (1995). Growth regulation of epithelial ovarian cancer by hormones, peptide growth factors, and cytokines. In Pasqualini, J. R. and Katzenellenbogen, B. S. (eds.) *Hormone Dependent Cancer*, in press. (New York: Marcel Dekker)

17. Schally, A. V. (1994). Hypothalamic hormones: from neuroendocrinology to cancer therapy. *Anticancer Drugs*, **5**, 115–30

18. Schally, A. V., Comaru-Schally, A. M. and Hollander, V. (1993). Hypothalamic and other peptide hormones. In Holland, J.-F., Frei, E., Bast, R. C., Kufe, D. W., Morton, D. L. and Weichselbaum, R. R. (eds.) *Cancer Medicine*, 3rd edn, pp. 827–40. (Philadelphia: Lea & Febiger)

19. Mortel, R., Satyaswaroop, P. G., Schally, A. V., Hamilton, T. and Ozols, R. (1986). Inhibitory effect of GnRH superagonist on the growth of human ovarian carcinoma NIH:OVCAR-3 in the nude mouse. *Gynecol. Oncol.*, **23**, 254–5

20. Peterson, C. M. and Zimniski, S. J. (1990). A long acting gonadotropin-releasing hormone agonist inhibits the growth of a human ovarian epithelial carcinoma (BG-1) heterotransplanted in the nude mouse. *Obstet. Gynecol.*, **76**, 264–7

21. Parmar, H., Nicoll, J., Stockdale, A., Cassoni, A., Phillips, R. H., Lightman, S. L. and Schally, A. V. (1985). Advanced ovarian carcinoma: response to the agonist D-Trp[6]LHRH. *Cancer Treat. Rep.*, **69**, 1341–2

22. Kullander, S., Rausing, A. and Schally, A. V. (1987). LH-RH agonist treatment in ovarian cancer. In Klijn, J. G. M. (ed.) *Hormonal Manipulation of Cancer: Peptides, Growth Factors and New (Anti)Steroidal Agents*, pp. 353–6. (New York: Raven Press)

23. Parmar, H., Rustin, F., Lightman, S. L., Phillips, R. H., Hanham, J. W. and Schally, A. V. (1988). Response to D-Trp[6]-luteinizing hormone-releasing hormone (Decapeptyl) microcapsules in advanced ovarian cancer. *Br. Med. J.*, **296**, 1229

24. Parmar, H., Phillips, R. H., Rustin, F., Lightman, S. L., Hanham, J. W. and Schally, A. V. (1988). Therapy of advanced ovarian cancer with D-Trp[6]LH-RH (Decapeptyl) microcapsules. *Biochem. Pharmacother.*, **42**, 531–8

25. Jäger, W., Wildt, L. and Lang, N. (1989). Some observations on the effects of a GnRH analog in ovarian cancer. *Eur. J. Obstet. Gynecol. Reprod. Biol.*, **32**, 137–48

26. Bruckner, H. W. and Motwani, B. T. (1989). Treatment of advanced refractory ovarian carcinoma with a gonadotropin-releasing hormone analogue. *Am. J. Obstet. Gynecol.*, **161**, 1216–18

27. Kavanagh, J. J., Roberts, W., Townsend, P. and Hewitt, S. (1989). Leuprolide acetate in the treament of refractory or persistent epithelial ovarian cancer. *J. Clin. Oncol.*, **7**, 115–8

28. Vavra, N., Barrada, M., Fitz, R., Sevelda, P., Baur, M. and Dittrich, C. (1990). Goserelin – eine neue Form der Hormontherapie beim Ovarialkarzinom. *Gynakol. Geburtshilfliche. Rundsch.*, **30** (Suppl. 1), 61–3

29. Lind, M. J., Cantwell, B. M. J., Millward, M. J., Robinson, A., Proctor, M., Simmons, D., Carmichael, J. and Harris, A. L. (1992). A phase II trial of goserelin (Zoladex) in relapsed epithelial ovarian cancer. *Br. J. Cancer*, **65**, 621–3

30. van der Burg, M. E. L., ten Bokkel Huinink, W. W., Kobiersky, A., Namer, M., Vermorken, J. B., Tumolo, S., Aapro, M., Neijt, J. P., Veenhof, C. N. N., van Oosterom, A. T., Renard, J., Buyse, M. and Pecorelli, S. (1993). Chemotherapy and hormonal treatment in ovarian cancer: experiences of the EORTC gynecological cancer cooperative group. In Meerpohl, H. G., Pfleiderer, A. and Profous., C. Z. (eds.) *Das Ovarialkarzinom*, Vol. 2, pp. 114–31. (Heidelberg, Berlin, New York: Springer Verlag)

31. Emons, G., Ortmann, O., Pahwa, G. S., Hackenberg, R., Oberheuser, F. and Schulz, K.-D. (1992). Intracellular actions of gonadotropic and peptide hormones and the therapeutic value of GnRH-agonists in ovarian cancer. *Acta Obstet. Gynecol. Scand.*, **71** (Suppl. 155), 31–8

32. Emons, G., Ortmann, O., Pahwa, G. S., Oberheuser, F. and Schulz, K.-D. (1992). LH-RH agonists in the treatment of ovarian cancer. *Recent Results Cancer Res.*, **124**, 55–68

33. Erickson, L. D., Hartmann, L. C., Su, J. Q., Nielsen, S. N. J., Pfeifel, D. M., Goldberg, R. M., Levitt, R. and Stanhope, C. M. (1994). Cyclophosphamide, cisplatin and leuprolide acetate in patients with debulked stage III or IV ovarian carcinoma. *Gynecol. Oncol.*, **54**, 196–200

34. Emons, G., Pahwa, G. S., Brack, C., Sturm, R., Oberheuser, F. and Knuppen, R. (1989). Gonadotropin releasing hormone binding sites in human epithelial ovarian carcinomata. *Eur. J. Cancer Clin. Oncol.*, **25**, 215–21

35. Pahwa, G. S., Vollmer, G., Knuppen, R. and Emons, G. (1989). Photoaffinity labelling of gonadotropin releasing hormone binding sites in human epithelial ovarian carcinomata. *Biochem. Biophys. Res. Commun.*, **161**, 1086–92

36. Emons, G., Ortmann, O., Becker, M., Irmer, G., Springer, B., Laun, R., Hölzel, F., Schulz, K.-D. and Schally, A. V. (1993). High affinity binding and direct antiproliferative effects of LH-RH analogues in human ovarian cancer cell lines. *Cancer Res.*, **54**, 5439–46

37. Irmer, G., Bürger, C., Müller, R., Ortmann, O., Peter, U., Kakar, S. S., Neill, J. D., Schulz, K.-D. and Emons, G. (1995). Expression of the messenger ribonucleic acids for luteinizing hormone releasing hormone and its receptors in human ovarian epithelial carcinoma. *Cancer Res.*, **55**, 817–22

38. Kakar, S. S., Musgrove, L. C., Devar, D. C., Sellers, J. C. and Neill, J. D. (1992). Cloning, sequencing, and expression of human gonadotropin releasing hormone (GnRH) receptor. *Biochem. Biophys. Res. Commun.*, **189**, 289–95

39. Imai, A., Ohno, T., Iida, K., Fuseya, T., Furui, T. and Tamaya, T. (1994). Gonadotropin-releasing hormone receptor in gynecological tumors. *Cancer*, **74**, 2555–61

40. Yano, T., Pinski, J., Radulovic, S. and Schally, A. V. (1994). Inhibition of human epithelial ovarian cancer cell growth *in vitro* by agonistic and antagonistic analogues of luteinizing hormone-releasing hormone. *Proc. Natl. Acad. Sci. USA*, **91**, 1701–4

41. Kakar, S. S., Grizzle, W. E. and Neill, J. D. (1994). The nucleotide sequences of human GnRH receptors in breast and ovarian tumors are identical with that found in pituitary. *Mol. Cell. Endocrinol.*, **106**, 145–9

42. Peterson, C. M., Jolles, C. J., Carrell, D. T., Straight, R. C., Parker-Jones, K., Poulson, A. M. Jr. and Hatasaka, H. (1994). GnRH agonist therapy in human ovarian epithelial carcinoma (OVCAR-3) heterotransplanted in the nude mouse is characterized by latency and transience. *Gynecol. Oncol.*, **52**, 26–30

43. Connor, J. P., Buller, R. E. and Conn, P. M. (1994). Effects of GnRH analogs on six ovarian cancer cell lines in culture. *Gynecol. Oncol.*, **54**, 80–6

44. Ohno, T., Imai, A., Furui, T., Takahashi, K. and Tamaya, T. (1993). Presence of gonadotropin-releasing hormone and its messenger ribonucleic acid in human ovarian epithelial carcinoma. *Am. J. Obstet. Gynecol.*, **169**, 605–10

45. Slotman, B. J., Poels, L. G. and Rao, B. R. (1989). A direct LH-RH agonist action on cancer cells is unlikely to be the cause of response to LH-RH agonist treatment. *Anticancer Res.*, **9**, 77–80

46. Thompson, M. A., Adelson, M. D. and Kaufman, L. M. (1991). Lupron retards proliferation of ovarian tumor cells cultured in serum-free medium. *J. Clin. Endocrinol. Metab.*, **72**, 1036–41

47. Manetta, A., Gamboa-Vujicic, L., Paredes, P., Emma, D., Liao, S., Leong, L., Asch, B. and Schally, A. V. (1995). Inhibition of growth of human ovarian cancer in nude mice by luteinizing hormone-releasing hormone antagonist cetrorelix (SB-75). *Fertil. Steril.*, **6**, 282–7

48. Emons, G., Schröder, B., Ortmann, O., Westphalen, S., Schulz, K.-D. and Schally, A. V. (1993). High affinity binding and direct antiproliferative effects of luteinizing hormone releasing homone analogs in human endometrial cancer cell lines. *J. Clin. Endocrinol. Metab.*, **77**, 1458–64

49. Irmer, G., Bürger, C., Ortmann, O., Schulz, K.-D. and Emons, G. (1994). Expression of luteinizing hormone releasing hormone and its m-RNA in human endometrial cancer cell lines. *J. Clin. Endocrinol. Metab.*, **79**, 916–9

50. Srkalovic, G., Wittliff, J. R. and Schally, A. V. (1990). Detection and partial characterization of receptor for [D-Trp^6] luteinizing hormone releasing hormone and epidermal growth factor in human endometrial carcinoma. *Cancer Res.*, **50**, 1841–6

51. Pahwa, G. S., Kullander, S., Vollmer, G., Oberheuser, F., Knuppen, R. and Emons, G. (1991). Specific low affinity binding sites for gonadotropin releasing hormone in human endometrial carcinomata. *Eur. J. Obstet. Gynecol. Reprod. Biol.*, **41**, 135–42

52. Yano, T., Pinski, J., Halmos, G., Szepeshazi, K., Groot, K. and Schally, A. V. (1994). Inhibition of growth of OV-1063 human epithelial ovarian cancer xenografts in nude mice by treatment with luteinizing hormone-releasing hormone antagonist SB-75. *Proc. Natl. Acad. Sci. USA*, **91**, 7090–4

53. Shirahige, Y., Cook, C. B., Pinski, J., Halmos, G., Nair, R. and Schally, A. V. (1994). Treatment with luteinizing hormone-releasing hormone antagonist SB-75 decreases levels of epidermal growth factor receptor and its mRNA in OV-1063 human epithelial ovarian cancer xenografts in nude mice. *Int. J. Oncol.*, **5**, 1031-5

Investigation of mechanisms responsible for the successful treatment of endometrial cancer with GnRH analogs

21

C. M. R. Bax, E. Chatzaki and C. J. Gallagher

INTRODUCTION

Endometrial cancer is the second most common pelvic malignancy in the United Kingdom. Although endometrial cancer usually presents at an early stage when it can be cured by primary surgery, approximately 25% of all women diagnosed with endometrial cancer die within 5 years, often having presented with apparently early-stage disease. Many of those at high risk of recurrence can be recognized by the already well described prognostic factors of depth of myometrial invasion, histological grade and cell type, and lymphatic invasion, so that local adjuvant radiotherapy can be applied to reduce the risk of local recurrence. However, there are many for whom the current prognostic factors are inadequate and in whom a better understanding of the biology predicting metastatic potential may be provided by the presence of molecular biological markers such as activated *ras* and *myc* oncogenes.

It has long been appreciated that the cyclical response of the uterine epithelium to variations in estrogen and progesterone concentrations during the menstrual cycle reflect the sensitivity of the mechanisms controlling its proliferation to stimulation by estrogen or inhibition by progesterone. A proportion of endometrial cancers retain the growth-controlling mechanisms of the normal endometrium and can be partly identified by their possession of estrogen and progesterone receptors. However, the correlation is not exact and, as has been appreciated with immuno-histological studies, there is considerable heterogeneity of expression of the receptors by cells within any one tumor. It may be their relative preponderance that determines whether there is tumor regression and a response to progesterone, and for how long that is maintained before the hormone-independent tumor cells grow and reform the tumor.

With the advent of long-lasting synthetic progestogens, several early series in the 1960s reported clinical response rates of 30–40% in recurrent endometrial carcinoma[1,2]. The response rate can be correlated with both tumor differentiation and expression of progestogen receptors, but does not appear to be affected by the type of progestogen administered, the route or the dose above a threshold value of 300 mg/day of medroxyprogesterone acetate or 160 mg/day of megestrol acetate. However, more recent reports have documented a lower response rate of 17–20%, perhaps reflecting a changing patient population, as in one series the response rate for well differentiated tumors was 40–60% compared with 0–10% in poorly differentiated receptor-negative tumors. The overall long-term survival, however, is only 10%, with the median duration of response of 8 months in the more recent reports. Both tamoxifen and aromatase inhibitors have been tested in recurrent endometrial cancer with variable results, from 30% response in one small series to 0% in a subsequent larger series, suggesting that responses are possible but probably uncommon. Attempts at receptor modulation by alternating tamoxifen and progestogens have also been tested, without obvious advantage.

CLINICAL STUDY OF GnRH ANALOG TREATMENT OF ENDOMETRIAL CANCER

The use of gonadotropin releasing hormone (GnRH) analogs to produce medical castration in the treatment of hormone-sensitive carcinomas of the breast and prostate is well known. However, for some time it has been suggested that there is direct extrapituitary role for GnRH, particularly in tissues of the reproductive tract. Reports of responses to GnRH in 10% of women with recurrent ovarian cancer, and the laboratory data for the presence of GnRH binding in ovarian and prostatic tissue support the idea of a possible direct effect of GnRH on tumor growth. We began to examine the effect of GnRH analogs on recurrent endometrial cancer in 1989[3] and, together with colleagues in the London Gynaecological Oncology Group, have now treated 32 postmenopausal women with recurrent metastatic endometrial carcinoma.

The aim of the study was to document the changes in gonadotropins and sex hormones associated with GnRH analog treatment in post-menopausal women using an appropriately sensitive assay[4], and the response to GnRH analog treatment in measurable lesions according to standard Union Internationale Contre Cancer criteria. In order to be eligible, patients had to have had locally recurrent or metastatic endometrial cancer following primary surgery and/or radiation treatment with or without progestogens. If they were currently receiving progestogens, these were stopped for a minimum of 4 weeks prior to GnRH analog treatment and all patients had measurable disease with no other primary malignancy. All patients gave informed written consent according to local ethical committee requirements.

The results of treatment are available in 32 patients, in 17 of whom previous progestogen therapy had failed. The serum hormonal analysis showed the rapid and expected fall in gonadotropins within the first 2 weeks of treatment, but no significant change in serum estradiol levels in these postmenopausal women, apart from in one patient who had not had a bilateral salpingo-oophorectomy at primary diagnosis but had received radiation treatment with retention of her ovarian stroma. In this patient, serum estradiol levels fell from the postmenopausal level of 100 pmol/l to 40 mol/l, consistent with the level found in the other oophorectomized women. No toxicity was experienced, apart from minor injection site reactions in two women. Response was rapid and prolonged remission of 5 or more years have been seen in 25% of women.

LABORATORY STUDY OF THE ACTION OF GnRH ANALOGS ON ENDOMETRIAL CANCER

The number of responses occurring in women who had previously failed to respond to progestogens stimulated our interest in the underlying mechanism by which the GnRH analogs might inhibit tumor growth. We undertook to investigate the hypothesis that the GnRH analogs were acting directly on the tumor cells by investigating the evidence for the presence of biologically active GnRH receptors on the surface of the endometrial cancer cells. Such an extrapituitary site of action had been previously postulated to exist in the placenta and ovary and there had been one previous report of GnRH analog binding to endometrial cancer cells[5]. We initially investigated the effects of GnRH analogs upon the secretory activity of Ishikawa endometrial cancer cells and of freshly cultured placental trophoblast, and upon the growth of the endo-metrial cancer lines HEC-1A and Ishikawa. In order to investigate the mechanism further, we compared GnRH analog binding in these cells and compared it to that in the GnRH receptor-positive αT3-1 pituitary cell line[6].

GROWTH AND SECRETION EXPERIMENTS

Experiments were performed with the Ishikawa endometrial cancer cell line. The effects of GnRH upon growth in cell number, DNA content and DNA [^{3}H]thymidine incorporation were measured, along with the effect upon secretion by the cells of placental alkaline phosphatase[7].

We observed significant differences in the effect of GnRH and its analogs, depending upon the conditions under which the cell lines or freshly derived cultures were prepared. In the presence of fetal calf serum, GnRH and its analog leuprorelin inhibited the number of viable Ishikawa cells. This effect was also observed when the cells were cultured in the presence of the serum substitute Ultraser G (Gibco, Paisley, United Kingdom) along with a stimulation of placental alkaline phosphatase secretion by the Ishikawa cells (Figure 1). However, no change was observed in total DNA content of the cultures (Figure 2B) in the absence of serum, and with charcoal stripped serum in phenol red free medium only a transient and inconsistent suppression of [³H]thymidine uptake was observed (Figure 2A).

These results, while tending to support the hypothesis that GnRH analogs may exert a direct effect upon endometrial cancer growth, are also open to alternative interpretations in view of the dependence of the effect upon the presence of fetal calf serum. Simple replacement of estradiol and epidermal growth factor did not restore the effect of the charcoal-stripped fetal calf serum and, in order to establish whether we were observing a GnRH receptor mediated event, further experiments were performed to examine ligand binding and GnRH receptor signal transduction in these cultures.

Standard displacement binding curves were obtained using freshly labelled high specific activity with native GnRH or the GnRH analogs goserelin, leuprorelin or D-Trp⁶-ethylamide. Membrane preparations from αT3-1 pituitary cells were used to standardize the assay and were compared with the binding to trophoblast and Ishikawa cell membranes. Using the membranes prepared from the αT3-1 cells an dissociation constant (K_d) of 6.6×10^{-9} mol/l was obtained with a B_{max} of 1.35×10^{-9} mol/mg for native GnRH whilst the values for the goserelin analog were K_d 2×10^{-9} mol/l and B_{max} 1.79×10^{-12} mol/mg (Figure 3). These values were within the expected range for pituitary gonadotropes and compare with the low affinity extrapituitary binding sites on the placental trophoblast: K_d 1.5×10^{-7} mol/l and B_{max} 9.4×10^{-8} mol/mg for GnRH and K_d 5.8×10^{-7} mol/l with B_{max} 63.9×10^{-12} mol/mg for goserelin (Figures 4 and 5). Membranes prepared from the Ishikawa cells demonstrated similar total binding to that observed with the trophoblast membranes, some of which was displaceable by cold GnRH or GnRH analog. However, it was of such low affinity in

(A)

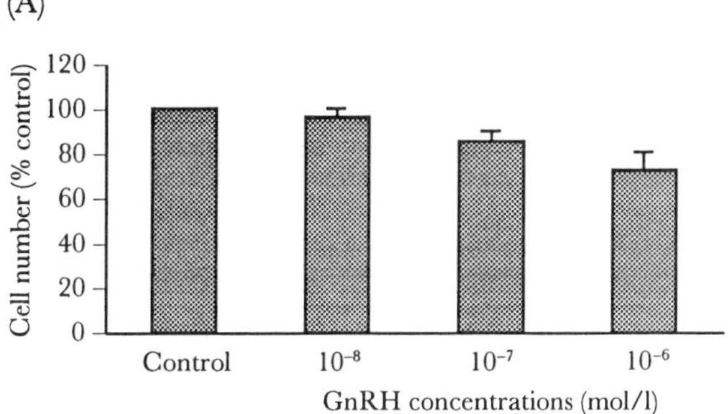

(B)

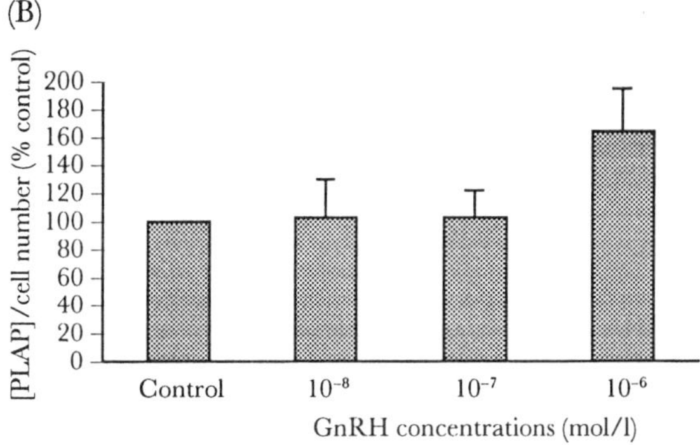

(C)

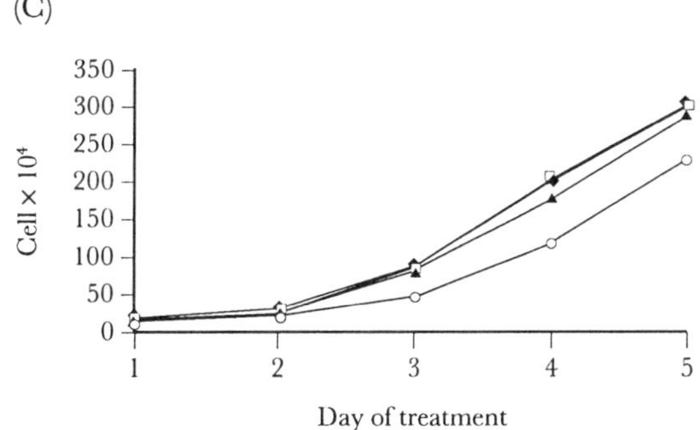

Figure 1 Ishikawa cells were cultured in DMEM (Dulbecco's modified Eagle's medium)/F10 with 10% Ultraser G and viable cells harvested and counted after 4 days of exposure to varying concentrations of GnRH (mean and SD of three measurements) (A). Culture supernatant from the same Ishikawa cells was assayed by radioimmunoassay for placental alkaline phosphatase (PLAP) after 4 days' exposure to varying concentrations of GnRH (B). Changes in Ishikawa cell number were assessed with serial estimations over 5 days at varying concentrations of GnRH in the presence of DMEM/F10 and Ultraser G (C). $\blacklozenge$, Control; $\square$, GnRH, (10^{-8} mol/l); $\blacktriangle$, GnRH (10^{-7} mol/l); $\bigcirc$, GnRH (10^{-6} mol/l).

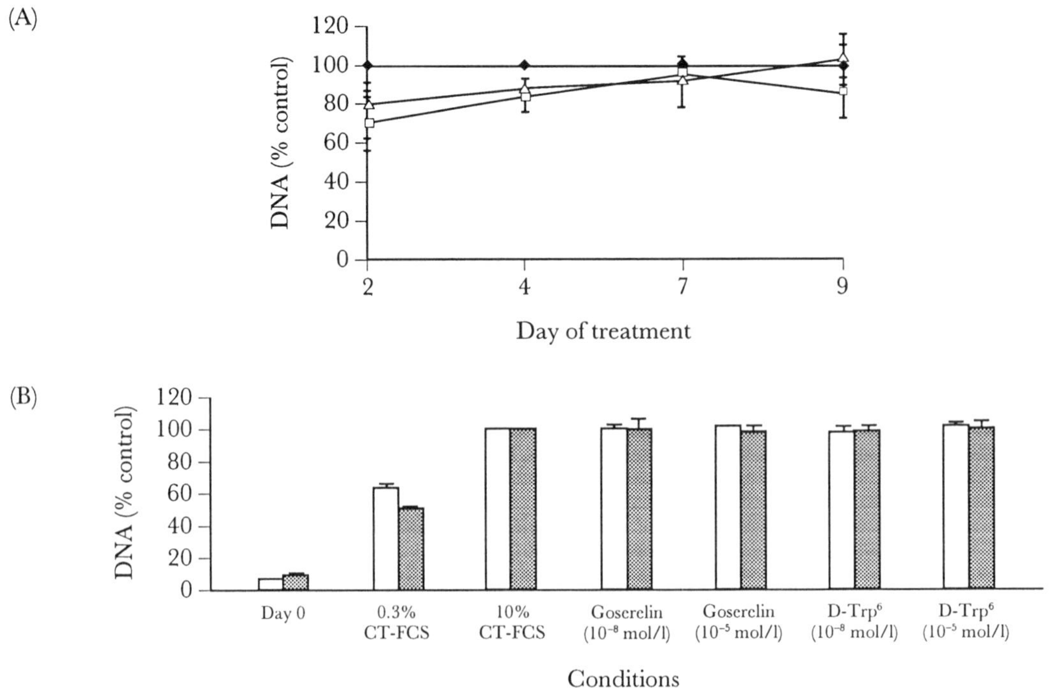

Figure 2 Changes in Ishikawa cell [³H]thymidine uptake (A) with serial estimation over 9 days at varying concentrations of leuprorelin when cultured without serum (mean and SD of three measurements). ◆, Control; △, leuprolide (10^{-7} mol/l); □, leuprolide (10^{-8} mol/l). Changes in Ishikawa and HEC-1A total DNA content (B) after exposure to varying concentrations of goserelin and D-Trp⁶-ethylamide when cultured with charcoal stripped serum in phenol red free DMEM/F12 medium. CT-FCS, charcoal-treated fetal calf serum; □, HEC-1A; ▨, Ishikawa.

comparison with the αT3-1 cells or the trophoblast cells that no reliable measurement could be made of either K_d or B_{max} by Scatchard analysis. These findings were unaffected by whether early or late passage cell lines were used, whether the cells were in log phase growth or confluent quiescent state, and whether they were cultured in the presence or absence of fetal calf serum and a variety of other medium supplements.

GnRH RECEPTOR SIGNAL TRANSDUCTION

In parallel with the binding experiments we also investigated whether GnRH or its analogs produced any evidence of receptor-mediated signal transduction in whole cells, in case the membrane binding experiments had failed to detect the expression of variant receptor sites in the

extrapituitary tissues by which ligand might still be able to have a biological effect.

The GnRH receptor belongs to a family of small peptide hormone receptors with seven transmembrane domains, but no integral tyrosine kinase activity. Signalling is believed to be mediated by G-proteins coupled to phosphoinositide-specific phospholipase C or adenylate cyclase. In this way either the second messenger inositol 1,4,5-triphosphate (IP_3) is produced to elevate cytoplasmic calcium concentrations or cyclic AMP is generated to activate other protein kinases and transcription factors. In the pituitary, gonadotropin secretion is a calcium-dependent process linked to the production of IP_3, whereas the role of cyclic AMP is still unclear. Even less has been previously described about the postulated effect of GnRH on the secretion of human chorionic gonadotropin (hCG) by the trophoblast.

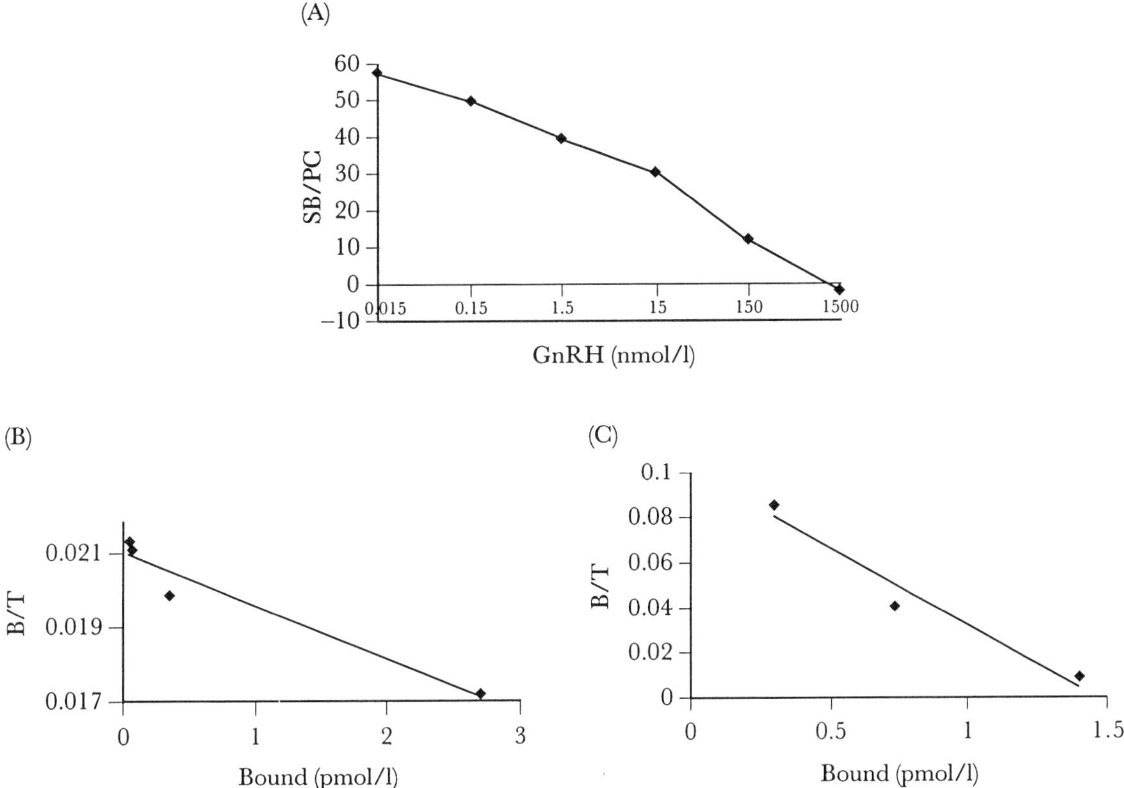

Figure 3 Displacement binding curve for freshly labelled [^{125}I]GnRH and the membrane fraction of pituitary αT3-1 (A). Scatchard plots for GnRH (B) and goserelin (C) binding to αT3-1 cell membranes. B/T, bound/total; SB/PC, specific binding per unit of membrane protein (c.p.m./μg)

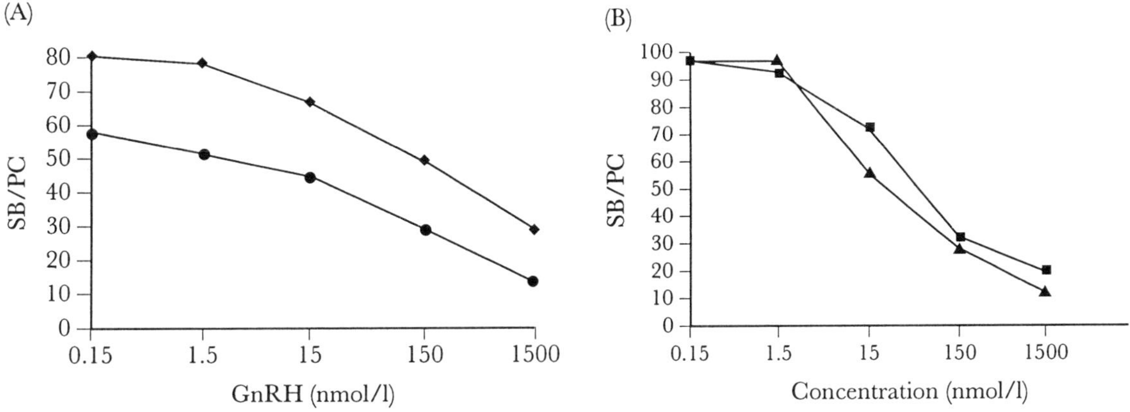

Figure 4 Displacement binding curve for [^{125}I]GnRH and whole membrane fraction of cytotrophoblast and syncytiotrophoblast (A). ♦, Cytoblast; ●, syncytiotrophoblast. Displacement binding curve comparing GnRH and leuprorelin binding to syncytiotrophoblast membranes (B). SB/PC defined in Figure 3. ▲, GnRH; ■, leuprolide

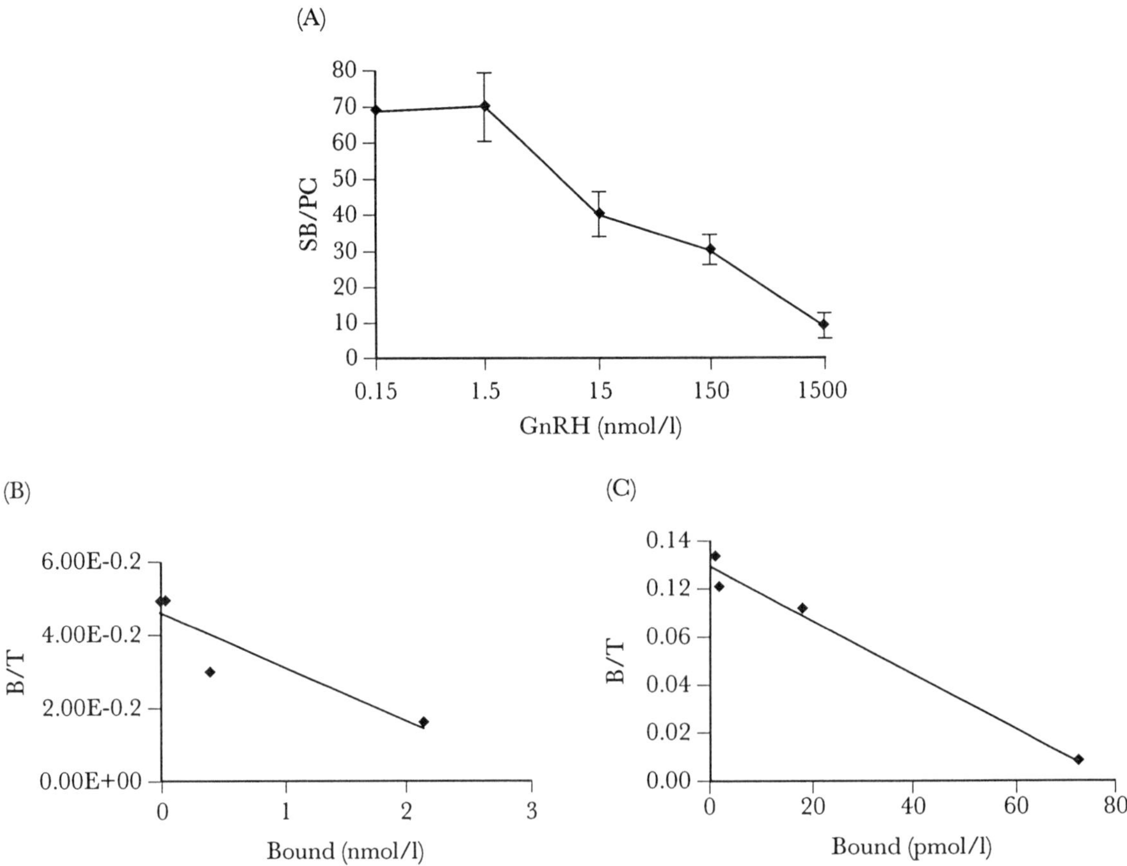

Figure 5 Displacement binding curve for [^{125}I]GnRH and trophoblast membranes (A). Scatchard plots for GnRH (B) and goserelin (C) binding to trophoblast membranes. B/T and SB/PC defined in Figure 3

Cytosolic calcium concentration was measured in fura-2 loaded cell suspensions of endometrial cancer cell lines and trophoblast cells and compared with the pituitary αT3-1 cells. In the αT3-1 cells GnRH at 10^{-9} mol/l and GnRH analog at 10^{-10} mol/l were able to elevate cytoplasmic calcium concentration from a resting level of 62 nmol/l to a peak of 110 nmol/l in a characteristic receptor-mediated response. No such response could be established in the Ishikawa cells. In addition, even though we could confirm that GnRH stimulated the production of free β-hCG by cultured trophoblasts (Figure 6), we could not show evidence for signal transduction by calcium concentration modulation that would support the hypothesis that this was a receptor-mediated event (Figure 7). All cells, however, retained their ability to respond to either ATP or fetal calf serum, confirming that their signal transduction mechanisms were intact. Further variations in culture conditions with respect to the presence or absence of fetal calf serum, growth factors or estrogens did not influence these findings.

DISCUSSION

GnRH analogs continue to provide some women with recurrent endometrial cancer a prolonged-relapse-free survival and excellent quality of life. We have found that on examination of endometrial cancer cell lines certain culture conditions may permit GnRH or its analogs to inhibit cell growth

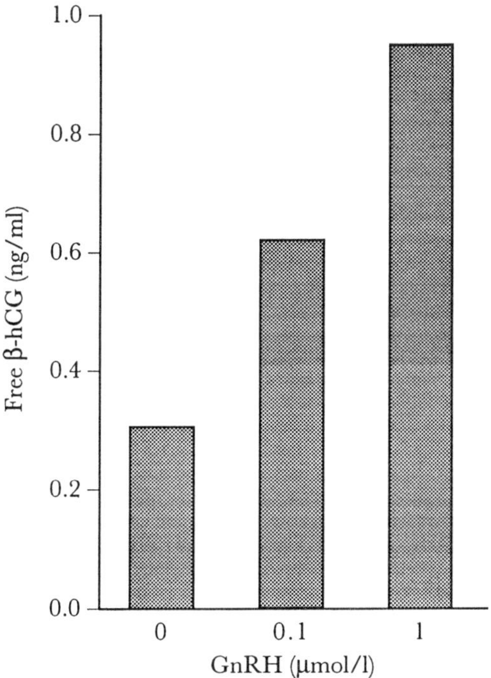

Figure 6 Secretion of free β-hCG by trophoblast in response to GnRH

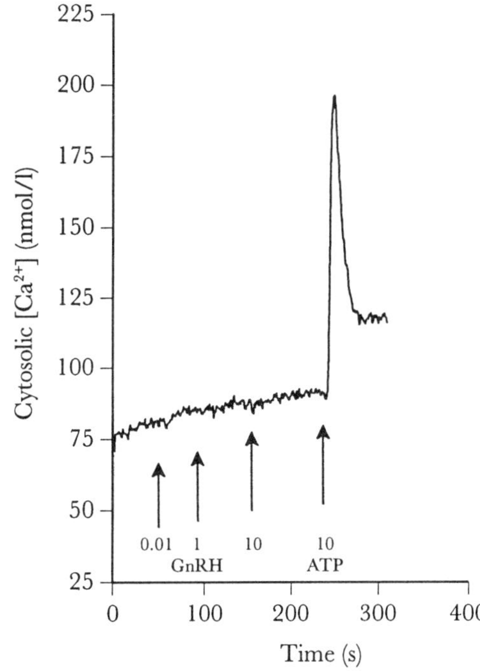

Figure 7 Cytosolic [Ca^{2+}] of cytotrophoblast cells following additions of GnRH (0.01–10 μM) or ATP (10 μM)

or stimulate their secretion of placental alkaline phosphatase. Similarly, GnRH is able to stimulate the secretion of hCG by cultured trophoblast cells. However, we could find no convincing evidence that these effects were mediated by GnRH receptors in comparison with pituitary GnRH receptor-positive cells. The pituitary cells expressed high-affinity binding sites and upon exposure to ligand there was intracellular calcium release. In contrast, the normal trophoblast and Ishikawa cells exhibited low-affinity binding with no associated intracellular signalling.

Therefore, we were unable to demonstrate a mechanism by which GnRH could exert a direct extrapituitary action and it remains to be seen whether the stimulation of secretion can be explained by some alternative pathway.

These results are in contrast with previous reports of high-affinity binding sites in freshly prepared endometrial cell membranes and the suppression of growth of endometrial cancer cell lines by GnRH analogs[5,8]. Expression of GnRH receptors may vary according to culture conditions that we were unable to reproduce or be a property of a minority population of the epithelial or accompanying cells. However, we are sure that with the quality of the positive controls included in our experiments we found no convincing evidence for a direct GnRH receptor-mediated effect of GnRH or its analogs upon tropohoblastic or Ishikawa cells. The study serves to emphasize the importance of constructing a complete chain of evidence before construing the presence of binding to cell membranes or the expression of receptor RNA as evidence for a biologically significant receptor-mediated mechanism by which cell behavior may be modulated in an autocrine or a paracrine manner. Further experiments are in progress to investigate alternative mechanisms by which GnRH analogs may suppress endometrial cancers *in vivo* and afford successful treatment for women with recurrent disease.

References

1. Kelley, R. M. and Baker, W. H. (1965). Progestational agents in the treatment of carcinoma of the endometrium. *N. Engl. J. Med.*, **246**, 216–22

2. Reifenstein, E. C. (1974). The treatment of advanced endometrial cancer with hydroxyprogesterone caproate. *Gynecol. Oncol.*, **2**, 377–414

3. Gallagher, C. J., Oliver, R. T. D., Oram, D. H., Fowler, C. G., Blake, P. R., Mantell, B. S., Slevin, M. L. and Hope-Stone, H. F. (1991). A new treatment for endometrial cancer with gonadotrophin releasing-hormone analogue. *Br. J. Obstet. Gynaecol.*, **98**, 1037–41

4. Dowsett, M., Gross, P. E, Powles, T. J., Hutchinson, G. and Brodie, A. M. (1987). Use of aromatase inhibitor 4-hydroxyandrosteredione in postmenopausal breast cancer: optimisation of therapeutic dose and route. *Cancer Res.*, **47**, 1957–61

5. Srkalovic, G., Witliff, J. C. and Schally, A. V. (1990). Detection and partial characterization of receptors for (D-Trp6)-luteinizing-hormone releasing hormone and epidermal growth factor in human endometrial carcinoma. *Cancer Res.*, **50**, 1841–6

6. Windle, J. J., Weiner, R. I. and Mellon, P. L. (1990). Cell lines of the pituitary gonadotrope lineage derived by targeted oncogenesis in transgenic mice. *Mol. Endocrinol.*, **4**, 597–603

7. Chatzaki, E., Gallagher, C. J., Iles, R. K., Ind, T. E. J., Nouri, A. M. E., Bax, C. M. R. and Grudzinkas, J. G. (1994). Characterization of the differential expression of marker antigens by normal and malignant endometrial epithelium. *Br. J. Cancer*, **69**, 1010–14

8. Emons, G., Schroder, B., Ortmann, O., Westphalen, S., Schulz, K. D. and Schally, A. V. (1993). High affinity binding and direct antiproliferative efects of luteinizing hormone-releasing hormone analogs in human endometrial cancer cell lines. *J. Clin. Endocrinol. Metab.*, **77**, 1458–64

Section 6

Ovulation induction

Endocrine and clinical characteristics of different GnRH agonist regimens used for gonadotropin ovulation induction

M. Filicori, G. E. Cognigni, R. Arnone, A. Falbo, P. Pocognoli, C. Tabarelli,
F. Carbone, W. Ciampaglia, C. Pari and P. Casadio

INTRODUCTION

Ovulation induction has been used for over three decades for the treatment of anovulatory infertility; in these patients the goal of therapy is the achievement of the maturation and ovulation of a single follicle. However, the more recent introduction of assisted reproduction techniques has created the need for ovulation induction regimens that consistently result in the development of multiple follicles and high-quality oocytes for otherwise normally ovulatory women. In addition, standardization of treatment and easy scheduling are critical features when many patients are treated within the same ovulation induction cycle that culminates with complex assisted reproduction procedures such as *in vitro* fertilization (IVF) or intracytoplasmic sperm injection.

In the mid-1980s it was recognized that supplementing gonadotropin ovulation induction with gonadotropin releasing hormone (GnRH) agonists may result in the improved response of some patients[1] and in better endocrine features[2]. Since then, several studies have compared the outcome of assisted reproduction ovulation induction cycles conducted with and without GnRH agonist supplementation. A recent meta-analysis of 1636 cycles in ten trials[3] demonstrated that GnRH agonist cycles were associated with a significantly decreased rate of cycle cancellations due to follicular luteinization or premature ovulation. This cause of treatment discontinuation, which used to occur in one-third of cycles in which gonadotropin alone was used, was almost abolished by the use of GnRH

agonists. Additional advantages of this approach[3] include increased clinical pregnancy rates per assisted reproduction cycle commenced and per embryo transfer. The spontaneous abortion rate was not increased by the addition of GnRH agonists.

Because of these and other advantages[4], GnRH agonists have been adopted in virtually every assisted reproduction program worldwide. However, several different administration schedules have been devised. This paper reviews the endocrine and clinical characteristics of these regimens.

GnRH AGONIST REGIMENS

Numerous GnRH agonist and gonadotropin administration schedules have been devised. All of these regimens share the goal of preventing the endogenous preovulatory luteinizing hormone (LH) surge, thus avoiding the risk of premature follicular luteinization and ovulation. Additional specific features are discussed in the following sections. Treatment regimens can be grouped into four major categories (Figure 1).

Long regimens

The use of long regimens represents the earliest and most commonly applied schedule. The finding that beginning GnRH agonist administration in the luteal phase causes faster pituitary desensitization suggested that starting GnRH agonist administration about a week before expected menses could result in sufficient therapeutic efficacy. Several published studies

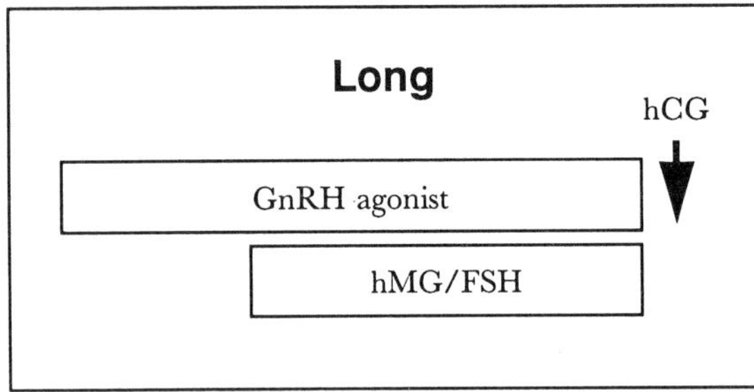

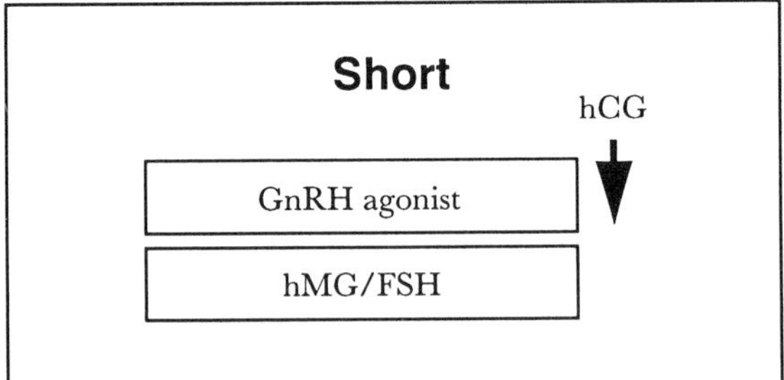

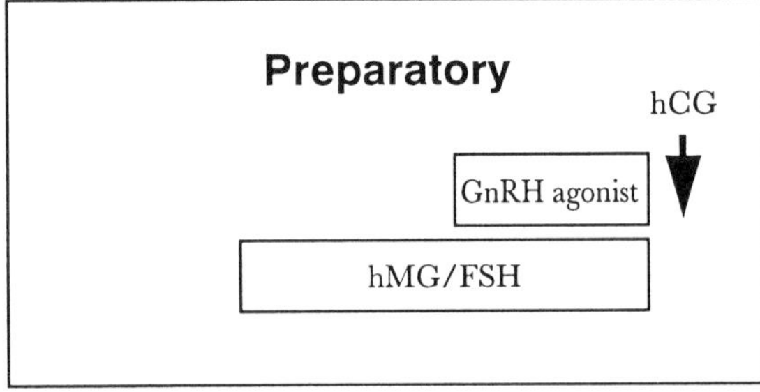

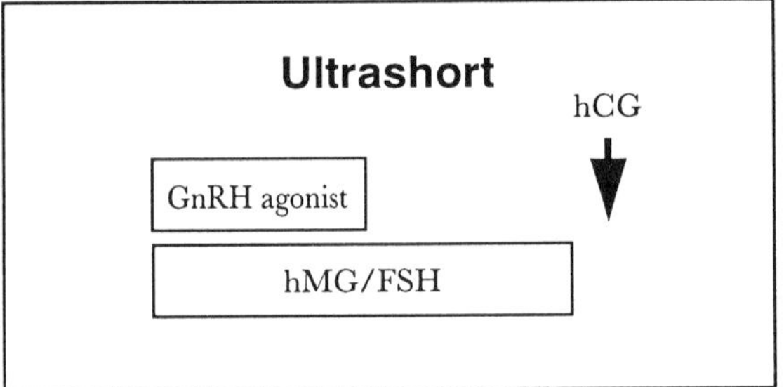

Figure 1 Schematic representation of the different ovulation induction regimens that combine exogenous gonadotropins and GnRH agonists

have demonstrated that this approach achieves very low LH levels across the follicular phase and abolishes the spontaneous mid-cycle LH surge[2,4] (Table 1). In addition, the start of GnRH agonist administration several days before the beginning of gonadotropin administration allows a fair degree of flexibility in the choice of the actual start of ovulation induction and better patient synchronization. The major drawback of this regimen is the more prolonged GnRH agonist administration and the greater amounts of exogenous gonadotropins sometimes required that render this approach more costly. Nevertheless, the better follicle yield reported in long cycles by most investigators[5–7] and the improvement in patient scheduling more than offset these economic considerations and have contributed to making this approach the most widely used in assisted reproduction.

Short (or flare-up) regimens

Early studies suggested that the high endogenous gonadotropin levels resulting from follicular phase GnRH agonist administration could be exploited to complement and enhance exogenous gonadotropins[8]. It was postulated that this could result in comparable or greater folliculogenesis with reduced exogenous gonadotropin requirements; thus, a saving could be obtained both in gonadotropin and GnRH agonist costs (due to shorter GnRH agonist administration). Unfortunately, more recent studies showed that short regimens, when compared to long regimens, are associated with a lower follicle yield[6,9], reduced embryo number and viability[9], and lower pregnancy rates[3,10,11]. Because of these disadvantages, the short GnRH agonist regimen is now employed by few centers and the number of these procedures is decreasing.

Table 1 Endocrine characteristics of different GnRH agonist regimens

Regimen	Follicular phase LH levels	Suppression of LH surge
Long	low	good
Short	high	good
Ultrashort	high	?
Preparatory	low	?

Ultrashort and preparatory regimens

Both these approaches derive from the observation that pituitary desensitization may outlast actual GnRH agonist administration by several days. Therefore, it was suggested that a shorter course of GnRH agonist could be adequate to abolish the mid-cycle LH surge[12]. In ultrashort regimens GnRH agonist administration is started in the early follicular phase and continued for just 3 days[13], whereas in preparatory regimens GnRH agonist administration is begun in the mid-luteal phase of the preceding cycle and discontinued at the start of gonadotropin administration[14]. It was recently shown that the ultrashort regimen when compared to the long regimen provided a lower follicle yield and pregnancy rate[13]. Insufficient information still exists on the preparatory regimen. For these reasons the use of ultrashort and preparatory regimens is still limited.

FORMULATIONS OF GnRH ANALOGS

GnRH agonists for ovulation induction are usually administered in short-acting preparations given through the subcutaneous route. Intranasal administration is also employed, in spite of the limited drug absorption typical of this route, as even low amounts of GnRH agonist are usually sufficient to prevent the mid-cycle LH surge. More recently, depot GnRH agonist preparations have also been used within ovulation induction programs. The major advantages of depot GnRH agonists include patient compliance and profound LH suppression for at least 28 days[15]. However, the greater cost of these preparations and concerns regarding early pregnancy exposure to GnRH agonists in conception cycles have limited their application.

Recent studies have shown that accidental GnRH administration during early pregnancy did not increase the risk of abortion or birth defects[16]. The use of depot GnRH agonists in assisted reproduction procedures did not result in an increment of abortion rates over the use of short-acting GnRH agonist preparations[17]. The development of children born after IVF conducted with GnRH agonist regimens was normal[18]. Finally, when GnRH agonists were intentionally given at high doses in the first trimester of pregnancy for the medical induction of abortion[19], progesterone and β-human chorionic gonadotropin (β-hCG) levels were unaffected and abortion had to be induced with traditional surgical procedures. Therefore, it appears that the use of long-acting depot GnRH agonist preparations is a feasible and safe way of administering these drugs in ovulation induction.

ENDOCRINE CHARACTERISTICS

We recently analyzed the clinical and endocrine characteristics of different GnRH agonist and gonadotropin regimens[6]. Four groups of ten normal women each received the following: purified follicle stimulating hormone (FSH) only (group A), purified FSH and a short GnRH agonist regimen (group B), purified FSH and a long GnRH agonist regimen (group C), and human menopausal gonadotropin (hMG) and a long GnRH agonist regimen (group D). Pelvic ultrasound scans, daily blood samples and pre-hCG follicular fluid samples were obtained in all women. Group B was associated with the lowest number of preovulatory follicles as well as high follicular phase LH, FSH, progesterone and testosterone, and high follicular fluid LH, testosterone and β-inhibin levels. No significant difference was found between purified FSH and hMG cycles (groups C and D). These findings provide a rationale for the improved clinical performance of long GnRH agonist cycles. Elevated LH levels found in short cycles are probably responsible for granulosa cell luteinization and elevated intrafollicular testosterone levels that may negatively affect folliculogenesis by increasing follicle atresia. Conversely, the use of long regimens was associated with both increased folliculogenesis and an improved endocrine milieu.

CONCLUSIONS

In the last decade GnRH agonists have proven their efficacy and safety as a complement of gonadotropins in assisted reproduction ovulation induction. Although both short and long regimens are effective for the block of the endogenous LH surge, the latter appears to be preferable, as it provides an improved follicle yield and endocrine milieu. Efficacy of shorter regimens is still controversial and their widespread use is unlikely. Finally, depot GnRH agonist preparations appear to be safe for ovulation induction in assisted reproduction.

ACKNOWLEDGEMENTS

We wish to thank Mrs Silvia Arsento for outstanding secretarial assistance.

References

1. Fleming, R., Haxton, M. J., Hamilton, M. P. R., McCune, G. S., Black, W. P., Macnaughton, M. C. and Coutts, J. R. T. (1985). Successful treatment of infertile women with oligomenorrhea using a combination of an LHRH agonist and exogenous gonadotrophins. *Br. J. Obstet. Gynaecol.*, **92**, 369–73

2. Dodson, W. C., Hughes, C. L., Whitesides, D. B. and Haney, A. F. (1987). The effect of leuprolide acetate on ovulation induction with human menopausal gonadotropins in polycystic ovary syndrome. *J. Clin. Endocrinol. Metab.*, **65**, 95–100

3. Hughes, E. G., Fedorkow, D. M., Daya, S., Sagle, M. A., Van de Koppel, P. and Collins, J. A. (1992). The routine use of gonadotropin-releasing hormone agonists prior to *in vitro* fertilization and gamete intrafallopian transfer: a meta-analysis of randomized controlled trials. *Fertil. Steril.*, **58**, 888–96

4. Filicori, M. (1994). Gonadotrophin-releasing hormone agonists. A guide to use and selection. *Drugs*, **48**, 41–58

5. Tan, S. L., Kingsland, C., Campbell, S., Mills, C., Bradfield, J., Alexander, N., Yovich, J. and Jacobs, H. S. (1992). The long protocol of administration of gonadotropin-releasing hormone agonist is superior to the short protocol for ovarian stimulation for *in vitro* fertilization. *Fertil. Steril.*, **57**, 810–14

6. Filicori, M., Flamigni, C., Cognigni, G. E., Falbo, A., Arnone, R., Capelli, M., Pavani, A., Mandini, M., Calderoni, P. and Brondelli, L. (1996). Different gonadotropin and leuprorelin ovulation induction regimens markedly affect follicular fluid hormone levels and folliculogenesis. *Fertil. Steril.*, **65**, 387–93

7. Chetkowski, R. J., Kruse, L. R. and Nass, T. E. (1989). Improved pregnancy outcome with the addition of leuprolide acetate to gonadotropins for *in vitro* fertilization. *Fertil. Steril.*, **52**, 250–5

8. Frydman, R., Belaisch Allart, J., Parneix, I., Forman, R., Hazout, A. and Testart, J. (1988). Comparison between flare up and down regulation effects of luteinizing hormone-releasing hormone agonists in an *in vitro* fertilization program. *Fertil. Steril.*, **50**, 471–5

9. Tummon, I.S., Daniel, S.A.J., Kaplan, B.R., Nisker, J.A. and Yuzpe, A.A. (1992). Randomized, prospective comparison of luteal leuprolide acetate and gonadotropins versus clomiphene citrate and gonadotropins in 408 first cycles of *in vitro* fertilization. *Fertil. Steril.*, **58**, 563–8

10. Abdalla, H. I., Ahuja, K. K., Leonard, T., Morris, N. N., Honour, J. W. and Jacobs, H. S. (1990). Comparative trial of luteinizing hormone-releasing hormone analog/human menopausal gonadotropin and clomiphene citrate/human menopausal gonadotropin in an assisted conception program. *Fertil. Steril.*, **53**, 473–8

11. Polson, D. W., MacLachlan, V., Krapez, J. A., Wood, C. and Healy, D. L. (1991). A controlled study of gonadotropin-releasing hormone agonist (buserelin acetate) for folliculogenesis in routine *in vitro* fertilization patients. *Fertil. Steril.*, **56**, 509–14

12. Macnamee, M. C., Howles, C. M., Edwards, R. G., Taylor, P. J. and Elder, K. T. (1989). Short-term luteinizing hormone-releasing hormone agonist treatment: prospective trial of a novel ovarian stimulation regimen for *in vitro* fertilization. *Fertil. Steril.*, **52**, 264–9

13. Ron El, R., Herman, A., Golan, A., Soffer, Y., Nachum, H. and Caspi, E. (1992). Ultrashort gonadotropin-releasing hormone agonist (GnRH-a) protocol in comparison with the long-acting GnRH-a protocol and menotropin alone. *Fertil. Steril.*, **58**, 1164–8

14. Pantos, K., Meimeth-Damianaki, T., Vaxevanoglou, T. and Kapetanakis, E. (1994). Prospective study of a modified gonadotropin-releasing hormone agonist long protocol in an *in vitro* fertilization program. *Fertil. Steril.*, **61**, 709–13

15. Filicori, M., Flamigni, C., Cognigni, G., Dellai, P., Arnone, R., Falbo, A. and Capelli, M. (1993). Comparison of the suppressive capacity of different depot gonadotropin-releasing hormone analogs in women. *J. Clin. Endocrinol. Metab.*, **77**, 130–3

16. Wilshire, G.B., Emmi, A.M., Gagliardi, C.C. and Weiss, G. (1993). Gonadotropin-releasing hormone agonist administration in early human pregnancy is associated with normal outcomes. *Fertil. Steril.*, **60**, 980–3

17. Porcu, E., Filicori, M., Dal Prato, L., Fabbri, R., Seracchioli, R., Colombi, C. and Flamigni, C. (1995). Comparison between depot leuprorelin and daily buserelin in IVF. *J. Assist. Reprod. Gen.*, **12**, 14–18

18. Ron El, R., Lahat, E., Golan, A., Lerman, M., Bukovsky, I. and Herman, A. (1994). Development of children born after ovarian superovulation induced by long-acting gonadotropin-releasing hormone agonist and menotropins, and by *in vitro* fertilization. *J. Pediatr.*, **125**, 734–7

19. Skarin, G., Nillius, S. J. and Wide, L. (1982). Failure to induce early abortion by huge doses of a superactive LRH agonist in women. *Contraception*, **26**, 457–63

GnRH agonists and assisted reproduction outcome

E. Porcu, L. Dal Prato, R. Seracchioli, R. Fabbri, S. Petracchi and C. Flamigni

INTRODUCTION

A substantial improvement of *in vitro* fertilization (IVF) organization and outcome has been achieved with the use of gonadotropin releasing hormone (GnRH) analogs in order to obtain pituitary desensitization before and during induction of multiple follicular growth. The control of endogenous secretion of luteinizing hormone (LH) by GnRH agonists prevents premature luteinization and the LH surge, reduces the cancellation rate, and improves follicular recruitment.

On the other hand, a number of potential disadvantages have been pointed out, including lower and slower ovarian response, impaired luteal function, the development of ovarian cysts, increased incidence of the ovarian hyperstimulation syndrome, embryo toxicity, fetal toxicity and impaired child development. These problems may be related to various parameters such as dose of analog, type of compound, protocol of administration, duration of administration and type of formulation.

The dose of analog necessary to avoid the LH surge and premature luteinization has been progressively reduced in the past few years, and very recently microdoses have been proposed, particularly for low responders, in order to avoid the excessive ovarian suppression[1-2].

Several compounds are at present commercially available: no major differences have been documented among them in terms of efficacy or side effects. On the other hand, the protocol of administration, i.e. long, short or ultrashort, seems to affect the treatment outcome. Loumaye and colleagues[3] have elegantly demonstrated that the short protocol gives rise to embryos of lower quality, probably because of the negative effects on follicular development of the LH peak induced by the analog at the beginning of stimulation.

The recent development of sustained-release formulations of GnRH analogs has increased patient compliance and has further improved the routine organization of assisted reproduction. However, some concern has been raised by the persistence of unnecessary and potentially unfavorable effects during the luteal phase and early pregnancy[4]. This concern led our group to investigate the safety of these compounds in several prospective studies.

DEPOT *VS.* SUSTAINED RELEASE

The first study[5] compared depot triptorelin (3.75 mg intramuscularly in a single dose) and standard release triptorelin (0.1 mg subcutaneously daily). In the cycle preceding that of IVF, in 11 patients, a series of GnRH tests was performed before and after depot or daily triptorelin administration to investigate pituitary desensitization.

This study showed no difference in the time necessary to reach pituitary desensitization (11.3 ± 1.03 vs. 11.3 ± 1.45 days). On the other hand, resumption of pituitary activity occurred about 7 days after the last dose of the daily analog and 2 months after the single injection of the depot form. Therefore, the effects of the depot forms are likely to persist in the luteal phase and in the early phases of pregnancy, at least in the majority of patients. Two problems may be related to this: the possible unfavorable effects on the luteal phase (due to the loss of the gonadotropin luteal support and/or a direct inhibition of luteal steroidogenesis), and the possible teratogenic effects. A GnRH challenge test before administration of human chorionic gonadotropin (hCG)

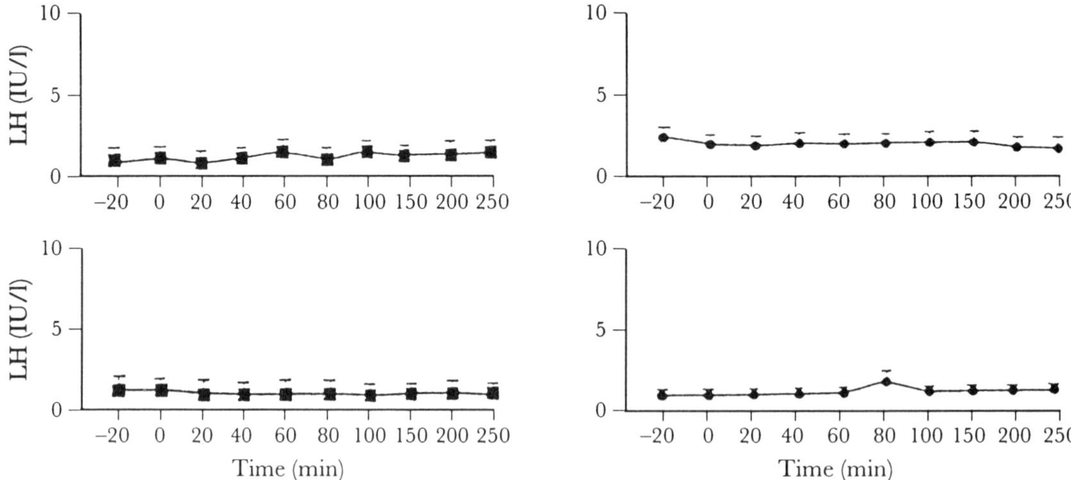

Figure 1 Late follicular (top) and midluteal (bottom) GnRH test in induction of superovulation: comparison between patients (nine in the late follicular phase and four in the luteal phase) treated with the long-acting analog triptorelin 3.75 mg intramuscularly (left) and patients (eight in the late follicular phase and three in the luteal phase) treated with the standard direct-release analog triptorelin 0.1 mg subcutaneously (right). From Porcu, E., Dal Prato, L., Seracchioli, R. *et al.* (1994). Comparison between depot and standard release triptorelin in *in vitro* fetilisation: pituitary sensitivity, luteal function, pregnancy outcome and perinatal results. *Fertil. Steril.*, **62**, 126–32. Reproduced with permission of the American Society of Reproductive Medicine (formerly The American Fertility Society)

and in the luteal phase in a group of volunteers showed a similar degree of persisting desensitization with both formulations (Figure 1). The luteal support is therefore impaired equally, although controversy still exists as to the necessity of LH in maintaining corpus luteum function.

As regards the second mechanism, direct effects of GnRH analogs on ovarian steroidogenesis have been hypothesized and a possible inhibitory action has been proposed on the basis of *in vitro* studies[6]. However, the question of direct action of GnRH on ovarian steroidogenesis is still unclear and conflicting data are reported in the literature[7-8]. The most recent results of our *in vitro* investigations[9] suggest that human granulosa cells are not acutely sensitive to direct action on steroidogenesis by GnRH analogs.

Moreover, our clinical investigation did not find any clear-cut difference in the luteal steroid levels when comparing the daily and depot formulations. In addition, in the patients undergoing IVF, the long-acting analogs did not seem to interfere with the percentage of pregnancies (28.6%) and of miscarriages (30%), which was not significantly different from that

observed with the daily forms (25.6% and 30%) and no significant differences were found in these patients in the obstetric and perinatal outcome (Table 1) with both formulations.

An additional study[10] comparing depot leuprorelin (3.75 mg in a single dose) and daily

Table 1 Obstetric and perinatal outcome of 196 IVF cycles randomized between daily and depot triptorelin treatment (triptorelin). Reproduced with permission from Porcu *et al.* (1994)[5]. Full copyright details appear in the legend to Figure 1

	3.75 mg i.m.	*0.1 mg s.c.*
Deliveries	16	14
Singletons	10 (62%)	8 (57.1%)
Twins	5 (31.2%)	6 (42.8%)
Triplets	1 (6.2%)	0
Preterm	5 (31.2%)	3 (21.4%)
Cesarean	8 (50%)	6 (42.8%)
Alive at birth	23	20
Weight (g)	2458 ± 839	2729 ± 566
Malformations	0	0
Alive at 1 month	20	20

i.m., intramuscular; s.c., subcutaneous

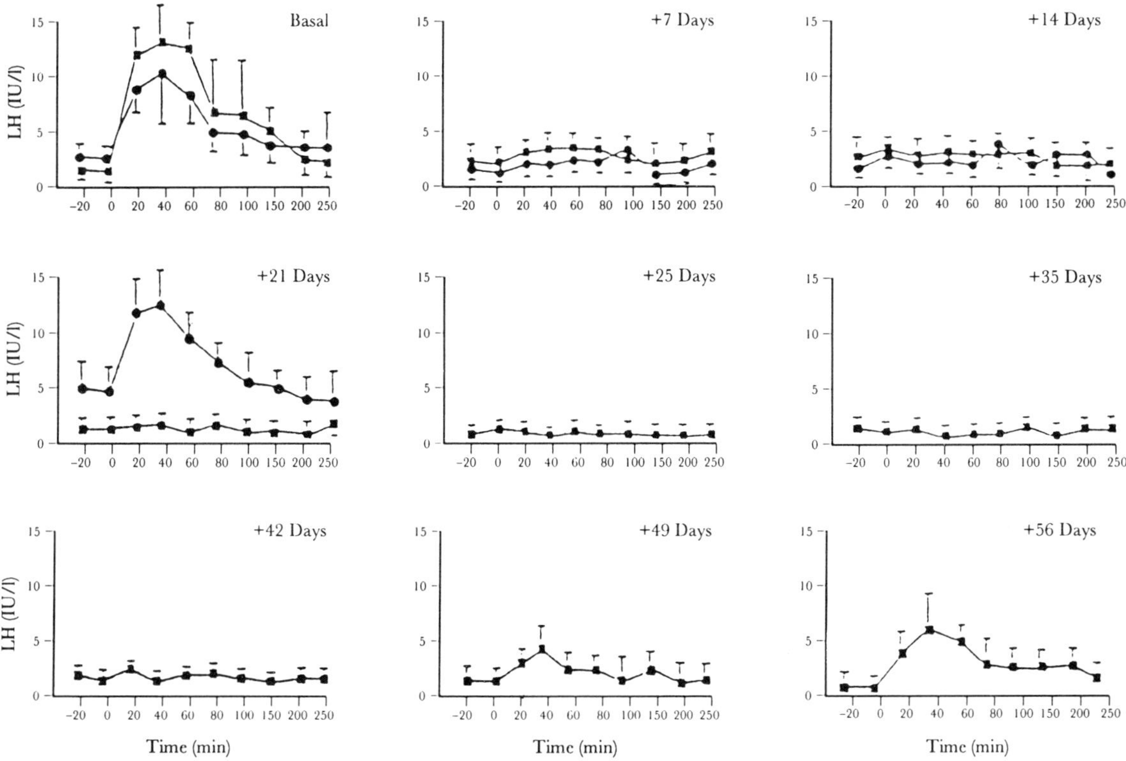

Figure 2 Study of the onset and duration of desensitization. ■ GnRH test before and after depot leuprorelin intramuscular administration in group A (five patients). ● GnRH test (basal), during (+7 and +14) and 7 days after discontinuation (+21) of daily buserelin subcutaneous administration in group B (five patients). From Porcu, E., Filicori, M., Dal Prato *et al.* (1995). Comparison between depot leuprorelin and daily buserelin in IVF. *J. Assist. Reprod. Genet.*, **12**, 14–18. Reproduced with permission of Plenum Press

Table 2 Clinical IVF results in comparison between daily and depot analog treatment. Reproduced with permission from Porcu *et al.* (1995)[10]. Full copyright details appear in the legend to Figure 2

	Leuprorelin	*Buserelin*
Cycles	65	64
Cancelled cycles	9 (13.8%)	6 (9.4%)
Cysts	3 (4.6%)	2 (3.1%)
Retrievals	56	58
Transfers	51	54
Pregnancies/cycle	23.1% (15/65)	21.8% (14/64)
Pregnancies/retrieval	26.8% (15/56)	24.1% (14/58)
Pregnancies/transfer	29.4% (15/51)	25.9% (14/54)
Implantation rate (%)	11.9	12.3
Miscarriages	26.6% (4/15)	28.5% (4/14)

buserelin (0.3 mg subcutaneously twice daily) confirmed our previous results as far as time to reach desensitization and resumption of pituitary activity were concerned (Figure 2). The pregnancy rate per transfer was slightly, but not significantly, better in the depot group (29.4% *vs.* 25.9%). No significant differences were found in the pattern of stimulation, oocyte quality, implantation rate (11.9% *vs.* 12.3%) and miscarriages (26.6% *vs.* 28.5%) (Table 2).

TYPE OF ANALOG

Taking into consideration the type of depot compound, in our experience a direct comparison of long-acting triptorelin and leuprorelin did not show any clear difference in the pattern of stimulation and in the IVF outcome between the

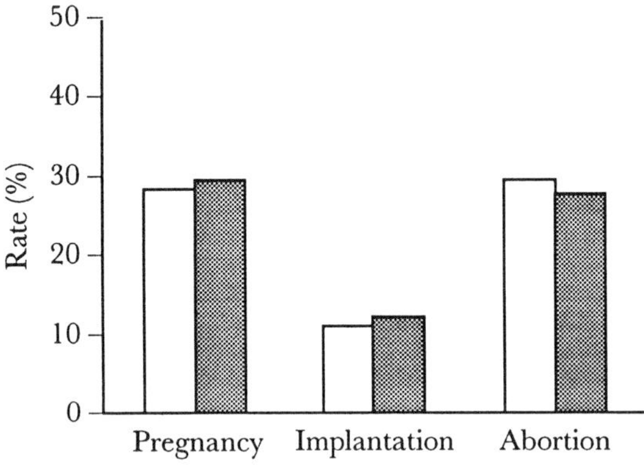

Figure 3 Comparison of pregnancy, implantation and abortion rates between triptorelin (□) and leuprorelin (▒) treatment in IVF cycles

two analogs (Figure 3). Hence, according to our results, both the long-acting and daily forms of GnRH analogs give rise to similar results in patients undergoing assisted reproduction.

Ovarian cysts

Several authors have reported the development of cysts in varying percentages after GnRH analog administration[11–13]. In our experience the incidence of ovarian cysts is low with every kind and formulation of GnRH analog[5,10] (Table 3), even lower than that found to occur spontaneously in normal women of different ages[14,15]. The presence of cysts did not impair our IVF results.

Ovarian hyperstimulation syndrome

It has been suggested that analogs increase the incidence of ovarian hyperstimulation syndrome[16,17]. One of the desired effects induced by the analogs is the recruitment of a higher number of follicles, which obviously implies a higher risk of overstimulated ovaries. However, the use of analogs also allows the achievement of a higher pregnancy rate, which is often linked to a higher percentage of hyperstimulation syndrome. It is then very difficult to conclude that the use of analogs in itself is responsible for a higher risk of this undesired effect.

Teratogenetic effects

Some concern about possible teratogenetic effects of GnRH analogs in human offspring has been raised because of the ability of these compounds to cross the placenta and cause a reduction of testicular weight in male Rhesus monkeys, as found by Sopelak and Hodgen[18]. However, several studies have shown that neither IVF procedures, nor GnRH analogs are associated with an increased risk of congenital malformations[19,20]. In our perinatal results no malformation has been detected at birth nor at 1 month, with every kind and formulation of GnRH analog. This confirms and adds more strength to the results obtained in various infertility centers[11–20].

Furthermore, several reports of the inadvertent administration of long-acting analogs during

Table 3 Incidence of ovarian cysts after GnRH analog administration in IVF

Authors	Analog	Administration	% Cysts
Feldberg et al. (1989)[11]	triptorelin, daily	follicular	29.0
	buserelin, depot	follicular	22.0
Caspi et al. (1989)[12]	triptorelin, depot	follicular	11.0
Herman et al. (1990)[13]	triptorelin, depot	follicular	13.6
	triptorelin, depot	luteal	15.4
Porcu et al. (1994)[5]	triptorelin, daily	luteal	2.1
	triptorelin, depot	luteal	5.8
Porcu et al. (1995)[10]	buserelin, daily	luteal	3.1
	leuprorelin, depot	luteal	4.6

pregnancy, documenting subsequent normal births, are reassuring (Table 4)[4,21–26]. Recently a report from the Centre de Reinseignements sur les Agents Teratogenes of Paris about the follow up of 28 pregnancies exposed to triptorelin showed no malformation, except a trisomy 13, which cannot be related to triptorelin, because the drug was administered 15 days after fertilization[24].

In all these studies the children were examined only during the first weeks of life, so any possible delayed effect, particularly on reproductive function, cannot be evaluated. Furthermore, the wide use of GnRH agonists, especially the long-acting GnRH agonists, raises the question of whether these drugs have any influence on the late physical, neurological and mental development of the infants born after an assisted reproduction procedure. In a recent comparative study, Ron-El and associates[27] showed that up to the age of 36 months, the children whose mothers were treated with long-acting GnRH analogs, had no physical, neurological or mental

Table 4 Pregnancy outcome after GnRH analog exposure

Author	Pregnancies	Malformations	Miscarriages
Golan *et al.* (1990)[22]	1	0	0
Smitz *et al.* (1991)[25]	13	—	3
Herman *et al.* (1992)[4]	11	—	4
Har-Toov *et al.* (1993)[23]	1	0	0
Balasch *et al.* (1992)[21]	14	—	1
Cahill *et al.* (1994)[26]	25	0	3
Elefant *et al.* (1995)[24]	28	1*	4

*Probably not related to the drug

impairment compared with control subjects from spontaneous pregnancies.

CONCLUSION

Although no definitive statement can yet be made, further studies being necessary, these data seem to confirm the efficacy and safety of long-acting GnRH agonists in assisted reproduction.

References

1. Scott, R. T. and Navot, D. (1994). Enhancement of ovarian responsiveness with microdoses of gonadotropin-releasing hormone agonist during ovulation induction for *in vitro* fertilization. *Fertil. Steril.*, **61**, 880–5
2. Feldberg, D., Farhi, J., Ashkenazi, J., Dicker, D., Shalev, J. and Ben-Rafael, Z. (1994). Minidose gonadotropin-releasing hormone agonist is the treatment of choice in poor responders with high follicle stimulating hormone levels. *Fertil. Steril.*, **62**, 343–6
3. Loumaye, E., Vankrieken, L., Depreester, S., Psalti, I., De Cooman, S. and Thomas, K. (1989). Hormonal changes induced by short-term administration of a gonadotropin releasing hormone agonist during ovarian hyperstimulation for *in vitro* fertilization and their consequences for embryo development. *Fertil Steril*, **51**, 105–11
4. Herman, A., Ron-El, R., Golan, A., Nachum, H., Soffer, Y. and Caspi E. (1992). Impaired corpus luteum function and other undesired results of pregnancies associated with inadvertent administration of long-acting agonist of gonadotropin-releasing hormone. *Hum. Reprod.*, **7**, 465–8
5. Porcu, E., Dal Prato, L., Seracchioli, R., Fabbri, R., Longhi, M. and Flamigni, C. (1994). Comparison between depot and standard release triptorelin in *in vitro* fertilization: pituitary sensitivity, luteal function, pregnancy outcome and perinatal results. *Fertil. Steril.*, **62**, 126–32.
6. Tureck, R. W., Mastroianni, L. Jr, Blasco, L. and Strauss J. F. (1982). Inhibition of human granulosa cell progesterone secretion by a gonadotropin-releasing hormone agonist. *J. Endocrinol. Metab.*, **54**, 1078–80
7. Parinaud, J., Beaur, A., Bourreau, E., Vieitez, G. and Pontonnier G. (1988). Effect of a luteinizing hormone-releasing hormone agonist (buserelin) on steroidogenesis of cultured human preovulatory granulosa cells. *Fertil. Steril.*, **50**, 597–602
8. Casper, R. F. and Yen, S. S. C. (1979). Induction of luteolysis in the human with a long acting analogue of luteinizing hormone-releasing factor. *Science*, **205**, 408–10
9. Fabbri, R., Porcu, E., Pession, A., Bonu., M. A.,

Sereni, E., Marsella, T., Soriani, P., Magrini, O., Seracchioli, R. and Flamigni, C. (1995). The effect of triptorelin and leuprorelin on steroidogenesis by human preovulatory granulosa cells *in vitro*. *IX Congress on In Vitro Fertilization and Assisted Reproduction*, Vienna, April 3–7, p. 331–7

10. Porcu, E., Filicori, M., Dal Prato, L., Fabbri, R., Seracchioli, R., Colombi, C. and Flamigni, C. (1995). Comparison between depot leuprorelin and daily buserelin in IVF. *J. Assist. Reprod. Genet.*, **12**, 14–18.

11. Feldberg, D., Ashkenazi, J., Decker, D., Yeshaya, A., Goldman, G. A. and Goldman, J. A. (1989). Ovarian cyst formation: a complication of gonadotropin-releasing hormone agonist therapy. *Fertil. Steril.*, **51**, 42–5

12. Caspi, E., Ron-El, R., Golan, A., Nachum, H., Herman, A., Soffer, Y. and Wieneraub, Z. (1989). Results of *in vitro* fertilization and embryo transfer by combined long acting gonadotropin releasing hormone and gonadotropins. *Fertil. Steril.*, **51**, 95–9

13. Herman, A., Ron-El, R., Golan, A., Nahum, H., Soffer, Y. and Caspi, E. (1990). Follicle cysts after menstrual versus midluteal administration of gonadotropin-releasing hormone analog in *in vitro* fertilization. *Fertil. Steril.*, **53**, 854–8.

14. Tayob, Y., Adams, J., Jacobs, H. S. and Guilleband, D. (1985). Ultrasound demonstration of increased frequency of functional ovarian cysts in women using progestogen only oral contraception. *Br. J. Obstet. Gynecol.*, **92**, 1003–9

15. Porcu, E., Venturoli, S., Dal Prato, L., Fabbri, R., Paradisi, R. and Flamigni, C. (1994). Frequency and treatment of ovarian cysts in adolescence. *Arch. Gynecol. Obstet.*, **255**, 69–72

16. Forman, R. G., Frydman, R., Egan, D., Ross, C. and Barlow, D. H. (1990). Severe ovarian hyperstimulation syndrome using agonists of gonadotropin-releasing hormone for *in vitro* fertilization: a european series and a proposal for prevention. *Fertil. Steril.*, **53**, 502–8

17. Golan, A., Ron-El, R., Herman, A., Wienraub, Z., Soffer, Y. and Caspi, E. (1988). Ovarian hyperstimulation following D-Trp-6 luteinizing hormone-releasing hormone microcapsules and menotropin for *in vitro* fertilization. *Fertil. Steril.*, **50**, 912

18. Sopelak, W. M. and Hodgen, G.(1987). Infusion of gonadotropin releasing hormone agonist during pregnancy: maternal and fetal responses in primates. *Am. J. Obstet. Gynecol.*, **156**, 755–60

19. Lancaster, P. (1987). Congenital malformations after *in vitro* fertilization. *Lancet*, **2**, 1392–3

20. Rizk, B., Doyle, P., Tan, S.L., Rainsbury, P., Betts, J., Brinsden, P. and Edwards, R. (1991). Perinatal outcome and congenital malformations in *in vitro* fertilization babies from the Bourn–Hallam group. *Hum. Reprod.*, **9**, 1259–64

21. Balasch, J., Jovè, I.C., Moreno, V., Civico, S., Puerto, B. and Vanrel, J. A. (1992). The comparison of two gonadotropin releasing hormone agonists in an *in vitro* fertilization program. *Fertil. Steril.*, **58**, 991–4

22. Golan, A., Ron-El, R., Herman, A., Weinraub, Z., Soffer, Y. and Caspi, E. (1990). Fetal outcome following inadvertant administration of long-acting DTRP6GnRH microcapsules during pregnancy. A case report. *Hum. Reprod.*, **5**, 123–4

23. Har-Toov, J., Brenner, S. H., Jaffa, A., Yavetz, H., Peyser, M. R. and Lessing, J. B. (1993). Pregnancy during long term gonadotropin releasing hormone therapy associated with clinical pseudomenopause. *Fertil. Steril.*, **59**, 446–7

24. Elefant, E., Biour, B., Blumberg-Tick, J., Roux, C. and Thomas, F. (1995). Administration of a gonadotropin-releasing hormone agonist during pregnancy: follow up of 28 pregnancies exposed to triptoreline. *Fertil. Steril.*, **63**, 1111–13

25. Smitz, J., Camus, M., Devroey, P., Bollen, N., Tournaye, H. and Van Steirteghem, A. C. (1991). The influence of inadvertent intranasal buserelin administration in early pregnancy. *Hum. Reprod.*, **6** (2), 290–3

26. Cahill, D. J., Fountain, S. A., Fox, R., Fleming, C. F., Brinsden, P. R. and Hull, M. G. (1994). Outcome of inadvertent administration of a gonadotrophin-releasing hormone agonist (buserelin) in early pregnancy. *Hum. Reprod.*, **9** (7), 1243–6

27. Ron-El, R., Lahat, E., Golan, A., Lerman, M., Bukovsky, I. and Herman, A. (1994). Development of children born after ovarian superovulation induced by long-acting gonadotropin-releasing hormone agonist and menotropins, and by *in vitro* fertilization. *J. Pediatr.*, **125**, 734–7

Perspectives on the use of GnRH antagonists in ovulation induction 24

P. Bouchard, I. Leroy, S. Christin-Maitre, F. Olivennes, B. Charbonnel and R. Frydman

INTRODUCTION

The menstrual cycle is driven by the gonadotropins follicle stimulating hormone (FSH) and luteinizing hormone (LH), that in association with local growth factors, modulate the ovarian function and, in particular, rescue small antral follicles from the process of follicular atresia during the reproductive life[1,2]. Gonadotropin secretion is under the control of the hypothalamic hormone gonadotropin releasing hormone (GnRH) secreted in the hypophyseal portal circulation in a pulsatile manner[1].

The understanding of the role of GnRH during the menstrual cycle has been hampered by the difficulties involved in monitoring the patterns of GnRH secretion during the menstrual cycle[3]. Our information about GnRH secretion during the human cycle has been obtained by analysis of pulsatile LH secretion in the peripheral circulation. This reflects a GnRH pulse frequency of every 60–90 min during the early and midfollicular phase[1]. During the luteal phase pulse frequency is slowed by the negative feedback effect of progesterone on the GnRH pulse generator. The role of GnRH during the midcycle LH peak is poorly defined[3]. Based upon the frequency and amplitude of LH pulses, it would appear that GnRH output should increase during the LH surge and represent the primary driving force as it is during the other phases of the menstrual cycle. However, there are several observations which have detracted from this concept. In women with hypogonadotropic hypogonadism and in monkeys in which GnRH secretion has been prevented by arcuate nucleus lesions, normal ovulatory cycles can be re-initiated by pulses of exogenous GnRH. Clearly, a rise in GnRH output is not required to induce the LH surge; indeed,

there is evidence to suggest that the monkey pituitary can still produce an LH surge in response to estradiol (E_2) when the pituitary has been deprived of GnRH for up to 48 hours. Also, radiotelemetric monitoring of the GnRH pulse generator shows that the multiunit activity precedes LH pulses throughout the menstrual cycle except during the LH surge when it appears to cease. Crucial experiments on measuring GnRH output directly in monkeys have produced equivocal results, but, recently, it seems that convincing demonstration of a GnRH surge has at last been obtained as it has been described previously in the ewe and in the rat[3,4]. Further, it has been suggested recently that the local application of E_2 to the ventromedial nucleus of the hypothalamus is sufficient to trigger the GnRH surge (A. Caraty, unpublished results). The LH surge is therefore under the influence of several factors, including the positive feedback of E_2 at the pituitary and hypothalamic levels, as well as the increased sensitivity of gonadotroph cells to GnRH.

GnRH antagonists are competitive inhibitors of GnRH for its receptors on the membranes of gonadotroph cells. Although the first antagonist was synthesized as early as 1972, one year after the elucidation of the structure of the native hormone, it has taken 20 years to synthesize compounds with potent antiovulatory activity and low histamine release[5,6]. The reason why antagonist compounds release histamine is still not fully understood. The presence of a basic amino acid in position 6 seems to play a role in this matter[5]. The more recent antagonists developed are substituted by D-amino acids on 5 or 6 positions. These compounds (e.g. Cetrorelix, Ganirelix, azaline B and Antarelix) have little or no histamine release properties and are being studied in clinical trials. All GnRH antagonists share similar properties: they are competitive inhibitors of GnRH for its receptors and, indeed, their suppressive effects are overridden by native GnRH administered in a pulsatile fashion. The fact that native GnRH can displace antagonists from their receptors may explain the escape phenomenon observed with weak antagonists. They also have a relatively long half-life due to their resistance to proteolysis and, in some circumstances, storage of the compound. This is observed with the more hydrophobic antagonists. However, they are efficient in milligram doses which clearly limits their present use because of the cost of synthesis.

GnRH antagonist administration induces an hypogonadotropic status by causing a rapid fall of bioactive gonadotropin secretion, creating a reversible 'gonadotropin deficiency'. This property allows the use of GnRH antagonists as a probe to study the physiology of GnRH/gonadotropin-dependent events in the menstrual cycle. We shall envisage the administration of GnRH antagonists in the follicular phase, and in the periovulatory period, especially in controlled ovarian hyperstimulation (COH) where we believe that GnRH antagonists can successfully replace GnRH antagonists.

FOLLICULAR PHASE ADMINISTRATION

Early data obtained with weak GnRH antagonists supported the concept that transient gonadotropin deprivation during the follicular phase could alter the functional capacity of developing follicles. Indeed, it was suggested that GnRH antagonist administration during the follicular phase of the cycle to both women and monkeys resulted in 'medical ablation' of the dominant follicle.

Although the use of GnRH antagonists as potential contraceptives in women is still questionable, the antagonists do seem more promising than the agonists because they do not appear to produce complete suppression of circulating E_2 levels. Human clinical data are, nonetheless, scarce and inconclusive. This is, related to the delayed introduction of GnRH antagonists in women's fertility control, due to the side effects resulting from histamine release which was observed with the first-generation

antagonists. Obviously, all the data obtained thus far needs to be re-evaluated with newer, more potent antagonists.

We have investigated the effect of a potent, new, long-acting, second-generation GnRH antagonist, [Ac-d2-Nal[1], 4CID-Phe[2], D3Pal[3], Arg[5], D-Glu[6](AA), Dala[10]] GnRH (Nal-Glu) on follicular development in normal women. Unlike early antagonists, Nal-Glu has only 10% of the histamine releasing potency of the earlier analogs. Our results suggest that this Nal-Glu antagonist has the ability to delay ovulation.

Twelve normal women aged between 20 and 30 years with regular menstrual cycles (mean length 28.5 days, range 26 to 31 days) were enrolled. Five women received Nal-Glu (10 mg subcutaneously) on day 10 of the follicular phase (group I). Plasma E_2 levels on the day of Nal-Glu administration were less than 200 pmol/l. When compared to the control cycles, all five treated women had a significantly ($p < 0.05$) increased length of the cycle (36.2 ± 1.8 versus 29.8 ± 1.1 days in controls). This was a reflection of an increased length of the follicular phase (22.8 ± 2.0 versus 16 ± 0.8 days, $p < 0.05$). However, the luteal phase length remained unchanged. In all women, a single injection of Nal-Glu on day 10 of the cycle resulted in a suppression of plasma LH, FSH and E_2 levels. Mean plasma LH levels decreased significantly by approximately 45% ($p < 0.02$) 24 hours after antagonist administration from 4.6 ± 0.8 mIU/ml to 2.6 ± 0.8 mIU/ml. By the second day following the Nal-Glu injection, plasma LH levels had returned to pretreatment values. LH was thus suppressed for only 24 hours. Plasma radioimmunoassay FSH fell from 2.8 ± 0.9 to 2.3 ± 0.3 mIU/ml on the day following Nal-Glu administration. This was not significant. Mean plasma E_2 levels were 444 ± 80 pmol/l prior to Nal-Glu administration and decreased to 210 ± 63 pmol/l and 196 ± 59 pmol/l on the first and second day after antagonist administration. Plasma E_2 levels returned to base line within 4 days following antagonist administration.

A transient bleeding episode of 2 to 3 days occurred in one subject 24 hours after Nal-Glu administration. In the other four women there was bleeding 3 days after Nal-Glu administration. In all these cases, bleeding occurred when plasma E_2 levels were at their lowest values.

A further group of five women received 10 mg of Nal-Glu subcutaneously on days 1, 7, 14 and 21 of their cycle (group II). The weekly administration regimen resulted in the absence of ovulation in four of five subjects as shown by the lack of elevation of E_2 and progesterone (P), and the absence of an LH surge significantly less than in controls. E_2 levels were suppressed for 48 hours after the second and third injections, but only for 24 hours after the final injection. Immunoreactive FSH plasma levels were not significantly suppressed at anytime during the treated cycle. Transient bleeding during Nal-Glu treatment occurred in three women, 3 days after the third Nal-Glu injection. The LH surge occurred 7–19 days after the last Nal-Glu injection. The length of the luteal phase was normal when compared to the control cycles. This study clearly shows that GnRH antagonists immediately suppress gonadotropin secretion and block ovulation. These data are in accordance with animal physiology: pituitary stalk section, lesions of the arcuate nucleus and GnRH immunoneutralization studies have indeed established the pivotal role that pulsatile GnRH plays in gonadotropin and steroid secretion and cyclical ovarian activity.

These data suggest that GnRH antagonists, in contrast to agonists, have an immediate and sustained suppressive effect on gonadotropin secretion.

PERIOVULATORY ADMINISTRATION

Several studies have shown that this positive feedback of E_2 acts at the pituitary level, but it is not yet known if GnRH is involved. As discussed before, recent studies in ewes and in monkeys have shown that the LH surge is accompanied by a 50-fold increase in secretion of GnRH in the portal circulation and the use of GnRH antagonists in these models suppress the LH surge.

We therefore investigated the role of GnRH during the periovulatory period in normal women by treating them with the GnRH antagonist Nal-Glu [Ac-D2Nal[1], D4-ClPhe[2], D3Pal[3], Arg[5], DGlu[6](AA), DAla[10]]when E_2 levels exceeded

550 pmol/l[7]. Nal-Glu was administered in five regimens: a single subcutaneous injection of 10 mg; a single injection of 20 mg; and an injection of 10 mg subcutaneously on two, three and five consecutive days. Gonadotropin suppression resulted in a transient decline in E_2 in groups 1 and 2. Relative to control cycles, the LH surge occurred with a delay of 24–48 hours following one injection of Nal-Glu, and 24–120 hours following two injections. Multiple injections of Nal-Glu resulted in degeneration of the dominant follicle in one-half of the women in each group. The remaining women showed a profile similar to that of a single injection (i.e. a transient decline in E_2 levels followed by a recovery). Simultaneous administration of Nal-Glu and estradiol benzoate (EB) induced a rise in E_2 levels and none of the women showed a rise in LH in response to the EB injection. However, the co-administration of pulsatile GnRH with the antagonist triggered the LH surge.

USES OF GnRH ANTAGONISTS IN CONTROLLED OVARIAN HYPERSTIMULATION

During COH, premature LH surges are deleterious since they may occur when follicular maturation is inadequate and the subsequent premature rise in P has negative effect on the endometrium and oocytes. GnRH agonists are now used widely to prevent the premature LH surges, but this treatment is expensive, the gonadotroph cells desensitization may require 1–3 weeks and high doses of human menopausal gonadotropin (hMG) are needed inducing high risk of ovarian hyperstimulation.

Several publications have shown that the administration of GnRH antagonists does prevent premature LH surge and subsequent luteinization in COH[9–13].

We have initially reported the observation that the administration of the GnRH antagonist Nal-Glu at the presumed time of the LH surge in women undergoing COH was able to postpone the surge[8–10].

However, the clinical use of the first generations of GnRH antagonists was impaired by the short biological half-life of the compounds, their relative low potency and, more significantly, histamine release. Therefore, the development of these compounds was slower than that of GnRH agonists. Recently, new potent, safer third-generation GnRH antagonists became available. GnRH antagonists are more potent at suppressing gonadotropins, particularly LH and, in contrast to GnRH agonists, no flare-up (initial stimulation of gonadotropins and sex hormones) occurs after the first injection. GnRH antagonists have already been successfully used in women to inhibit the endogenous surge of LH. GnRH antagonists are usually administered as a single or repeated injections when plasma E_2 levels reach a level that might trigger the LH surge. The antagonist administration thus prevents the LH surge while follicular maturation is completed with the continuation of hMG administration. Ovulation may then be triggered when follicular maturation is completed. This is usually achieved with a single injection of human chorionic gonadotropin (hCG). Alternatively, ovulation may be triggered by a single injection of a GnRH agonist which would override the antagonist occupation of the GnRH receptors at the pituitary level. This possibility could be of interest in cases of high risk of ovarian hyperstimulation. Preliminary studies have shown that injection of antagonists are useful in *in vitro* fertilization and embryo transfer (IVF-ET), with report of several pregnancies. At this stage of development, and although new antagonists may be developed, the use of GnRH antagonists in COH seems to be a very attractive indication. Obviously, new antagonists such as Cetrorelix, Ganirelix, Antarelix, or azaline B will probably be the compounds of choice, because of their absence of significant histamine release. Our results with Cetrorelix ([Ac-D-Nal(2)[1], D-Phe (4Cl)[2], D-Pal(3)[3], D-Cit[6], D-Ala[10]] GnRH) suggests a bright future for these compounds[8,11,13].

We have reported the use of a GnRH antagonist (Cetrorelix) both in spontaneous cycles and in an IVF program. In spontaneous cycles, a single administration of 3 mg Cetrorelix (subcutaneously) during the late follicular phase significantly delayed LH surges by 6–17 days. Moreover, the same study showed that the LH surge was interrupted even when the antagonist was administered after the beginning of the surge. Thus, so far we have not observed any spontaneous LH surges in any of the IVF-ET cycles that received a single or dual administration of Cetrorelix. The only difficulty that remained is the timing of the administration of the antagonist. Indeed, in relation with the speed of follicular growth, a repeated injection of Cetrorelix is necessary in 64% of cases. The only difficulties left are the precise timing of the first injection, the timing of the second injection (if it is necessary) and, theoretically, the possibility that D-amino acids would remain in circulation at the time of conception.

In further studies we could show that provided that COH is induced with no more than two ampules of hMG, a single injection of 3 mg Cetrorelix on day 8 of the stimulation cycle was enough to terminate follicular development; a repeat injection was necessary in only three of 11 subjects (slower responders). In all subjects, the dose of hMG is 40% less than in agonist-treated cycles.

At this stage more than 80 cycles have been studied using one or two injections of Cetrorelix with no endogenous LH surges. The dose of Cetrorelix can probably be decreased to 2 mg per injection. An alternative protocol has been described by Diedrich *et al.*[12] that uses daily administration of Cetrorelix starting on day 7 of the COH cycle. While this protocol seems very effective, we favor the single or dual injection protocol for reasons of simplicity, cost and the reduced dose of gonadotropins and the subsequent risk of hyperstimulation. The results of plasma Cetrorelix measurement in both protocols are still pending. Unpublished results show that the triggering of ovulation with GnRH agonist (0.1 mg of D-Trp[6] GnRH) is perfectly adequate to trigger ovulation. The absolute requirement of a progesterone substitution in the luteal phase has not been studied.

CONCLUSION

Our results clearly suggest that premature LH surges can be successfully prevented with a very simple GnRH antagonist administration protocol in the majority of women undergoing IVF. A comparison on a large scale remains to be performed on the effect of GnRH agonists versus antagonists in IVF-ET cycles. It is also quite remarkable that the use of GnRH antagonists will probably allow the development of IVF in spontaneous cycles where the occurrence of an LH surge is the cause of cancellation. The co-administration of antagonist and low doses of hMG at the end of the follicular phase will certainly allow a full follicular development without LH surges.

References

1. Knobil, E. (1980). The neurocrine control of the menstrual cycle. *Rec. Prog. Horm. Res.*, **36**, 53–88
2. Bouchard, P., Wolf, J. P. and Hajri, S. (1988). Inhibition of ovulation: comparison between the mechanism of action of steroids and GnRH analogues. *Hum. Reprod.*, **3**, 503–6
3. Fraser, H. and Bouchard, P. (1994). Uses of GnRH antagonists in gynecology: a critical review. *Trends Endocrinol. Metab.*, **5**, 87–93
4. Caraty, A., Antoine, C., Delaleu, B., Locatelli, A., Bouchard, P., Gautron, J. P., Evans, N. P., Moenter, S. M. and Karsch, F. J. (1993). The preovulatory surge of GnRH in the ewe. In Bouchard, P., Caraty, A., Coelingh Bennink, H. and Pavlou, S. N. (eds.) *GnRH, GnRH Analogs, Gonadotropins, Gonadal Peptides.* (Carnforth, UK: Parthenon Publishing Group)
5. Schimdt, F., Sundaram, K., Thau, R. B. and Bardin, C. W. (1984). {Ac-Nal(2)1,4FD-Phe2,D-Trp3,Arg6}LHRH, a potent antagonist of LHRH produces transient edema and behavioural changes in rats. *Contraception*, **29**, 283–9
6. Karten, M. J., Hoeger, C. A., Hook, W. A., Lindberg, M. C. and Naqvi, R. H. (1990). The development of safer antagonists: strategy and status. In Bouchard, P., Haour, F., Franchimont, P. and Schatz, B. (eds.) *Recent Progress on GnRH and Gonadal Peptides*, pp. 147–58. (Paris: Elsevier)
7. Dubourdieu, S., Charbonnel, B., d'Acremont, M. F., Carreau, S., Spitz, I. M. and Bouchard, P. (1994). Effect of administration of a GnRH antagonist (Nal-Glu) during the preovulatory period: the LH surge requires the secretion of GnRH. *J. Clin. Endocrinol. Metab.*, **78**, 343–7
8. Leroy, I., d'Acremont, M. F., Brailly-Tabard, S., Frydman, R., de Mouzon, J. and Bouchard, P. (1994). A single injection of a gonadotropin-releasing hormone (GnRH) antagonist (Cetrorelix) postpones the luteinizing hormone (LH) surge: further evidence for the role of GnRH during the LH surge. *Fertil. Steril.*, **62**, 461–7
9. Frydman, R., Cornel, C., de Ziegler, D., Taieb, J., Spitz, I. M. and Bouchard, P. (1991). Prevention of premature luteinizing hormone and progesterone rise with a gonadotropin-releasing hormone antagonist, Nal-Glu, in controlled ovarian hyperstimulation. *Fertil. Steril.*, **56**, 923–32
10. Frydman, R., Cornel, C., de Ziegler, D., Taïeb, J., Spitz, I. M. and Bouchard, P. (1992). Spontaneously luteinizing hormone surge can be reliably prevented by timely administration of a gonadotropin-releasing hormone antagonist (Nal-Glu) during the late follicular phase. *Hum. Reprod.*, **7**, 930–3
11. Olivennes, F., Fanchin, R., Bouchard, P., de Ziegler, D., Taïeb, J., Selva, J. and Frydman, R. (1994). The single or dual administration of the GnRH antagonist Cetrorelix prevents premature LH surges in an IVF-ET program. *Fertil. Steril.*, **62**, 468–76
12. Diedrich, K., Diedrich, E., Santos, E., Zoll, C., Al-Hasani, Reissman, T. (1994). Suppression of the endogenous LH surges by the GnRH antagonist Cetrorelix during ovarian hyperstimulation. *Hum. Reprod.*, **9**, 788–91
13. Olivennes, F., Fanchin, R., Bouchard, P., Taïed, J., Selva, J. and Frydman, R. (1995). Scheduled administration of a GnRH antagonist (Cetrorelix) on day 8 of IVF cycles; a pilot study. *Hum. Reprod.*, **10**, 1382–6

Comparison between human chorionic gonadotropin and human luteinizing hormone (LH) to produce a midcycle LH surge

25

E. Loumaye, A. Piazzi, A. Munafo and I. Martineau

INTRODUCTION

The midcycle luteinizing hormone (LH) surge is a key event in the menstrual cycle. Appropriate timing and adequate duration and amplitude of this surge are prerequisites for human female fertility. An adequate surge will lead to several changes at the follicle level that are pivotal for obtaining a pregnancy. First, the surge induces the cumulus oophorus mucinification, allowing the oocyte to be released subsequently from the follicular wall. Second, it provokes the resumption of the oocyte meiosis, that is from germinal vesicle stage to metaphase II. Reaching the metaphase II meiotic stage is a mandatory step for allowing proper fertilization of the oocyte and embryonic development. Third, the LH surge triggers follicular rupture, expelling the oocyte from the follicle and leading to its capture by the fallopian tube. Finally, it induces a shift in the granulosa cell steroidogenic process, changing it from a dominating estradiol secretory process towards a progesterone secretory process, forming an active corpus luteum.

Three major regulatory factors have been identified as playing a role in the induction of the midcycle LH surge: the hypothalamic gonadotropin releasing hormone (GnRH), the ovarian steroids (estradiol [E_2] and progesterone [P_4]) and some less well characterized peptide hormones (e.g. gonadotropin surge-attending factor)[1].

THE NEED FOR A SURROGATE LH SURGE

In several clinical situations a surrogate LH surge must be produced, as the endogenous feedback mechanisms that produce an endogenous LH surge are absent or impaired.

In anovulation resulting from severe gonadotropin deficiency (World Health Organization [WHO] group I anovulation; hypogonadotropic hypogonadism), follicular growth induced by a combined administration of follicle stimulating hormone (FSH) and LH is usually not followed by a spontaneous LH surge. In anovulation resulting from a hypothalamic pituitary dysfunction, which is characterized by residual gonadotropin and E_2 secretion (WHO group II anovulation; polycystic ovary disease [PCOD]), the restoration of follicle growth by FSH administration does not usually lead to correct timing and adequate amplitude of the LH surge[2]. Treatment of anovulations with gonadotropins thus requires the production of a surrogate LH surge.

In ovulatory patients undergoing stimulation of multiple follicular development by administration of pharmacological doses of FSH prior to assisted reproductive technology (ART), it has been shown that feedback mechanisms are often disrupted. This leads to mistimed LH surges that are often also blunted[3,4]. The administration of a surrogate LH surge has therefore become a standard procedure in ART. Moreover, as mistimed LH surges have been regarded as a cause of failure of the ART treatment, most patients are now pretreated with a GnRH agonist. This treatment abolishes pituitary responsiveness to endogenous GnRH and prevents the occurrence of a spontaneous endogenous LH surge[4]. This has resulted in a significant improvement of ART treatment outcome[5].

A third indication for a surrogate LH surge could be in patients undergoing intrauterine insemination (IUI) with washed sperm; in such patients the probability of conception appears to be related to the duration of the surge[6]. In this study, an LH surge lasting for 1 day was associated with a pregnancy rate three times lower than that obtained when the surge lasted for 2 days. It is, however, not established whether the abnormal surge is the primary defect or if in these infertile patients it is the consequence of an impaired follicular development or a mistimed feedback mechanism. Moreover, the clinical efficacy of administering a surrogate LH surge to prolong the LH signal remains to be established.

THE NATURAL LH SURGE

The main characteristics of a natural LH surge as reported in the literature are summarized in Table 1. The natural surge lasts for about 2 days and is composed of an ascending phase, a plateau and a descending phase. LH serum levels, when measured by radioimmunoassay (RIA), are about 10–20 times the basal LH levels. Figure 1 shows mean values for serum immunoreactive LH concentrations, assayed with an immuno-radiometric assay (IRMA: MAIAclone LH) in four female volunteers who underwent frequent blood sampling around the midcycle period. In this study the mean peak value was 46 ± 16 IU/l. The absolute peak value was somewhat lower than that reported in the published data using an RIA but the relative increase on baseline secretion was essentially similar (around 10-fold). When frequent sampling is performed during the surge, a clear-cut pulsatile pattern for the LH secretion is observed. The LH pulse frequency appears to be the same as that of the late follicular phase LH secretion. The amplitude of the pulse is, however, very significantly increased[7].

Studies analyzing the LH surges show relatively large variations between individuals in terms of duration and amplitude of the LH surge. This might result partially from insufficiently high sampling frequency. From a clinical point of view, this variation also suggests that patients may have different threshold levels for the LH surge, as is the case for FSH in terms of follicular development. This should be taken into account when designing a therapeutic regimen for inducing a surrogate LH surge that must be effective in most patients. Indeed, in contrast to FSH therapy, no dose adjustment is possible.

In perfused rat ovaries, different thresholds have been identified for the different physiological roles of the surge[8]. Only 5% of the LH peak concentrations is sufficient to trigger the resumption of oocyte meiosis. A significant dose–response relationship was recorded for the P_4 secretion, but 5% of the LH peak value concentrations is also sufficient to trigger significant luteinization. By contrast, more than 85% of the LH surge peak concentration is required to trigger follicular rupture and ovulation. The practical consequence of this is that a regimen for inducing a surrogate surge needs to be designed based on the therapeutic objective. The regimen for provoking oocyte maturation and luteinization in patients for whom no follicular rupture is required (i.e. prior to ovum pick up [OPU] for ART), could be different from one aiming to provoke the full process of ovulation for *in vivo* conception.

In terms of steroid profiles at the time of the natural LH surge, P_4 has been shown to increase in two steps – an initial rise ending in a plateau at about 12 hours, followed by a second increase. Androstenedione and testosterone also surge at the time of the LH surge. Their peak values are four times and two times higher than before the surge for androstenedione and testosterone, respectively[9].

THE hCG SURGE

Human chorionic gonadotropin shares with LH the common biological property of recognizing and activating the same receptor. It is, however, somewhat different from LH in terms of receptor affinity. The binding affinities of urinary human chorionic gonadotropin (uhCG) and of recombinant hCG (rhCG) are about two to four times higher than those of pituitary derived human LH (hLH) and rhLH (Serono internal report). In addition, there are significant differences in terms of pharmacokinetic characteristics; hCG has a terminal half-life about three times longer than uhLH and rhLH. Together these differences

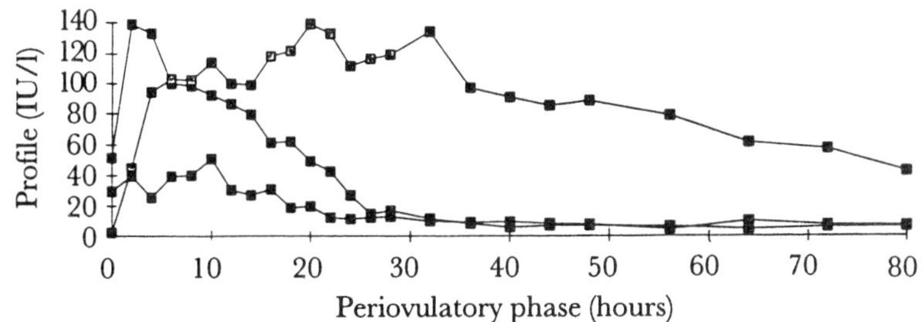

Figure 1 Mean LH and hCG profiles of four female volunteers who were monitored during three cycles. A spontaneous LH surge was recorded during cycle A. An endogenous surge was triggered by one injection of 250 μg buserelin acetate subcutaneously when the dominant follicle reached a mean diameter of 18 mm in cycle B. During cycle C, 5000 IU hCG was administered when the leading follicle reached 18 mm. Luteinizing hormone MAIAclone IRMA was used to measure serum LH levels in cycle A and B. Human chorionic gonadotropin MAIAclone IRMA was used to measure serum hCG in cycle C (Serono study GF 6113, data on file). ■, GnRH analog induced LH surge (*n* = 4); ▨, hCG surge (*n* = 4); ■, spontaneous LH surge (*n* = 4)

Table 1 Summary of LH surge characteristics

LH surge characteristics	Natural midcycle LH surge	hCG (5000 IU)	GnRH agonist-induced surge
Surge duration (hours)	49 ±9	> 96	24–28
Ascending phase (hours)	≅ 14	≅ 20	≅ 4
Plateau	≅ 14	0	0
Descending phase	≅ 20	> 72 hours	20–36
LH peak value (I-LH)	100–200	—	50–250
Peak/baseline ratio	10–20	—	10–20

indicate that administration of an equal dose of LH and hCG (in terms of molarity), assuming all other pharmacokinetic properties to be similar (e.g. rate and extent of absorption, distribution) will lead to a higher and more prolonged biological signal with hCG than with LH.

The use of uhCG instead of LH to mimic the preovulatory LH surge has been historically justified by the fact that uhCG was easier to obtain than LH. For the last 30 years, therapeutic preparations of hCG were extracted from the urine of pregnant women. Initially, having a preparation with a prolonged activity was an advantage, as ultrasound was not available for timing the surge administration, and patients were generally WHO group I anovulators who require a luteal phase support. Recently, hCG produced *in vitro* by recombinant DNA technology has entered the clinical phase of evaluation (rhCG, Ovidrel®). The pharmacokinetic characteristics of rhCG are very similar to those of the urinary-derived hCG. Their terminal half-lives are about 30 hours. (Serono, data on file). Based on the extended experience with uhCG, its efficacy and its safety, it is anticipated that rhCG will become the reference preparation for inducing a surrogate LH surge in most patients.

The main characteristics of a standard hCG surge as reported in the literature are summarized in Table 1. Figure 1 shows mean values for immunoreactive hCG serum concentrations assayed with an immunoradiometric assay (IRMA: MAIAclone hCG) in four female volunteers. They received 5000 IU hCG intramuscularly during a spontaneous cycle, when the dominant follicle reached a diameter of 18 mm. It should be noted that the units used for measuring hCG cannot be directly compared with the units used for LH serum concentrations, as assays are specific and do not use the same reference preparation. In addition, the units used to express the potency of a preparation (e.g. on an ampoule of hCG for therapeutic use) cannot be directly converted into immunoactivity as they represent a biological activity in terms of *in vivo* activity, as determined by an *in vivo* bioassay (Van Hell assay).

The widely accepted dose range for hCG is 5000–10 000 IU as a single injection. One dose-finding study has indicated that 2000 IU is insufficient for the requirements of the *in vitro* fertilization (IVF) population, as no oocytes were retrieved at the OPU in 23% of patients receiving that dose. Successful oocyte retrieval was recorded in more than 95% of patients treated with 5000 and 10 000 IU hCG[10].

The surge profile obtained after a single injection of hCG is definitively more prolonged than the natural LH surge (Figure 1 and Table 1). Practically, after an injection of 10 000 IU hCG, serum levels of the hormone were found to be above baseline in all patients up to day 10 postinjection[11].

The efficacy and safety of the surrogate hCG surge are well established and to date there are no arguments for questioning its use at least in most patients. However, the occurrence of ovarian hyperstimulation syndrome (OHSS), of multiple pregnancies and of a somewhat low implantation rate after human menopausal gonadotropin (hMG)-FSH/hCG therapy has drawn the interest of clinicians to the putative contribution of the prolonged activity of hCG to these adverse outcomes. It is well established that the amplitude of the response to FSH (i.e. the number of growing follicles) will determine the risk of OHSS and of multiple pregnancy[12]. Therefore, the development of 'soft' protocols, which use the minimal effective dose of FSH with careful adjustment steps and monitoring of the ovarian response to the gonadotropin, have led to a significant reduction in the incidence of these adverse outcomes. Using a 'chronic low dose protocol' for treating WHO group II anovulation, the incidence of significant OHSS is less than 1% and that of multiple pregnancy rate is around 5%[13]. Although these figures are low, and better than the figures obtained with standard regimen, a significant proportion of cycles still have to be cancelled. Therefore, further improvement of these figures would be medically relevant. In ART, severe OHSS is recorded in less than 0.5–2% of the treated cycles[14]. Using this indication the incidence of multiple pregnancy is related to the number of embryo replaced.

In addition, in patients receiving hCG after controlled ovarian hyperstimulation (COH), preliminary data suggest that P_4 rises more abruptly than in the natural cycle, which may accelerate the secretory changes in the endometrium to the point of phasing out endometrial receptivity, and thus in some cases impair the implantation process[15]. In this preliminary study, no significant relative changes in the androgen levels were recorded, contrasting with what is observed in the natural cycle. Further assessment of these differences in the steroid profiles between the natural surge and the hCG surge are needed to establish if they have a clinical relevance in terms of success rate after gonadotropin therapy.

ALTERNATIVES TO THE hCG SURGE

The theoretical and unproven therapeutic benefit of using LH instead of hCG, thus providing a short lasting, more physiological surrogate surge for those patients presenting a high risk of adverse outcome, has been addressed by clinicians since gonadotropin therapy was first developed. In the early years, only pituitary-derived human LH was available, and very limited experience was gained. More recently, clinicians have used GnRH agonists as well as native GnRH for triggering an endogenous LH surge. Very recently some preclinical works using human LH produced *in vitro* by recombinant DNA technology have been published.

Pituitary LH

Human LH preparations derived from cadaver pituitary glands were used in the 1960s to trigger final follicular maturation and ovulation in WHO group I anovulation treated with hMG. Repeated administrations of pituitary LH were used (i.e. 800–1200 IU every 8 hours for 24 hours). Continuation of LH administration throughout the luteal phase was shown to be necessary to obtain a pregnancy[16]. This is not surprising considering that these patients are profoundly deficient in both LH and FSH. The

Table 2 GnRH agonist-induced LH surge in WHO group II/polycystic ovarian disease patients

Study	Patient eligibility criteria	Analog	Luteal support	No. of cycles	Moderate or severe OHSS	Pregnancy	Multiple pregnancy
Emperaire et al. 1991[18]	E_2 > 1200 pg/ml and/or > 3 follicles > 17 mm	buserelin 3 × 200 µg i.n.	none	48	0	8	1
van der Meer et al. 1993[25]	E_2 > 1200 pg/ml and/or > 3 follicles > 18 mm	buserelin 3 × 200 µg i.n.	vaginal progesterone 300 mg/day	27	3	NA	—
Corson et al. 1993[26]	≥ 2 follicles > 17 mm	nafarelin 1 or 2 × 400 µg i.n.	none	22	0	3	0
Lanzone et al. 1994[27]	E_2 > 1200 pg/ml and/or > 3 follicles > 15 mm	buserelin 200 µg s.c.	progesterone 50mg/day/i.m.	20	0	3	0
Shalev et al. 1994[28]	E_2 > 2500 pg/ml and/or ≥ 20 follicles > 14 mm	Decapeptyl 0.5 mg s.c.	progesterone 50 mg/day/i.m.	12	0	6	0
Blumenfeld et al. 1994[29]	E_2: 2800 ± 681 pg/ml ≥ 8 follicles > 16 mm	GnRH 200 µg i.v.	hCG 2 × 2500 IU	44	2	10	2
Balasch et al. 1994[30]	E_2 > 1000 pg/ml and/or ≥ 4 follicles ≥ 14 mm	leuprolide 0.5 mg s.c.	none	23	0	4	0
Total				196	5 (2.5%)	34 (17%)	3 (9%)

i.n., intranasally; s.c., subcutaneously; i.v., intravenously; i.m., intramuscularly

pituitary-derived preparations are obviously no longer acceptable as therapeutic preparations because of the risk of infectious agent transmission[17].

GnRH agonists

The GnRH agonist-induced LH surge works through an indirect mechanism that relies on the patient's own pituitary response to GnRH. The main characteristics of a standard GnRH agonist-induced LH surge, as reported in the literature, are summarized in Table 1. Published data suggest that multiple administrations of a GnRH agonist does not lead to a prolonged surge when compared with a single administration[18,19]. Figure 1 shows mean values for immunoreactive LH serum concentrations assayed with an immuno-radiometric assay (IRMA: MAIAclone LH) in four female volunteers who received 250 µg buserelin subcutaneously during a spontaneous cycle, when the dominant follicle reached a diameter of 18 mm. In this study the mean peak value was 127 ± 55 IU/l LH. The induced LH surge has a sharper profile and a higher peak value than the naturally occurring surge. Its duration is smaller than the natural surge and the hCG surge.

The GnRH agonist-induced LH surge efficacy and safety have been investigated in two clinical situations. The first is WHO group II/PCOD patients who are over-responding to hMG/FSH and therefore would, in most cases, have not received hCG because of the risk of OHSS and multiple pregnancy. Table 2 summarizes these studies. Experience is still limited. Pregnancies

Table 3   GnRH agonist-induced LH surge in ART patients

Study	Patient eligibility criteria	Analog	Luteal support	No. of cycles	Moderate or severe OHSS	Pregnancy
Bentick et al. 1990[31]	—	buserelin 100 μg i.n.	vaginal progesterone 400 mg/day	1	—	1
Gonen et al. 1990[32]	regular IVF cycles	leuprolide 0.5 mg s.c.	none	9	—	3
Itskowitz et al. 1991[19]	moderate and over-response	buserelin 250–1000 μg s.c.	progesterone i.m. E$_2$ valerate p.o.	14	—	3
Imoedemhe et al. 1991[33]	regular IVF cycles	buserelin 100 μg i.n.	vaginal progesterone 400 mg/day	36	—	15
Segal et al. 1992[34]	regular IVF cycles	leuprolide 0.5 mg s.c.	vaginal progesterone	84	—	17
Total				144	0	39 (27%)

i.n., intranasally; s.c., subcutaneously; i.m., intramuscularly; p.o., oral administration

can be obtained and the pregnancy rate is 17% per cycle. Some twins and triplets have been reported, the multiple pregnancy rate is around 10%. Some significant OHSS was reported after the GnRH-agonist induced surge, with an incidence of 2.5%. At least one OHSS was reported in a cycle without conception. Finally, a high incidence of luteal phase deficiency has been observed, which indicates a luteal phase support when triggering an endogenous LH surge with a GnRH agonist[20,21]. The second clinical indication in which GnRH agonist-induced surges have been used is to trigger final follicular maturation prior to ART. This applies to cycles that are not pretreated with a GnRH agonist, or to cycles treated with a GnRH antagonist. Table 3 summarizes the published clinical experience of this indication. Contrasting with the WHO group II indication, studies have not been focused on patients who are over-responding. No definitive conclusions can be drawn in terms of differences from hCG surges. Absence of OHSS in 144 patients does not indicate whether the incidence of severe OHSS will be less or greater than 1%. The pregnancy rate appears to be acceptable. A luteal phase support is recommended.

Recombinant human LH

Human LH produced by DNA recombinant technology (LHadi®, Serono) appears to have essentially similar pharmacokinetic characteristics to the pituitary-derived hLH. In monkeys, the distribution half-life after intravenous administration was found to be less than 1 hour, and the terminal half-life to be 11.0 ± 0.9 hours[22]. In humans, rhLH was also found to have a terminal half-life after intravenous administration of around 10 hours. This is similar to urine-derived LH (hMG) terminal half-life (Serono internal report). Some experience with rhLH for producing a surrogate LH surge has been gained in the monkey and the rabbit. In monkeys, rhLH has been compared with pituitary LH and hCG in an IVF model[23]. Two injections of rhLH (2500 IU) at 18 hours apart elicit LH surge levels for 36–48 hours and induces periovulatory events similar to those elicited by a hCG injection (1000 IU). Attenuated LH surges of 18–24 hours reinitiate oocyte meiosis and promote granulosa cell luteinization but fail to promote corpus luteum development. In the rabbit, rhLH (50 IU) was compared with uhCG (50 IU) to induce ovulation[24]. In the rhLH treated group, the ovulation rate was lower but the implantation rate was higher than in the group treated with hCG.

CONCLUSIONS

Human chorionic gonadotropin is expected to remain the reference preparation for promoting final follicular maturation and triggering ovulation, both for induction of ovulation and for triggering final follicular maturation prior to ART.

Patients at risk of adverse outcomes such as OHSS and multiple pregnancies, despite the use of an appropriate FSH administration regimen and careful treatment monitoring, could benefit from a more physiological LH surge. Current experience suggests that a surge should last for about 48 hours to promote full corpus luteum formation. The requirements for the surge amplitude vary according to the therapeutic objectives; that is, final follicular maturation or ovulation. A luteal phase support by progesterone appears to be necessary for both indications. The clinical superiority of such surges over the hCG surge remains to be established. Only large-scale well controlled studies will provide a definitive answer.

The hypothesis linking the relatively low implantation rate after FSH/hCG with the prolonged activity of hCG is relevant but at this stage remains speculative. Appropriate clinical research work is necessary to elucidate this question.

References

1. Shoham, Z., Schachter, M., Loumaye, E., Weissman, A., Macnamee, M. and Insler, V. (1995). The luteinizing hormone surge – the final stage in ovulation induction: modern aspects of ovulation triggering. *Fertil. Steril.*, **64**, 237–51
2. Seibel, M. M., Kamrava, M. M., McArdle, C. and Taymor, M. L. (1984). Treatment of polycystic ovary disease with chronic low-dose follicle stimulating hormone: biochemical changes and ultrasound correlation. *Int. J. Fertil.*, **29**, 39–43
3. Glasier, A., Hillier, S. G., Thatcher, S. S., Baird, D. T. and Wickings, E. J. (1988). Superovulation with exogenous gonadotropins does not inhibit the luteinizing hormone surge. *Fertil. Steril.*, **49**, 81–5
4. Loumaye, E. (1990). The control of endogenous secretion of LH by gonadotropin-releasing hormone agonists during ovarian hyperstimulation for *in-vitro* fertilisation and embryo transfer. *Hum. Reprod.*, **5**, 357–76
5. Hughes, E. G., Fedorkow, D. M., Daya, S., Sagle, M. A., Van de Koppel, P. and Collins, J. A. (1992). The routine use of gonadotropin-releasing hormone agonists for IVF and gamete intra-fallopian transfer: a meta-analysis of randomised controlled trials. *Fertil. Steril.*, **58**, 888–96
6. Cohlen, B. J., te Velde, E. R., Scheffer, G., van Kooij, R. J., de Brouwer, C. P. M. and van Zonneveld, P. (1993). The pattern of the luteinizing hormone surge in spontaneous cycles is related to the probability of conception. *Fertil. Steril.*, **60**, 413–17
7. Adams, J. M., Taylor, A. E., Schoenfeld, D. A., Crowley, W. F. and Hall, J. E. (1994). The midcycle gonadotropin surge in normal women occurs in the face of an unchanging gonadotropin-releasing hormone pulse frequency. *J. Clin. Endocrinol. Metab.*, **79**, 858–64
8. Peluso, J. J. (1990). Role of the amplitude of the gonadotropin surge in the rat. *Fertil. Steril.*, **53**, 150–4
9. Hoff, J. D., Quigley, M. and Yen, S. S. C. (1983). Hormonal dynamics at midcycle. A reevaluation. *J. Clin. Endocrinol. Metab.*, **57**, 792–6
10. Abdalla, H. I., Ah-Moye, M., Brinsden, P., Howe, D. L., Okonofua, F. and Craft, I. (1987). The effect of the dose of human chorionic gonadotropin and the type of gonadotropin stimulation on oocyte recovery rates in an in vitro fertilization program. *Fertil. Steril.*, **6**, 958–63
11. Damewood, M. D., Shen, W., Zacur, H. A., Wallach, E. E., Rock, J. A. and Schlaff, W. D. (1989). Disappearance of exogenously administered human chorionic gonadotropin. *Fertil. Steril.*, **52**, 398–400
12. Pride, S. M., James, C. S. J. and Yuen, B. H. (1990). The ovarian hyperstimulation syndrome. *Semin. Reprod. Endocrinol.*, **8**, 247–60

13. Hamilton-Fairley, D., Kiddy, D., Watson, H., Sagle, M. and Franks, S. (1991). Low-dose gonadotrophin therapy for induction of ovulation in 100 women with polycystic ovary syndrome. *Hum. Reprod.*, **6**, 1095–9

14. Rizk, B. and Smitz, J. (1992). Ovarian hyperstimulation syndrome after superovulation using GnRH agonists for IVF and related procedures. *Hum. Reprod.*, **7**, 320–7

15. Fanchin, R., Castracane, D., Taieb, J., Freidtas, S., Olivennes, F., Frydman, R., Bouchard, P. and De Ziegler, D. (1993). The post-hCG hormonal profile in IVF-ET: plasma P increases 3 times more rapidly than in the menstrual cycle but androgens are unaffected. *Am. Fertil. Soc.* (suppl.), October (abstr.)

16. Van de Wiele, R., Bogumi, J., Dyrenfurth, I., Warren, M., Jewelewich, R. and Ferin, M. (1970). Mechanisms regulating the menstrual cycle in women. *Hormone Res.*, **26**, 63–103

17. Cochius, J. I., Burns, R. J., Blumbergs, P. C., Mack, K. and Alderman, C. P. (1990). Creutzfeldt–Jakob disease in a recipient of human pituitary-derived gonadotropin. *Aust. N.Z. J. Med.*, **20**, 592–3

18. Emperaire, J. and Ruffie, A. (1991). Triggering ovulation with endogenous luteinizing hormone may prevent the ovarian hyperstimulation syndrome. *Hum. Reprod.*, **6**, 506–10

19. Itskovitz, J., Erlik, Y., Boldes, R., Levron, J. and Brandes, J. M. (1991). Induction of preovulatory luteinizing hormone surge and prevention of ovarian hyperstimulation syndrome by gonadotropin releasing hormone agonist. *Fertil. Steril.*, **56**, 213–20

20. Balasch, J., Fábregues, F., Tur, R., Creus, M., Casamitjana, R., Peñarrubia, J., Barri, P. N. and Vanrell, J. A. (1995). Further characterization of the luteal phase inadequacy after gonadotrophin releasing hormone agonist induced ovulation in gonadotrophin stimulated cycles. *Fertil. Steril.*, **10**, 1377–81

21. Gerris, J., De Vits, A., Joostens, M. and Van Royen, E. (1995). Triggering of ovulation in human menopausal gonadotrophin-stimulated cycles: comparison between intravanously administered gonadotrophin-releasing hormone (100 and 500 μg), GnRH agonist (buserelin, 500 μg) and human chorionic gonadotrophin (10 000 IU). *Hum. Reprod.*, **10**, 56–62

22. Porchet, H. C., Le Cotonnec, J.-Y., Neuteboom, B., Canali, S. and Zanolo, G. (1995). Pharmacokinetics of recombinant human luteinizing hormone after intravenous, intramuscular, and subcutaneous administration in monkeys and comparison with intravenous administration of pituitary human luteinizing hormone. *J. Clin. Endocrinol. Metab.*, **80**, 667–73

23. Chandrasekher, Y. A., Hutchison, J. S., Zelinski-Wooten, M. B., Hess, D. L., Wolf, D. P. and Stouffer, R. L. (1994). Initiation of periovulatory events in primate follicles using recombinant and native human luteinizing hormone to mimic the midcycle gonadotropin surge. *J. Clin. Endocrinol. Metab.*, **79**, 298–306

24. Romeu, A., Molina, I., Tresguerres, J. A. F., Pla, M. and Peinado, J. A. (1995). Effect of recombinant human luteinizing hormone versus human chorionic gonadotrophin : effects on ovulation, embryo quality and transport, steroid balance and implantation in rabbits. *Hum. Reprod.*, **10**, 1290–6

25. van der Meer, S., Gerris, J., Joostens, S. and Tas, B. (1993). Triggering of ovulation using a gonadotrophin-releasing hormone agonist does not prevent ovarian hyperstimulation syndrome. *Hum. Reprod.*, **8**, 1628–31

26. Corson, S. L., Batzer, F. R., Gocial, B. and Maislin, G. (1993). The luteal phase after ovulation induction with human menopausal gonadotropin and one versus two doses of a gonadotropin-releasing hormone agonist. *Fertil. Steril.*, **59**, 1251–6

27. Lanzone, A., Fulghesu, A. M., Villa, P., Guida, C., Guido, M., Nicoletti, M. C., Caruso, A. and Mancuso, S. (1994). Gonadotropin-releasing hormone agonist versus human chorionic gonadotropin as a trigger of ovulation in polycystic ovarian disease gonadotropin hyperstimulated cycles. *Fertil. Steril.*, **62**, 35–41

28. Shalev, E., Geslevich, Y. and Ben-Ami, M. (1994). Induction of pre-ovulatory luteinizing hormone surge by gonadotrophin-releasing hormone agonist for women at risk for developing the ovarian hyperstimulation syndrome. *Hum. Reprod.*, **9**, 417–19

29. Blumenfeld, Z., Lang, N., Amit, A., Kahana, L. and Yoffe, N. (1994). Native gonadotropin-releasing hormone for triggering follicular maturation in polycystic ovary syndrome patients undergoing human menopausal gonadotropin ovulation induction. *Fertil. Steril.*, **62**, 456–60

30. Balasch, J., Tur, R., Creus, M., Buxaderas, R., Fábregues, F., Ballescá, J. L., Barri, P. N. and Vanrell, J. A. (1994). Triggering of ovulation by a gonadotropin releasing hormone agonist in gonadotropin-stimulated cycles for prevention of ovarian hyperstimulation syndrome and multiple pregnancy. *Gynecol. Endocrinol.*, **8**, 7–12

31. Bentick, B., Shaw, R. W., Iffland, C. A., Burford, G. and Bernard, A. (1990). IVF pregnancy after induction of an ovulatory endogenous gonadotrophin surge using an LHRH agonist nasal spray. *Hum. Reprod.*, **5**, 570–2

32. Gonen, Y., Balakier, H., Powell, W. and Casper, R. F. (1990). Use of gonadotropin-releasing hormone agonist to trigger follicular maturation for *in vitro* fertilization. *J. Clin. Endocrinol. Metab.*, **71**, 918–22

33. Imoedemhe, D. A. G., Sigue, A. B., Pacpaco, E. L. A. and Olazo, A. B. (1991). Stimulation of endogenous surge of luteinizing hormone with gonadotropin-releasing hormone analog after ovarian stimulation for *in vitro* fertilization. *Fertil. Steril.*, **55**, 328–32

34. Segal, S. and Casper, R. F. (1992). Gonadotropin-releasing hormone agonist versus human chorionic gonadotropin for triggering follicular maturation in *in vitro* fertilization. *Fertil. Steril.*, **57**, 1254–8

Section 7

Preparation for surgery in leiomyoma patients

Preparation for laparotomy or vaginal surgery in women with leiomyomas treated with GnRH agonists

26

A. J. Friedman

INTRODUCTION

Leiomyomas are the most common pelvic tumor in the female reproductive tract. It has been estimated that 20–30% of reproductive-age women have leiomyomas that may be detected at bimanual examination[1]. Histological sectioning of hysterectomy specimens at 2 mm intervals revealed subclinical leiomyomas in three-quarters of all women[2].

Approximately 20–50% of women with clinically palpable leiomyomas will have symptoms related to these tumors[1]. The most common symptoms are due to an enlarged pelvic mass (e.g. pelvic pressure, urinary frequency and pelvic discomfort) or excessive menstrual flow (e.g. menorrhagia, hypermenorrhea and anemia). In women with moderate-to-severe symptoms, surgical treatment is often recommended. There are two main surgical options: hysterectomy, which is the only known cure for leiomyomas, and myomectomy, which is carried out at about one-tenth of the frequency when the uterus is removed. Both procedures are highly successful in reducing, or relieving, preoperative symptoms[1,3].

HYSTERECTOMY

Leiomyomas are the leading single diagnosis for all hysterectomies performed in the United States, accounting for 34% of all cases[4]. Significant differences exist between Caucasians and Blacks in the proportion of women undergoing hysterectomy for leiomyomas; 29% of Caucasian women undergoing hysterectomy have a preoperative diagnosis of leiomyomas, compared to 61% of Blacks. Approximately 90% of hysterectomies performed for leiomyomas in the United States are performed via an abdominal route; the remainder are performed vaginally. Enlargement of the uterus is probably the primary reason why the vast majority of these hysterectomies are performed via the abdominal route.

When performed by a skilled surgeon, the intra- and postoperative morbidity for vaginal hysterectomy is approximately one-half that of abdominal hysterectomy[5]. In addition, women undergoing vaginal hysterectomy usually have shorter hospital stays and recovery times than those undergoing abdominal hysterectomy. For these reasons, hysterectomy via the vaginal route is preferred, when it is feasible.

Two goals of preoperative medical therapy are to decrease intra- and postoperative morbidity and to decrease the overall cost of treatment. It has been proposed that preoperative treatment of women with a gonadotropin releasing hormone (GnRH) agonist may help to achieve these goals in selected patients. The induction of profound hypoestrogenemia by GnRH agonists will lead to a mean decrease in uterine volume of 35–50% after 12 weeks of treatment[6–9]. It has been reported that 70% of women treated with a GnRH agonist for 12 weeks have a reduction in uterine volume by at least 25%[10]. In addition, GnRH agonist treatment causes menstrual suppression in the vast majority of women, leading to significant improvements in hemoglobin (Hgb) concentrations and hematocrit (Hct) in anemic patients[11,12].

CONVERSION OF ABDOMINAL HYSTERECTOMY TO VAGINAL HYSTERECTOMY

Although it is commonly believed that women with large leiomyomatous uteri who undergo abdominal hysterectomy have a higher morbidity rate than those with smaller uteri, supporting data are lacking[13]. However, shrinkage of a leiomyomatous uterus may enable the surgeon to 'convert' an abdominal hysterectomy to a vaginal hysterectomy. This hypothesis was tested in a clinical trial in which 50 women with symptomatic leiomyomatous uteri, whose uterine size ranged from that expected at 14 to 18 weeks' gestation, were randomized to receive either 3.75 mg of leuprolide acetate depot (Lupron depot, TAP Pharmaceuticals Inc., Deerfield, IL, USA) intramuscularly every 4 weeks for 2 weeks ($n = 25$) or no medical treatment ($n = 25$) before undergoing hysterectomy[14]. Vaginal hysterectomy was attempted in all women whose uterine size was similar to that found at 14 weeks' gestation or less after medical treatment. Nineteen (76%) women pretreated with leuprolide acetate met this criterion; 13 (52%) had successful vaginal hysterectomies. In contrast, four (16%) women who did not receive preoperative medical therapy were candidates for vaginal hysterectomy; two (8%) had successful vaginal hysterectomies ($p < 0.05$ between groups).

In this study, mean intraoperative blood loss was significantly less in women receiving leuprolide acetate (527 ± 74 ml versus 614 ± 108 ml, $p < 0.05$), although there was no difference in transfusion rates. Women receiving preoperative leuprolide acetate had a significantly shorter postoperative hospital stay (3.8 ± 1.9 days versus 5.2 ± 1.8 days, $p < 0.05$) and convalescence period (17.5 ± 4.5 days versus 28.5 ± 6.2 days, $p < 0.05$) which, in turn, led to lower overall treatment costs.

STUDY RESULTS

The results of this study suggest that treatment of women with enlarged leiomyomatous uteri with a GnRH agonist may decrease the uterine size below a critical threshold, enabling the surgeon

to perform a vaginal hysterectomy. Clearly, proper patient selection for preoperative GnRH agonist treatment will depend on multiple variables, including:

(1) Pretreatment uterine size;

(2) The anticipated reduction in uterine size;

(3) The surgeon's comfort with vaginal surgery;

(4) The surgeon's assessment of her uterine size 'threshold';

(5) An assessment of uterine mobility; and

(6) An assessment of the bony structure and soft tissues of the pelvis.

The efficacy of preoperative GnRH agonist treatment for women undergoing abdominal myomectomy is less clear. In one randomized, double-blind clinical trial[15], women with leiomyomas treated preoperatively with leuprolide acetate for 12 weeks had significantly less intraoperative blood loss compared to placebo-treated controls (189 ± 44 ml versus 390 ± 20 ml, $p < 0.01$) in women with pretreatment uterine volumes that were greater than 600 cm^3. There was no difference in mean blood loss in the two treatment groups with pretreatment uterine sizes that were less than 600 cm^3, nor was there a difference in transfusion rates. Other morbidity variables (e.g. febrile morbidity), duration of hospital stay and convalescence did not differ between groups. Although other studies[14,16–18] have reported decreased intraoperative blood loss in women pretreated with a GnRH agonist undergoing hysterectomy or myomectomy compared to controls, no study has reported a decrease in the transfusion rate. Since homologous transfusion rates for these surgical procedures are generally less than 10% a large, possibly multicenter, trial would be needed to determine whether preoperative medical treatment lowers the transfusion rate.

Another potential benefit of preoperative GnRH agonist therapy is the induction of menstrual suppression which, in turn, may correct anemia in women with menorrhagia. Approximately three-quarters of women with leiomyomas will have complete menstrual suppression (i.e. amenorrhea) after 3 months of treatment[19]; the majority of the remaining women will have light bleeding or irregular spotting. Menstrual suppression and repletion of iron stores are two medical treatment strategies to correct anemia in women with menorrhagia-associated anemia. One randomized, double-blind, placebo-controlled, multicenter study compared the efficacy of daily oral iron therapy with iron plus leuprolide acetate depot for 12 weeks[20]. Patients enrolled in the study were required to have a Hgb concentration of 10.2 g/dl or less and/or a Hct of 30% or less. Treatment success was defined as a Hgb concentration of greater than 12 g/dl and a Hct of greater than 36%. After 12 weeks of treatment, 74% of women treated with leuprolide plus iron ($n = 142$) had correction of anemia compared to 49% of women receiving iron alone ($n = 59$, $p < 0.01$). The proportion of women treated successfully was the same for those who received 3.75 mg or 7.5 mg leuprolide acetate depot at 4, 8 and 12 weeks of treatment. Mean Hgb concentration increased from 8.2 g/dl to 12.6 g/dl ($p < 0.001$) in women receiving 3.75 mg of leuprolide acetate depot plus iron compared to an increase from 8.0 g/dl to 11.5 g/dl in those receiving iron alone. Correspondingly, the mean Hct increased from 28.1% to 39.1% ($p < 0.001$) in leuprolide plus iron-treated subjects and from 27.6% to 35.7% in iron-treated controls. Not surprisingly, a higher proportion of leuprolide-treated women experienced adverse effects, including hot flushes, dizziness, depression, vaginitis and abdominal pain.

Thirty-three of 188 (17%) women receiving leuprolide plus iron donated autologous blood compared to seven of 77 (9%) of those receiving iron only. Hysterectomy was performed in 63% of patients and myomectomy was performed in 37%. Homologous blood transfusion occurred in ten of 188 (5%) women receiving leuprolide plus iron compared to ten of 77 (13%) women receiving iron only. As there was no standardization regarding autologous blood donation or transfusion guidelines, no conclusions can be made regarding the impact of these two treatments on the likelihood of transfusion.

SUMMARY

The decision to offer preoperative GnRH agonist treatment to a woman with leiomyomas must be individualized. The patient's goals, the surgeon's goals and level of skill, an understanding of the drug's expected beneficial and adverse effects, as well as consideration of the cost of therapy, must all be weighed before a decision is reached. In properly selected patients, preoperative treatment with a GnRH agonist may decrease intra- and postoperative morbidity, the duration of hospital stay and the convalescence period, as well as the overall cost of treatment.

References

1. Buttram, V. C. and Reiter, R. C. (1981). Uterine leiomyomata: etiology, symptomatology, and management. *Fertil. Steril.*, **36**, 433–45
2. Cramer, S. F. and Patel, A. (1990). The frequency of uterine leiomyomas. *Am. J. Clin. Pathol.*, **94**, 435–8
3. Carlson, K. J., Miller, B. A. and Fowler, F. J. Jr (1994). The Maine Women's Health Study: I. Outcomes of hysterectomy. *Obstet. Gynecol.*, **83**, 556–65
4. Wilcox, L. S., Koonin, L. M., Pokras, R., Strauss, L. T., Xia, Z. and Peterson, H. B. (1994). Hysterectomy in the United States, 1988–1990. *Obstet. Gynecol.*, **83**, 549–55
5. Dicker, R. C., Greenspan, J. R., Strauss, L. T., Cowart, M. R., Scally, M. J., Peterson, H. B., DeStefano, F., Rubin, G. L. and Ory, H. W. (1982). Complications of abdominal and vaginal hysterectomy among women of reproductive age in the United States. *Am. J. Obstet. Gynecol.*, **144**, 841–8
6. Friedman, A. J., Barbieri, R. L., Benacerraf, B. R. and Schiff, I. (1987). Treatment of leiomyomata with intranasal or subcutaneous leuprolide, a gonadotropin releasing-hormone agonist. *Fertil. Steril.*, **48**, 560–4
7. Friedman, A. J., Harrison-Atlas, D., Barbieri, R. L., Benacerraf, B., Gleason, R. E. and Schiff, I.

(1989). A randomized, placebo-controlled, double-blind study evaluating the efficacy of leuprolide acetate depot in the treatment of uterine leiomyomata. *Fertil. Steril.*, **51**, 251–6

8. Friedman, A. J., Hoffman, D. I., Comite, F., Browneller, R. W. and Miller, J. D (1991). Treatment of leiomyomata uteri with leuprolide acetate depot: a double-blind, placebo-controlled, multicenter study. *Obstet. Gynecol.*, **77**, 720–5

9. Schlaff, W. D., Zerhouni, E. A., Huth, J. A. M., Chen, J., Damewood, M. D. and Rock, J. A. (1989). A placebo-controlled trial of a depot gonadotropin-releasing hormone analogue (leuprolide) in the treatment of uterine leiomyomata. *Obstet. Gynecol.*, **74**, 856–62

10. Friedman, A. J., Daly, M., Juneau-Norcross, M. and Rein, M. S. (1932). Predictors of uterine volume reduction in women with myomas treated with a gonadotropin releasing-hormone agonist. *Fertil. Steril.*, **58**, 413–5

11. Candiani, G. B., Vercellini, P., Fedele, L., Arcaini, L., Bianchi, S. and Candiani, M. (1990). Use of goserelin depot, a gonadotropin-releasing hormone agonist, for the treatment of menorrhagia and severe anemia in women with leiomyomata uteri. *Acta Obstet. Gynecol. Scand.*, **69**, 413–15

12. Friedman, A. J., Barbieri, R. L., Doubilet, P. M., Fine, C. and Schiff, I. (1988). A randomized, double-blind trial of a gonadotropin releasing-hormone agonist (leuprolide) with or without medroxyprogesterone acetate in the treatment of leiomyomata uteri. *Fertil. Steril.*, **49**, 404–9

13. Reiter, R. C., Wagner, P. L. and Gambone, J. C. (1992). Routine hysterectomy for large asymptomatic uterine leiomyomata: a reappraisal. *Obstet. Gynecol.*, **79**, 481–4

14. Stovall, T. G., Ling, F. W., Henry, L. C. and Woodruff, M. R. (1991). A randomized trial evaluating leuprolide acetate before hysterectomy as a treatment for leiomyomas. *Am. J. Obstet. Gynecol.*, **164**, 1420–5

15. Friedman, A. J., Rein, M. S., Harrison-Atlas, D., Garfield, J. M. and Doubilet, P. M. (1989). A randomized, placebo-controlled, double-blind study evaluating leuprolide acetate depot treatment before myomectomy. *Fertil. Steril.*, **52**, 728–33

16. Golan, A., Bukovsky, I., Pansky, M., Schneider, D., Weinraub, Z. and Caspi, E. (1993). Pre-operative gonadotrophin-releasing hormone agonist treatment in surgery for uterine leiomyomata. *Hum. Reprod.*, **8**, 450–2

17. Smith, S. and Levi, C. (1991). On the utility of preoperative leuprolide acetate depot therapy prior to abdominal myomectomy. *Am. J. Gynecol. Health*, **5**, 11–15

18. Lumsden, M. A., West, C. P. and Baird, D. T. (1987). Goserelin therapy before surgery for uterine fibroids. *Lancet*, **1**, 36–7

19. Friedman, A. J., Daly, M., Juneau-Norcross, M., Rein, M. S., Fine, C., Gleason, R. and LeBoff, M. (1993). A prospective, randomized trial of gonadotropin releasing-hormone agonist plus estrogen–progestin or progestin 'add-back' regimens for women with leiomyomata uteri. *J. Clin. Endocrinol. Metab.*, **76**, 1439–45

20. Stovall, T. G., Muneyyirci-Detale, O., Summitt, R. L. Jr and Scialli, A. R. (1995). GnRH agonist and iron versus placebo and iron in the anemic patient before surgery for leiomyomas: a randomized controlled trial. *Obstet. Gynecol.*, **86**, 65–71

27

Combined GnRH agonists and laser endoscopy in the management of dysfunctional bleeding, submucous fibroids and large endometriomas

J. Donnez, M. Nisolle, F. Casanas-Roux, R. Polet, M. Smets and S. Bassil

INTRODUCTION

Dysfunctional bleeding and fibroids are the major reasons for hysterectomy in women aged > 40 years. Since 1985, gonadotropin releasing hormones (GnRH) agonists have been recognized as the medical management for these conditions[1]. Nevertheless, because of the bone loss induced by the hypoestrogenism, this therapy must be considered as either a temporary medical approach before endoscopic surgery or as a long-term therapy combined with a so-called 'add-back therapy'[2,3].

Endometriosis is one of the major causes of female infertility and GnRH agonist has also proved to be effective in its management[4-6]. Here also, a combined (medical and surgical) therapy has been proposed[7-10].

The aim of this review is to evaluate the place of GnRH agonists as a preoperative therapy before hysteroscopy in cases of dysfunctional bleeding or fibroids and before laparoscopic surgery in cases of endometriosis.

DYSFUNCTIONAL BLEEDING AND FIBROIDS

Hysteroscopic surgical techniques have proved to be successful in the control of menorrhagia[11,12]. The hysteroscope allows the destruction of the endometrium to be carried out under direct vision. Both the electrical current of the resectoscope[13-17] and the energy of the neodymium:yttrium–aluminium–garnet (Nd:YAG) laser[11,18-22] have been effective tools in the destruction of endometrial tissue to a sufficient depth to avoid regeneration.

The aim of this procedure is to decrease the menstrual flow sufficiently to allow patients to avoid hysterectomy. Indeed, amenorrhea and hypomenorrhea are recognized as sequelae of intrauterine adhesions; the laser ablation procedure is designed to create this condition. Other methods have been used in an attempt to create endometrial destruction and scarring: cryotherapy, superheated steam, intracavitary radium, rigorous curettage, quinocrine methylcyanoacrylate, oxalic acid, paraformaldehyde and silicone rubber. However, only the Ng:YAG[11,12,18,23] and the resectoscope[16,17] have had acceptable results.

Laser energy has some advantages in precision of tissue destruction that are not shared by the electrical energy used in the resectoscope. Unlike electricity, laser energy does not travel through tissue; its tissue effect depends on the amount of power used, and its effects are quite reproducible.

MATERIALS AND METHODS

A series of 746 patients treated for men metrorrhagia was analyzed.

Endometrial ablation

In a first group, only women without intrauterine lesions were considered. In this series of 380 women the authors tried to classify the uterine pathology in order to evaluate endometrial ablation in dysfunctional bleeding. Two groups of women were defined according to the size of the uterine cavity ($< 10\ \mathrm{cm}^2$; $> 10\ \mathrm{cm}^2$) prior to

GnRH agonist therapy. Women contemplating this procedure must be aware that further childbearing cannot be considered. These women should have a diagnostic hysteroscopy with endometrial sampling prior to laser ablation. Women with atypical endometrium should not be considered.

Having decided to proceed with surgery, the endometrium was brought into a resting phase by GnRH agonist therapy[8]. The implant (Zoladex, Zeneca, Cambridge, United Kingdom) was injected subcutaneously at the end of the luteal phase, to curtail the initial gonadotropin stimulation phase always associated with a rise in estrogens. The authors consider the ideal scheme of therapy to be as follows:

(1) Preoperative GnRH agonist therapy by injection at weeks 0 and 4.

(2) Hysteroscopic surgery at weeks 5 or 6.

Indeed, a period of 4–5 weeks of very low estradiol levels (after the well-known flare-up effect) is sufficient to reduce the endometrium to a very thin postmenopausal state.

Regional or general anesthesia is used, as local anesthesia is accompanied by considerable cramp. The authors prefer to perform all operative hysteroscopies with the uterine cavity well distended (the intrauterine pressure exceeding the venous pressure), so that bleeding cannot occur from the endometrial surface.

There are three techniques for applying laser energy to the endometrial cavity:

(1) The touch technique[11,24];

(2) The non-touch technique[12]; and

(3) A combination of both techniques.

The touch technique was used in our series. Endometrial ablation was carried out in the uterine cavity, except in an area 1 cm above the uterine isthmus, in order to avoid complete amenorrhea. In this group, the proposed goal was to obtain hypomenorrhea and not amenorrhea.

Hysteroscopic myomectomy

In the authors' department, 366 women aged between 23 and 43 years (mean age 33 years) with symptomatic submucous uterine fibroids were treated with a biodegradable GnRH agonist (Zoladex). One implant was systematically injected at weeks 0, 4 and 8. Hysteroscopic myomectomy was carried out at 8 weeks.

Classification of myomas[19,25]

According to hysterosalpingography data, submucosal fibroids were classified as:

(1) Submucosal fibroid whose greatest diameter is inside the uterine cavity;

(2) Submucosal fibroid whose largest portion is located in the myometrium; or

(3) Multiple (> 2) submucosal fibroids (myofibromatous uterus with submucosal fibroids and intramural fibroids) diagnosed by hysterography and echography.

In cases of submucosal fibroids whose *greatest diameter was inside* the uterine cavity, myomectomy was performed by hysteroscopy and Nd:YAG laser. The myometrium overlying the myoma was less vascular and the 'shrinkage' of the uterine cavity may have accounted for the relative ease of separating the myomas from the surrounding myometrium.

In cases of *very large submucous fibroids whose largest portion* was not inside the uterine cavity but inside the uterine wall a *two-step operative hysteroscopy* was proposed[10]. After an 8-week preoperative GnRH agonist therapy, a partial myomectomy was carried out by resecting the protruded portion of the myoma. Thereafter, the laser fiber was directed, as perpendicularly as possible, at the remaining (intramural) fibroid portion and was introduced into the fibroid to a depth of 5–10 mm. During the application of laser energy, the fiber was slowly removed so that the deeper areas were coagulated. The aim of this procedure was to decrease the size of the remaining myoma by decreasing the vascularity. This technique induces a myoma necrobiosis and can be called 'transhysteroscopic myolysis'[19]. GnRH agonist therapy was given for another 8 weeks and the second-look hysteroscopy was then performed. In all cases, the myoma was found to protrude inside the uterine cavity and appeared very white and

Table 1 Nd:YAG laser hysteroscopic endometrial ablation in two consecutive series of 380 patients who underwent partial endometrial laser ablation (PELA) for dysfunctional bleeding (myomas excluded)

	Uterine cavity			
	< 10 cm²		> 10 cm²	
No. of patients	280		100	
Results:				
amenorrhea	3	(11%)	1	(1%)
hypomenorrhea	264	(93%)	83	(83%)
normal flow	10	(4%)	10	(50%)
failed	6	(2%)	6	(6%)
Recurrence of menometrorrhagia (2-year follow-up)	5	(2%)	14	(14%)
Total of failures (2 years)	11	(4%)	20	(20%)

without any apparent vessels on its surface. The shrinkage of the uterine cavity allowed the residual myoma portion to be easily separated from the surrounding myometrium and dissected off. Myomectomy was then carried out. At the end of the procedure, the myoma can be left in the uterine cavity.

In cases of *multiple submucosal fibroids*, each myoma was either separated from the surrounding myometrium or totally photocoagulated. Each myoma was systematically destroyed and at the end of surgery, endometrial ablation with the Nd:YAG laser was carried out.

RESULTS

Table 1 shows the results of our series of patients treated by a touch technique for endometrial ablation.

In the first subgroup (uterine cavity less than 10 cm²) hypomenorrhea was achieved in 94% of cases. Amenorrhea occurred in only 1% of cases, and failures in 2% of cases. In the other subgroup (uterine cavity more than 10 cm², the failure rate was significantly ($p < 0.01$) higher (6/100; 6%). The operating time varied from 15 min to 25 min. Blood loss was minimal. No uterine perforation occurred.

When performed, hysterosalpingography revealed a shrinkage of the uterine cavity (Figure 1). In the subgroup of women with a uterine cavity of more than 10 cm², the recurrence rate of menometrorrhagia was significantly ($p < 0.01$) higher (14%) than that observed when the uterine cavity was < 10 cm² (2%) (Table 1). The total of failures was respectively 4% and 20% according to the uterine cavity area < 10 or > 10 mm². The difference was significant ($p < 0.001$).

Since GnRH agonist therapy was systematically administered and the continuous-flow hysteroscopic system used, fluid overload syndrome did not occur.

Using the method previously described[19,26,27], the reduction of very large submucous fibroid areas was calculated (Table 2). When more than one fibroid was present, only the largest was evaluated. In all cases except four, the fibroid area decreased by an average of 38%. However, the response was variable, ranging from 4% to 95%. The fibroid area was found to decrease significantly ($p < 0.01$) from the baseline area (7.2 ± 4.7 cm²) to 4.4 ± 3.5 cm² by 8 weeks of therapy. About 10% of myomas do not appear to respond well to the GnRH agonist. Table 3 shows the long-term results according to the myoma classification.

In cases of large submucous fibroids whose greatest diameter was inside the uterine cavity ($n = 233$), surgery was successfully carried out in 230 cases. In three cases, an endometrial stromal tumor was diagnosed by the histological

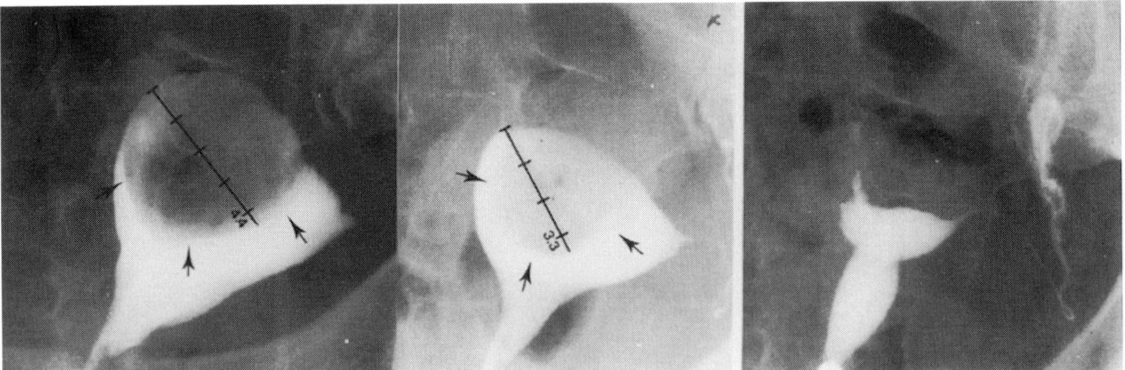

Figure 1 Left: preoperative aspect of the uterine cavity before GnRH agonist. Middle: preoperative aspect of the uterine cavity after GnRH agonist (on day before surgery). Right: shrinkage of the uterine cavity 6 months after the procedure

Table 2 Submucosal fibroid areas as assessed by hysterosalpingography before and after an 8-week GnRH agonist therapy

	Area (cm^2)		
	Pre-therapy	*Post-therapy*	*Reduction (%)*
> 10 cm^2 ($n = 34$)	14.5 ± 6.5	9.7 ± 5.6	34.4
> 10 cm^2 ($n = 36$)	6.9 ± 1.3	4.5 ± 1.9	34.9
> 10 cm^2 ($n = 80$)	2.5 ± 1.2	1.7 ± 0.9	34.4
Total ($n = 150$)	6.3 ± 5.8	4.7 ± 3.8	34.5

Table 3 Surgical procedures and long-term results according to the site of myomas

	Greatest diameter inside the uterine cavity	*Largest portion located in the uterine wall*	*Multiple submucosal myomas (myomectomy and endometrial ablation)*
Surgical procedures:			
patients (n)	233	78	55
successful	230	74	51
failed	3*	4[†]	4[‡]
Recurrence of menometrorrhagias	5 (2%)	4 (5%)	15 (27%)

*Stromal tumor. [†]A third-look hysteroscopy allowed the myoma to be removed. [‡]Myomectomy was not totally successful (in two cases, second-look laser hysteroscopy was performed successfully. In the other two cases, vaginal hysterectomy was proposed and successfully performed. Recurrence = recurrence of menorrhagia

examination of the removed 'myomas'. Hysteroscopically, they appeared as benign myomas. Thus, the incidence of 'stromal tumors' in apparently benign myomas is 1.2% (3/233). It is important to note that all three cases were observed in the subgroups of myomas which did not respond well (< 10% decrease) to GnRH agonist therapy. When successfully performed, myomectomy permits the restoration of normal menstrual flow. Long-term result evaluation[28] shows that recurrence of menorrhagia occurred more frequently (27%) in cases of multiple submucosal myomas than in cases of single submucosal myomas. Recurrence of menorraghia was provoked by the growth of myomas in other sites, as proved by hysterography and hysteroscopy.

DISCUSSION

Endometrial ablation

Numerous methods have been used in an attempt to create endometrial destruction and scarring: cryotherapy, superheated steam, intracavitary radium, rigorous curettage, quinacrine methyl-cyanoacrylate, oxalic acid, paraformaldehyde and silicone rubber. However, only the Nd:YAG laser and the resectoscope have had acceptable results.

Once the decision to proceed with surgery has been made, the endometrium is brought into a resting phase by treating with danazol (400 mg twice a day), beginning during the menses[12], or by GnRH agonist therapy[26]. Indeed, the use of GnRH analogs constitutes an interest in reducing uterine size to facilitate the surgical procedure[8,10,22,26]. In the authors' department, an implant of a biodegradable GnRH agonist was injected subcutaneously at the end of the luteal phase, to curtail the initial gonadotropin stimulation phase always associated with a rise in estrogens. Significant shrinkage was found to occur at 4–5 weeks of therapy. Indeed, as documented by hysterosalpingography imaging (using the short-line 'multipurpose test system' described by Weibel)[26] patients experienced a decrease in the uterine cavity area, with an average decrease of 35%[22,26]. The response was variable, however, ranging from 5% to 60%. The decrease in total uterine cavity area was greater in cases of a very enlarged uterine cavity (> 10 cm²) than in cases of an initial uterine cavity area of < 10 cm².

The advantages of a preoperative therapy are:

(1) Endometrial ablation is easily performed (thin endometrium, small uterine cavity); and

(2) The risk of fluid overload is decreased.[19,22,29]

In a series of 380 women, 'partial' endometrial laser ablation (PELA) was carried out in order to provoke hypomenorrhea, so that a little bleeding could be observed at the menstruation time[22]. Indeed, for psychological reasons hypomenorrhea could be preferred to amenorrhea. This procedure could be proposed in the future to women in their 40s in order to reduce menstrual flow, even in the absence of dysfunctional bleeding.

In the literature, most authors[11,12,18,22,23,30–32] have presented a high rate for 'immediate' good results, but only a few[22] have published the long-term results. Significant differences have been observed according to the uterine cavity area. If the uterine cavity area is > 10 cm², failure rates (6%) and recurrent menometrorrhagia rates (14%) are higher than those observed if the uterine cavity is < 10 cm² (2% and 2%, respectively). The significant differences related to the uterine cavity area account for some discrepancies in the results published and/or shown during the numerous congresses. The authors' results suggest proposing endometrial ablation only to women with a uterine cavity < 10 cm², and also reducing the preoperative therapy duration to 4–5 weeks. Indeed, the authors' results prove that a 4–5-week therapy is sufficient to reduce the uterine cavity and endometrial thickness. Postoperative bleeding and fluid overload leading to pulmonary edema did not occur in this second series. The problem is similar to that described in transurethral resection of the prostate[33]. Fluid absorption could be influenced by the thickness of the endometrium and vascularization of the chorion. These two parameters are influenced by GnRH agonist therapy. In the last series of > 700 cases no fluid overload occurred, since GnRH agonist therapy was systematically administered and the continuous flow hysteroscopic system used.

In conclusion, GnRH agonist therapy effects a decrease in the total uterine cavity area which facilitates surgical treatment and reduces the risk of fluid overload syndrome. Endometrial laser ablation (ELA) is quickly performed by experienced gynecologists. The morbidity rate and hospitalization time are reduced. Also, the primary advantage is that hysterectomy can be avoided in young women suffering from abnormal bleeding.

Submucous myomas

Because most leiomyomata return to pretreatment size within 4 months of cessation of GnRH agonist therapy, these agents cannot be used as definitive medical therapy[1,2,34,35]. Several reports have demonstrated reductions in uterine and fibroid volumes of 52–77% after 6 months of a GnRH agonist therapy, as assessed by ultrasound imaging. In the authors' study, as documented by hysterographic imaging, an average decrease of 35% was found in the uterine cavity[26,27]. Another study[19] demonstrated reductions in fibroid area of 38% after 8 weeks of GnRH agonist therapy. The response was variable, however, ranging from 2% to 95% . There was no difference in the extent of decrease according to the pretreatment fibroid area.

In cases of submucosal uterine fibroids, hysteroscopic myomectomy was carried out if the greatest diameter of the leiomyoma, as assessed by hysterography, was inside the uterine cavity. A treatment duration of 8 weeks was advised before hysteroscopic myomectomy. Indeed, in a previous study[26], a significant uterine shrinkage was observed after 8 weeks of therapy.

The peroperative blood loss was minimal, possibly because of the decreased vascularity of the myometrium, which was demonstrated by a significant reduction in the uterine arterial blood flow (Doppler) after treatment with a GnRH agonist[36]. In all cases (except when no decrease in the myoma size was observed), the myoma was left in the uterine cavity and there were no complications. Probably, after a necrotic phase, the myoma was ejected with the menstrual blood.

In cases of very large fibroids where the largest diameter was not inside the uterine cavity, the myomectomy was carried out in two stages. During the first surgical procedure, the protruding portion was removed and the intramural portion was devascularized by introducing the laser fiber into the myoma to a depth of 5–10 mm, depending on the depth of the remaining intramural portion. The distance between the deepest portion of the myoma and the uterine serosa was evaluated by echography. An interesting finding was that this intramural portion of the myoma became submucosal and protruded inside the uterine cavity, possibly because of the GnRH agonist induced uterine shrinkage, which provoked this protrusion of the remaining portion. In all cases, the largest diameter of the remaining portion of the myoma was inside the uterine cavity, so that myomectomy was easily performed by separating it from the surrounding myometrium with the help of the Nd:YAG laser.

In conclusion, the use of GnRH agonist represents an adjunct for preoperative reduction of tumor size, so that the subsequent surgical treatment by hysteroscopy is possible. In the authors' series, even when the largest diameter was in the myometrium, the two-step hysteroscopic therapy combined with GnRH agonist therapy[19,20,37] represented the ideal management of large submucous myomas, reducing the need for myomectomy by laparotomy, which is often accompanied by increased operative blood loss and postoperative adhesion formation.

Because of the cessation of uterine bleeding, preoperative therapy resulted in the restoration of a normal hemoglobin concentration, which allows for the possibility of a later autologous transfusion.

The amount of fluid absorbed was lower if the endometrium was atrophic. By reducing the amount of fluid absorbed, the preoperative GnRH agonist therapy reduced the risk of fluid overload and this represents another major advantage of this combined medical and surgical approach to therapy. The advantages of the preoperative use of a GnRH agonist are as follows:

(1) The reduction of the myoma size;

(2) The decreased risk of fluid overload;

(3) The restoration of a normal hemoglobin concentration; and

(4) Detection of a stromal tumor.

A stromal tumor was found in the authors' series in three (1.2%) cases. In all three cases, the 'myoma' was found not to be decreased by GnRH agonist therapy. In cases of numerous submucosal intramural myomas, a higher risk of recurrence was observed when compared to patients with only one submucosal myoma[28]. Because of this high rate of recurrence, the authors prefer to perform a laparoscopic supracervical hysterectomy (LASH)[20,38] instead of the hysteroscopic procedure.

Treatment of endometriosis

Hormonal therapy

During the last decade three new agents, danazol, gestrinone and GnRH agonist, have created further options in the hormonal treatment of endometriosis, but many studies have reported that medical therapy is insufficient to eradicate it[8–10,39–41]. In infertile patients, it has not been proved that medical therapy and/or surgical treatment of minimal endometriosis improve fertility, but pregnancies following medical, surgical or combined treatment often occur within the first month following treatment[42] and it has not been excluded that there is still a place for a combined short-term medical and surgical approach[25,43].

In asymptomatic patients, the treatment of endometriotic implants during diagnostic laparoscopy is debatable. While it is reasonable to leave the apparently inactive implant untreated in the older patient, it is probably justified to eliminate active implants in the young patient because they can extend and provoke adhesions[43]. Indeed, despite its relatively superior efficacy when compared to other drugs, GnRH agonist was unable to completely suppress endometriotic cells because the ectopic foci are not governed by the normal control mechanisms governing the uterine endometrial glands and stroma. The precise reason why a number of implants or cells do not respond to hormonal therapy is unknown, but four hypotheses[8] have been proposed.

(1) The drug does not gain access to the ovarian endometriotic foci because fibrosis surrounding the foci prevents access locally.

(2) Endometriotic cells may have their own genetic programming, while an endocrine influence appears to be only secondary and dependent on the degree of differentiation of the individual cell.

(3) The low number of endometriotic steroid receptors and their different regulatory mechanisms in ectopic and eutopic endometrium may result in deficient endocrine dependency. The nuclear estrogen binding sites seen in foci of endometriosis do not appear to change during the menstrual cycle, whereas these sites in the uterine endometrium down-regulate during the secretory phase[44].

(4) The steroids receptors are biologically inactive[44,45].

As suggested in a previous study[8], the advantage of an efficacious hormonal treatment is the reduction in pelvic vascularity and inflammation, often present around endometriotic foci. The improved pelvic environment facilitates the technical aspect of surgery and reduces the risk of postoperative adhesion formation. GnRH agonists have found numerous applications in the reversible control of gonadal steroid secretion.

There is probably no indication for the use of GnRH agonist before laparoscopic vaporization except in cases of very inflammatory and active disease, characterized by the presence of many well-vascularized red lesions. As suggested by Evers in the World Congress in Brussels in 1992[46], GnRH agonist can be given in such circumstances in order to achieve a better relief of the disease, but we have to have in mind that 'destruction', either by laser or by coagulation, remains the first step in the management of peritoneal endometriosis.

Rationale for surgery

The relationship between infertility and ovarian endometriomas is clear. Indeed, an ovarian endometriotic cyst can disturb the follicular maturation and the follicle rupture, and provoke adhesions.

Three different types of ovarian endometriosis[25,47,48] can be classified as:

(1) Superficial hemorrhagic lesions;

(2) Hemorrhagic cysts (endometriomas); and

(3) Deep-infiltrating ovarian endometriosis (infrequent).

Superficial lesions. Superficial ovarian lesions are small vesicular lesions covering the ovarian cortex, or small implants usually found on the lateral surface of the ovary. The endometrial cyst may be lined with free endometrial tissue similar histologically and functionally to eutopic endometrium[49], but in some instances atypical epithelium and ciliated cells are found[41].

Endometriosis. The term 'chocolate cyst' was applied by Sampson (1927)[50] to describe the endometrial cyst of the ovary. As pointed out by Hughesdon (1957)[51], the internal surface of a chocolate cyst is really the external surface of the ovary; the ovarian cortex is identifiable by the presence of primordial follicles. The mobilization of the cyst from its fixed position provokes the rupture and subsequent spillage of contents[7,52].

Three months after drainage of the endometrioma and GnRH therapy (which provokes amenorrhea), chocolate-colored fluid is still present[8], proving that endometrial shedding is not responsible for chocolate-colored fluid formation. In the author's opinion, its origin could be cyst wall exudation (Donnez), congested cyst wall blood vessels (Brosens[49]) or inflammation around persistent intracystic endometrial foci, which are resistant to medical therapy[10,41].

Deep-infiltrating ovarian endometriosis. This is characterized by the presence of very active endometrial glands which are completely hormonally independent and which invade the ovarian cortex. Areas of oviduct-like epithelium with ciliated cells were demonstrated in 62% of cases[9,41].

In the authors' series of patients with endometriosis, ovarian endometriomas > 3 cm in diameter were found in 481 patients. A three-step therapy was proposed because of the size of the endometriomas.

(1) During diagnostic laparoscopy, the endometrial cyst was washed out with irrigation fluid (saline solution), and a biopsy was taken;

(2) A GnRH agonist was given for 12 weeks to reduce the cyst size; and

(3) The residual endometrial cyst wall was then vaporized with the CO_2 laser, equipped with the Swiftlase (Figure 2).

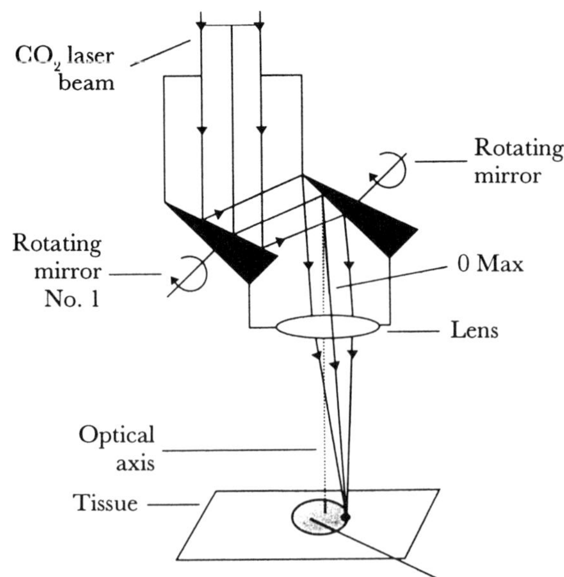

Figure 2 Swiftlase: a miniature opto-mechanical scanner. The mirrors constantly rotate at slightly different angular velocities, thereby rapidly varying with time, between zero and a maximum value 0 max. A focal spot which rapidly and homogenously scans and covers a round area of 2.5 mm diameter

The resolution of ovarian diseases depended on the decrease in size of endometrial cysts (Figure 3). Although GnRH agonist reduced endometriotic lesions in numerous cases[53], large ovarian cysts were never completely resolved by either treatment[37]. The authors' laparoscopic findings were confirmed by the histological study. In all cases, histological examination of residual ovarian endometriotic lesions after hormonal therapy revealed glandular epithelium and stroma. Although GnRH agonist therapy is effective in reducing endometriotic implant size to a greater extent than other drugs[10], this therapy was unable to suppress endometriotic cells completely because some ectopic foci are more or less autonomous and not governed by the normal control mechanisms governing the uterine endometrial glands. The lower incidence of active endometriosis observed in the authors' study in the GnRH agonist group probably explains the better resolution of the disease observed in this group. Laparoscopy was used to evaluate the effect of medical therapy, and a variable degree of

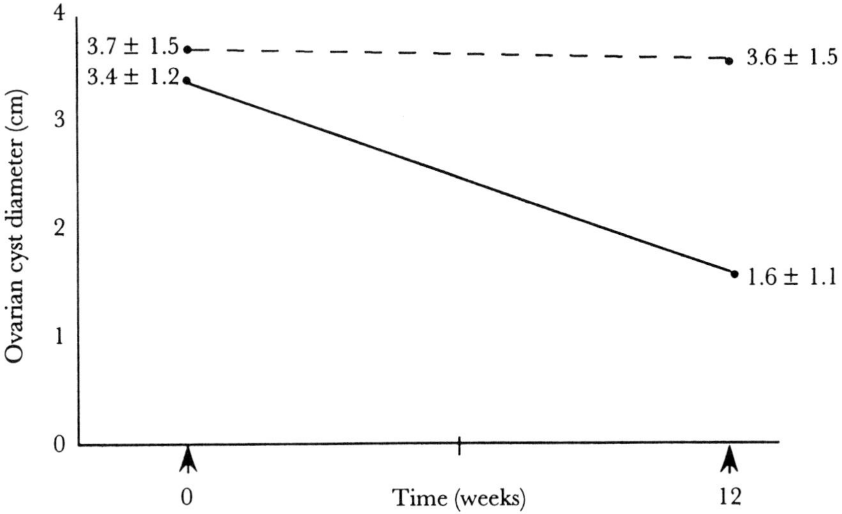

Figure 3 Decrease in ovarian cyst diameter after drainage, and after drainage and GnRH agonist for 3 months. – – –, drainage; ——, drainage + GnRH agonist

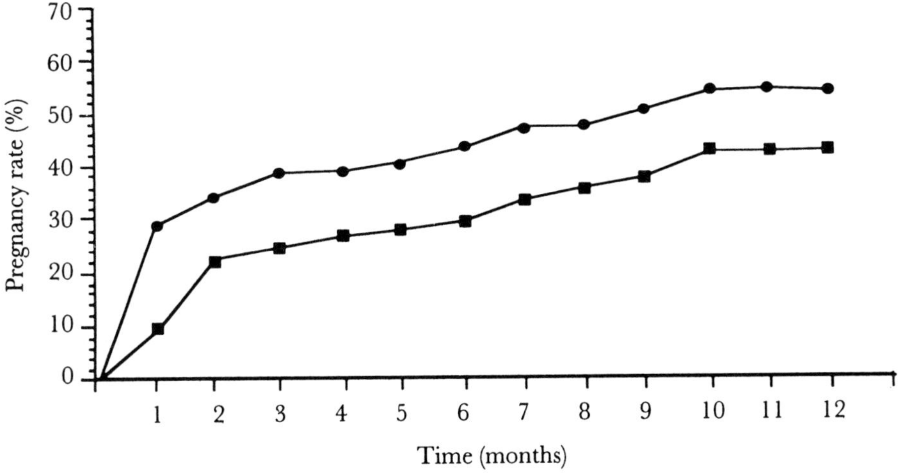

Figure 4 Pregnancy rate after combined (medical and surgical) therapy in moderate (●, $n = 305$) and severe endometriosis (■, $n = 102$)

resolution was described after long-term therapy. In moderate and severe endometriosis, when the scores before and after hormonal therapy were compared, the most significant difference was found among women treated with GnRH agonist[8–10]. The data were in agreement with a previous study in which a lower mitotic index was found in ectopic glandular epithelium after buserelin therapy than that observed after either lynestrenol or gestrinone therapy[41]. By reducing the cyst size and the internal wall thickness, GnRH agonist makes the laparoscopic management of large endometrial cysts possible. The cumulative pregnancy rate (51% for a 1-year follow-up) achieved after combined (GnRH agonist and endoscopy) therapy was similar to that obtained after microsurgery and allows us to propose this form of therapy in the management of large endometriomas (Figure 4). The advantages of the preoperative use of GnRH agonist are as follows:

(1) The significant reduction in endometrial cyst diameter;

(2) The thinner epithelial lining of the internal wall;

(3) The reduction of pelvic inflammation and hypervascularization often present around the endometriotic foci; and

(4) The absence of follicles or corpus luteum.

All these advantages make the endoscopic procedure easier but so far no randomized studies have demonstrated a significant difference in terms of pregnancy rates.

Moreover, the recurrence rate was low (7%) although Fayez and Vogel (1991)[54] reported a 22% incidence of deep ovarian endometriosis at second look laparoscopy after laparoscopic stripping of ovarian endometriomas in cases of very large cysts and/or friable cyst walls. Using the same laparoscopic procedure, Canis *et al.*[55] reported a 7% incidence of deep ovarian endometriosis at second-look laparoscopy in cases of endometriomas of > 3 cm. They suggest an additional vaporization or fulguration when the ovarian stripping is not satisfactory. To avoid loss of bone mineral content, a therapy of no longer than 3 months is suggested.

References

1. Maheux, R., Guilloteau, C., Lemay, A., Bastide, A. and Fazekas, A. T. A. (1985), Luteinizing hormone-releasing hormone agonist and uterine leiomyoma: pilot study. *Am. J. Obstet. Gynecol.*, **152**, 1034

2. Friedman, A. J., Barbieri, R. L., Doubilet, P. M, Fine, C. and Schiff, I. (1988). A randomized, double-blind trial of gonadotropin releasing-hormone agonist (leuprolide) with or without medroxyprogesterone acetate in the treatment of leiomyomata uteri. *Fertil. Steril.*, **49**, 404–35

3. Maheux, R., Lemay, A., Blanchet, P., Friede, J. and Pratt, X. (1991). Maintained reduction of uterine leiomyoma following addition of hormonal replacement therapy to a monthly luteinizing hormone-releasing hormone agonist implant: a pilot study. *Hum. Reprod.*, **6**, 500–5

4. Meldrum, D. R., Chang, R. J., Lu, J., Vale, W., Rivier, J. and Judd, H. L. (1982). 'Medical oophorectomy' using a long-acting GnRH agonist: a possible new approach to the treatment of endometriosis. *J. Clin. Endocrinol. Metab.*, **54**, 1081–3

5. Shaw, R. W., Fraser, H. M. and Boyle, H. (1983). Intranasal treatment with luteinizing hormone releasing hormone agonist in women with endometriosis. *Br. Med. J.*, **287**, 1167–9

6. Lemay, A., Maheux, R., Faure, N., Jean, C. and Fazekas, A. (1984). Reversible hypogonadism induced by a luteinizing hormone-releasing hormone (LHRH) agonist (buserelin) as a new therapeutic approach for endometriosis. *Fertil. Steril.*, **41**, 863–71

7. Donnez, J. (1987). CO$_2$ laser laparoscopy in infertile women with adhesions or endometriosis. *Fertil. Steril.*, **48**, 390–4

8. Donnez, J, Nisolle, M., Clerckx, F. and Casanas, F. (1989). Combined therapy in endometriosis: preoperative use of danazol, gestrinone, lynestrenol, buserelin spray and buserelin implant. In Boutaleb, Y. and Gzouli, Z. (eds.) *Treatment of Endometriosis – Recent Developments in Fertility and Sterility*. (Carnforth, UK: Parthenon Publishing)

9. Donnez J, Nisolle, M. and Casanas-Roux, F. (1989). Administration of nasal buserelin as compared with subcutaneous buserelin implant for endometriosis. *Fertil. Steril.*, **52**, 27–30

10. Donnez, J., Nisolle, M. and Casanas-Roux, F. (1990). Endometriosis-associated infertility: evaluation of preoperative use of danazol, gestrinone and buserelin. *Int. J. Fertil.*, **42**, 128

11. Goldrath, M. H. (1985). Hysteroscopic laser surgery. In Baggish, M. S. (ed.) *Basic and Advanced Laser Surgery in Gynecology*, p. 357. (Norwalk, CT: Appleton-Century-Crofts)

12. Loffer, F. D. (1988). Laser ablation of the endometrium. *Obstet. Gynecol. Clin. North Am.*, **15**, 17

13. Neuwirth, R. S. (1983). Hysteroscopic management of symptomatic submucous fibroids. *Obstet. Gynecol.*, **62**, 509

14. Decherney, A. and Polan, M. L. (1983). Hysteroscopic management of intrauterine lesions and intractable uterine bleeding. *Obstet. Gynecol.*, **61**, 392

15. Hallez, J. P., Netter, A. and Cartier, R. (1987).

Methodical intrauterine resection. *Am. J. Obstet. Gynecol.*, **156**, 1080

16. Van Caillie, T. (1989). Electrocoagulation of the endometrium with the ball-end resectoscope. *Obstet. Gynecol.*, **74**, 425

17. Hamou, J. (1993). Electroresection of fibroids in endoscopic surgery for gynecologists. In Sutton, C. and Diamond, M. (eds.) *Endoscopic Surgery for Gynecologists*, pp. 327–30. (London: W.B. Saunders)

18. Donnez, J., and Nisolle, M. (1989). Laser hysteroscopy in uterine bleeding: endometrial ablation and polypectomy. In Donnez, J. (ed.) *Laser Operative Laparoscopy and Hysteroscopy*, p. 277. (Louvain: Nauwelaerts)

19. Donnez, J., Gillerot, S., Bourgonjon, D, Clerckx, F. J. and Nisolle, M. D. (1990). Neodynium: YAG laser hysteroscopy in large submucous fibroids. *Fertil. Steril.*, **54**, 999

20. Donnez, J. and Nisolle, M. (1992). Hysteroscopic surgery. *Curr. Opin. Obstet. Gynecol.*, **4**, 439

21. Dequesne, J. (1989). Focal treatment of uterine bleeding and infertility with Nd:YAG laser and flexible hysteroscope. *J. Gynecol. Surg.*, **5**, 177

22. Nisolle, M., Grandjean, P., Gillerot, S. and Donnez, J. (1991). Endometrial ablation with the Nd-YAG laser in dysfunctional bleeding. *Min. Inv. Therap.*, **1**, 35–9

23. Garry, R., Erian, J. and Grochmal, S. (1991). A multicentre collaborative study into the treatment of menorrhagia by Nd-YA laser ablation of the endometrium. *Br. J. Obstet. Gynaecol.*, 48, 357–62

24. Goldrath, M. H., Fuller, F. A. and Segel, S. (1981). Laser photovaporization of endometrium for the treatment of menorrhagia. *J. Obstet. Gynecol.*, **140**, 14

25. Donnez, J., Nisolle, M., Casanas-Roux, F. and Clerckx, F. (1993). Rationale for surgery. In Brosens, I. and Donnez, J. (eds.) *The Current Status of Endometriosis Research and Management*, p. 385. (Carnforth, UK: Parthenon Publishing)

26. Donnez, J., Schrurs, B., Gillerot, S., Sandow, J. and Clerckx, F. (1989). Treatment of uterine fibroids with implants of gonadotropin-releasing hormone agonist: assessment by hysterography. *Fertil. Steril.*, **51**, 947

27. Donnez, J., Schrurs, B., Clerckx, F. and Nisolle, M. (1989). Les agonistes de la LH-RH une alternative dans le traitement de la myomatose utérine. *Contracep. Fertil. Sexual.*, **17**, 47

28. Donnez, J. (1993). Nd-YAG laser hysteroscopic myomectomy. In Sutton, C. and Diamond, M. (eds.) *Endoscopic Surgery for Gynecologists*, p. 331. (London: W.B. Saunders)

29. Donnez, J., Malvaux, V., Nisolle, M. and Casanas-Roux, F. (1990). Hysteroscopic sterilization with the Nd-YAG laser. *J. Gymecol. Surg.*, **6**, 149

30. Lomano, J. M. (1988) Photocoagulation of the endometrium with the Nd:YAG laser for the treatment of menorrhagia. *J. Reprod. Med.*, **31**, 148–50

31. Baggish M. S. and Baltoyannis, P. (1988). New techniques for laser ablation of the endometrium in high risk patients. *Am. J. Obstet. Gynecol.*, **159**, 287–92

32. Gallinat, A. (1993). Endometrial ablation using the Nd:YAG laser in CO_2 hysteroscopy. In Lueken, R. P. and Gallinat, A. (eds.) *Endoscopic Surgery in Gynecology*, p. 109. (Demeter Verlag GmbH)

33. Van Boven, M., Singelyn, F., Donnez, J. and Gribomont, B. (1989). Dilution hyponatrema associated with intrauterine endoscopic laser surgery. *Anesthesiology*, **3**, 71

34. Healy, D. L, Fraser, H. M. and Lawson, S. L. (1984). Shrinkage of a uterine fibroid after subcutaneous infusion of a LH-RH agonist. *Br. Med. J.*, **209**, 267

35. Andreyko, J. L., Blumenfeld, Z., Marschall, L. A., Monroe, S. E., Hricak, H. and Jaffe, R. B. (1988). Use of an agonistic analog of gonadotropin-releasing hormone (nafarelin) to treat leiomyomas: assessment by magnetic resonance imaging. *Am. J Obstet. Gynecol*, **158**, 903

36. Matta, W. H. M., Stabile, I., Shaw, R. S. and Campbell, S. (1988). Doppler assessment of uterine blood flow changes in patients with fibroids receiving the gonadotropin-releasing hormone agonist Buserelin. *Fertil. Steril.*, **49**, 1083

37. Donnez, J., Nisolle, M., Clerckx, F., Casanas-Roux, F., Saussoy, P. and Gillerot, S. (1994). Advanced endoscopic techniques used in dysfunctional bleeding, fibroids and endometriosis and the role of gonadotrophin-releasing hormone agonist treatment. *Br. J. Obstet. Gynaecol.*, **101** (Suppl. 10), 2–9

38. Donnez, J. and Nisolle, M. (1993). LASH: laparoscopic supracervical hysterectomy. *J. Gynecol. Surg.*, **9**, 91–4

39. Buttram, V., Reiter, R. and Ward, S. (1985). Treatment of endometriosis with danazol: report of a 6-year prospective study. *Fertil. Steril.*, **43**, 353

40. Evers, J. L. H. (1987). The second-look laparoscopy for evaluation of the result of medical treatment of endometriosis should not be performed during ovarian suppression. *Fertil. Steril.*, **47**, 502–4

41. Nisolle, M., Casanas-Roux, F. and Donnez, J. (1988). Histologic study of ovarian endometriosis

after hormonal therapy. *Fertil. Steril.*, **49**, 423–6

42. Tulandi, T. and Mouchawar, M. (1991). Treatment-dependent and treatment-independent pregnancy in women with minimal and mild endometriosis. *Fertil. Steril.*, **56**, 790–1

43. Brosens, I. (1993). Minimal endometriosis: should it be treated? *Gynecol. Obstet.*, **1**, 367

44. Nisolle, M., Casanas-Roux, F., Wyns, Ch., de Menten, Y., Mathieu, P. E. and Donnez, J. (1994). Immunohistochemical analysis of estrogen and progesterone receptors in endometrium and peritoneal endometriosis: a new quantitative method. *Fertil. Steril.*, **62**, 751–9

45. Metzger, D. A. (1993). Cyclic changes in endometriosis implants. In Brosens, I. and Donnez, J. (eds.) *The Current Status of Endometriosis. Research and Management*, pp. 89–108. (Carnforth, UK: Parthenon Publishing)

46. Evers, J. L. H. (1993). The immune system in endometriosis: introduction. In Brosens, I. and Donnez, J. (eds.) *The Current Status of Endometriosis. Research and Management*, p. 213–17. (Carnforth, UK: Parthenon Publishing)

47. Donnez, J. and Nisolle, M. (1991). Laparoscopic management of large ovarian endometrial cyst: use of fibrin sealant. *J. Gynedol. Surg.*, **7**, 163–7

48. Donnez, J., Nisolle, M., Gillerot, S., Anaf, V., Clerck, F. and Casanas-Roux, F. (1994). Ovarian endometrial cyst: the role of gonadotropin-releasing hormone agonist and/or drainage. *Fertil. Steril.*, 62, 63–6

49. Brosens, I. and Gordon, A. (1989). Endometriosis: ovarian endometriosis. In Brosens, I. and Gordon, A. (eds.) *Tubal Infertility*, pp. 313–17. (London, UK: Gower Medical Publishing)

50. Sampson, J. A. (1927). Peritoneal endometriosis due to the menstrual dissemination of endometrial tissue into the peritoneal cavity. *Am. J. Obstet. Gynecol.*, **14**, 422–69

51. Hughesdon, P. E. (1957). The structure of endometrial cysts of the ovary. *Obstet. Gynaecol. Br. Emp.*, **64**, 481–7

52. Donnez, J, Nisolle, M. and Casanas-Roux, F. (1989). CO_2 laser laparoscopy in infertile women with adnexal adhesions and women with tubal occlusion. *J. Gynecol. Surg.*, **5**, 47–53

53. Shaw, R. W. (1992). The role of GnRH analogues in the treatment of endometriosis. *Br. J. Obstet. Gyaecol.*, **99** (Suppl. 7), 9–12

54. Fayez, J. A. and Vogel, M. S. (1991). Comparison of different treatment methods of endometriosis by laparoscopy. *Obstet. Gynecol.*, **78**, 660–5

55. Canis, M., Mage, G., Wattiez, A., Chapra, C., Pouly, J. L. and Bassil, S. (1992). Second look laparoscopy after laparoscopic cystectomy of large endometriomas. *Fertil. Steril.*, **58**, 617–19

The risk of leiomyoma recurrence after myomectomy

28

L. Fedele, S. Bianchi, F. Parazzini, L. Tozzi and E. Cavalleri

INTRODUCTION

Uterine myoma affects about one in five women of reproductive age, and is the most common solid tumor of the pelvis. Myomectomy is the treatment of choice in symptomatic patients wanting to conserve reproductive and menstrual function. The success of this operation may, however, be impaired by recurrence which is reported after different intervals of time. The recurrence rate varies from 5 to 30% according to the series[1].

This wide range may be explained by the criteria used for the diagnosis of recurrence (clinical or ultrasound) and by the length of follow-up. Another factor that could influence recurrence rates is the preoperative use of hormonal drugs.

CLINICAL STUDY

We analyzed the risk of recurrence of uterine myomas in 622 patients who underwent myomectomy between 1970 and 1984[2]. The surgical indication was menorrhagia and pelvic pain in 59%, infertility in 36% and recurrent miscarriage in 5%, associated with the presence of at least one myoma of more than 5 cm diameter. The median follow-up was 102 months. The cumulative 10-year recurrence rate after myomectomy was 27% and this increased steadily during the period studied. The recurrence rate was similar in women of 30 years or over and those under 30 years (25% and 24%, respectively). Recurrence tended to be less frequent in women with a single myoma. Of the women who had a child after myomectomy, 16% had a recurrence compared with 28% of those who did not have children ($\chi^2 = 3.96$, $p = 0.05$). Being parous or nulliparous at myomectomy did not affect the risk of recurrence. These results agree with those of other clinical studies[3,4] which reported recurrence rates of 25–35%.

ULTRASOUND STUDY

In order to obtain more precise information on the role of surgery in the treatment of myomas we subsequently performed an ultrasound study on recurrence of the disorder[5]. This series consisted of 189 women who underwent myomectomy in our department between 1987 and 1991. Transvaginal ultrasonography was performed systematically before surgery to obtain a precise map of the uterus and myomas. After myomectomy, clinical examination and transvaginal ultrasonography were performed every 12 months. The median follow-up was 49 months. The cumulative probability of recurrence (CPR) increased during the study period, reaching 51% at 5 years. The 5-year CPR decreased with parity after myomectomy. Age at myomectomy, number of myomas removed and parity at the time of surgery did not affect the recurrence rate significantly.

PREOPERATIVE USE OF GnRH ANALOGS

Various authors have suggested that the preoperative use of analogs, by reducing the size of the neoformation and vascularization of the uterus, may facilitate myomectomy and decreased postoperative morbidity. With the aim of better defining the effects of such treatment on recurrence, we randomized 24 myomectomy candidates to preoperative treatment with buserelin (1200 µg/day) for 3 months (eight women) or immediate conservative surgery (16 women)[6]. Postoperative follow-up included a pelvic exploration at 3, 6 and 12 months and trans-abdominal and transvaginal ultrasonography at 6 and 12 months. At 6 months the pelvic examination was normal in all cases, whereas ultrasonography demonstrated residual myomas in five women (63%) treated with the analogs and two (13%) controls ($p < 0.05$). At 12 months one of the five patients of the buserelin group had a myoma more than 1.5 cm in diameter, another was pregnant, and in the other three the ultrasound findings were unchanged. In the control group no other recurrence was observed. The results of this study indicate that a period of hypoestrogenism preceding myomectomy may favor the recurrence of myomas in the short term. This phenomenon is probably due to the reduction in size and consistency of the myomas induced by the analog, so that the smallest myomas are not identified at the time of surgery.

COMMENTS

Consensus has not been reached on the significance of the reappearance of myomas after myomectomy.

Some authors consider it as persistence; that is, the result of an unintentionally incomplete intervention that left unappreciable nodular formations *in situ* in the myometrium. However, the possibility of *ex novo* formation of myomatous cellular clones cannot be excluded, and this may be favored by a genetic predisposition and/or the presence of hormonal and growth factors. The results of both our clinical and our ultrasound study seem to support the second hypothesis, as the probability of recurrence rose constantly with time; in the case of persistence there would be an initial peak and then a plateau. The use of analogs before myomectomy could favor reappearance of the disease due to persistence.

In conclusion, the risk of recurrence after myomectomy is relatively high. A term pregnancy after myomectomy considerably reduces the probability of this event. Although the biological mechanism of the association is not clear, this finding has also been confirmed in epidemiological studies which demonstrated a protective effect of parity on the risk of recurrence of uterine myomas[7,8].

References

1. Buttram, V. C. Jr and Reiter, R. C. (1981). Uterine leiomyomata: etiology, sympto-matology, and management. *Fertil. Steril.*,**36**, 433–45
2. Candiani, G. B., Fedele, L., Parazzini, F. and Villa L. (1991). Risk of recurrence after myomectomy. *Br. J. Obstet. Gynaecol.*, **98**, 385–9
3. Loeffler, F. E. and Noble, A. D. (1970). Myomectomy at the Chelsea Hospital for women. *J Obstet. Gynaecol. Br. Commonw.*, **77**, 167–71
4. Babaknia, A., Rock, J. A. and Jones, H. W. Jr (1978). Pregnancy success following abdominal myomectomy for infertility. *Fertil. Steril.* **30**, 644–7
5. Fedele, L., Parazzini, F., Luchini, L., Mezzopane, R., Tozzi, L. and Villa, L. (1995). Recurrence of fibroids after myomectomy: a transvaginal ultrasonographic study. *Hum. Reprod.*, **10**, 1795–6
6. Fedele, L., Vercellini, P., Bianchi, S., Brioschi, D. and Dorta, M. (1990). Treatment with GnRH agonists before myomectomy and the risk of short-term myoma recurrence. *Br. J. Obstet. Gynaecol.*, **97**, 393–6
7. Parazzini, F., LaVecchia, Negri, E., Cecchetti, G. and Fedele, L. (1988). Epidemiologic characteristics of women with uterine fibroids: a case control study. *Obstet. Gynecol.*, **72**, 853–7
8. Parazzini, F., Negri, E., LaVecchia, C., Fedele, L., Rabaiotti, M. and Luchini, L.(1992). Oral contraceptive use and the risk of uterine fibroids. *Obstet. Gynecol.*, **79**, 430–3

Section 8

Other applications

29

The use of GnRH analog in dysfunctional uterine bleeding

C. Bulletti, V. Polli, E. Giacomucci, S. Rossi, V. Negrini, A. Jama and C. Flamigni

INTRODUCTION

Metrorrhagia is a clinical sign often occurring in perimenopausal women[1]. It is mainly due to inadequate endogenous estrogen and/or progesterone production[2], or to disordered estrogen transportation from the blood into the endometrium[3,4]. The years before menopause represent the period of highest risk for development of endometrial hyperplasia, which in turn may result in endometrial cancer in about 10 years[5]. Endometrial hyperplasia may be part of a continuum that is ultimately manifested in the histological and biological pattern of the adenocarcinoma[6]. In the premenopausal years, an increase in estrogen production and/or a deficiency of progesterone plasma levels are often observed[7]. This hormonal production leads to endometrial overstimulation that may be a risk factor for endometrial cancer.

A therapeutic approach has been tested with a gonadotropin releasing hormone (GnRH) agonist (Zoladex), in a depot formulation, that induced a sustained and reversible hypogonadotropic hypogonadism[8,9]. Since the ovarian suppression was pharmacologically induced, a transdermal 17 β-estradiol and oral progestin were also administered to obtain adequate endometrial growth and to avoid the potential risk of osteoporosis when low plasma levels of estrogens and hypogonadism are maintained over 6 months[10].

MATERIALS AND METHODS

A total of 201 premenopausal women attended the Department of Obstetrics and Gynecology, S. Orsola University Hospital, Bologna for a clinical study on the therapeutic association of GnRH agonist (Zoladex depot) subcutaneously administered and sequential therapy with transdermal 17 β-estradiol and oral progestin. A total of 109 women were enrolled in the study but 25 dropped out before the end; 84 women completed the study. They were selected according to the following criteria: (1) age 42–49; (2) metrorrhagia with or without endometrial hyperplasia (without atypia); (3) hemoglobin < 11 mg/100 ml – anemia was established in close association with metrorrhagia in the last 12–60 months; (4) within 20% of ideal body weight (BMI)[11]; (5) no hormonal therapy for the last 2 years; (6) no uterine myomata at ultrasonography, (7) non-smoker; (8) medical history not including carcinomas, hypertension, liver disease, gallbladder disease, diabetes mellitus, cardiovascular diseases, alcoholism or corticosteroid therapy; and (9) osteoporosis excluded by dual photon computerized linear scanning of distal extremity ($^1/_{10}$) of radius of the not-dominant arm (Osteoden-P, source I125, A241, NIM srl, Verona, Italy). The women underwent thorough physical examination, electrocardiogram, mammography, endometrial biopsy and routine blood and urine chemistry tests including those to determine the luteinizing hormone (LH) surge (Clearplan, Farmades S.p.A. Roma). Symptoms and clinical signs were recorded by patients in a diary.

Forty-two women were considered for the study (group A) and the other 42 were included as controls (group B). The study protocol for groups A and B during the 12 months of observation has been previously reported[12]. Patients of both groups A and B were divided according to criteria of the same histological diagnosis of the endometrium. Endometrial samples were obtained by curettage or under hysteroscopic control at baseline (7th to 8th day of cycle), at the LH peak, after 6 months of steroid replacement therapy (7th to 8th day of transdermal 17 β-estradiol administration), after the beginning of oral progestin administration, after 12 months, and 3 months after the end of treatment. All tissue samples were processed for routine hematoxylin and eosin (H&E)-stained sections[13], and endometrial hyperplasia was evaluated using the criteria of DiSaia and Creasman[14]. Immunostaining for laminin was performed on the paraffin sections of all specimens, as described by Barsky and colleagues[15]. Paraffin sections were attached to slides by epoxy glue, deparaffinized in xylol, and rehydrated in graded alcohols and distilled water. Immunohistochemical evaluation for laminin was used to establish an adequate differentiation of human endometrium[3,16,17].

The transformed data and other data of both study groups were normally distributed as assessed by the Kolmogorov–Smirnov test[18]. Statistical analysis was performed by using multivariate (MANOVA) analysis of variance for all factors considered[19].

RESULTS

Both study groups (A and B) had similar baseline values. Fifteen days after the first GnRH agonist injection in group A, there was the expected reduction in the plasma levels of LH, follicle stimulating hormone (FSH) and estradiol.

There was a significant difference between 180 days and baseline for the reduction of bleeding and metrorrhagia and for the appearance of vasomotor symptoms in group A ($p < 0.001$), but not in group B (NS) (Table 1). In comparison of values between baseline and 360 days, there was a highly significant difference for bleeding, metrorrhagia and vasomotor symptoms in group A ($p < 0.001$), but not in Group B (NS) except for the hot flushes, which had increased after that length of time ($p < 0.01$) (Table 1).

In comparison of data obtained after 180 days and 360 days, there were no differences in vaginal bleeding, metrorrhagia and vasomotor symptoms in group A (NS) (Table 1). Bleeding and metrorrhagia had not changed in group B (NS), while vasomotor symptoms changed from 180 to 360 days ($p < 0.01$) (Table 1).

The immunohistochemical reaction to laminin was negative for both groups at the baseline, whereas group A showed a significant increase in the immunoreactions at 180 days and 360 days ($p < 0.001$ vs. baseline) (Table 2). There were no positive reactions in group B (Table 2). The significance of the comparison of the immuno-

Table 1 Variability of vaginal bleeding, metrorrhagia and vasomotor symptoms reported in the daily diary, and their significance

	Group A		Group B		
	n	*%*	*n*	*%*	*p-value (group A vs. group B)*
Vaginal bleeding:					
baseline	42	100	42	100	NS
180 days	1	2	40	95	< 0.001
360 days	1	2	32	95	< 0.001
Metrorrhagia:					
baseline	34	81	34	81	NS
180 days	0	0	15	36	< 0.001
360 days	2	5	17	40	< 0.001
Hot flushes and headaches:					
baselines	32	76	5	12	< 0.001
180 days	0	0	5	12	NS
360 days	6	14	20	48	NS

NS, not significant

Table 2 Positive immunoreaction to laminin of endometrial samples from group A patients compared with the positive immunoreaction of endometrial samples collected from group B patients. Positive immunoreaction represents the predecidualization of the endometrium that in turn corresponds to quiescence of endometrial epithelial cell mitosis

	Group A		Group B	
	n	%	n	%
Baseline	0	0	0	0
180 days	19	45	0	0
360 days	10	24	0	0

reaction to laminin with the baseline in both groups was $p < 0.001$ at 180 days and $p < 0.02$ at 360 days; the significance of the comparison of the immunoreaction to laminin between 180 and 360 days was $p < 0.003$.

Both groups had the same histological diagnosis at the baseline (NS) (Table 3). At 180 days the endometrial decidualization was the most represented histological feature encountered in group A; adenomatous hyperplasia persisted in only eight cases ($p < 0.001$) (Table 3). Comparison at the baseline and at 180 days between groups A and B showed a significance of $p < 0.001$ for histological diagnosis, as did the comparison between 360 days and the baseline, whereas the intergroup comparison at 180 and 360 days was not significant (NS) (Table 3).

DISCUSSION

The surgical treatment for women having dysfunctional uterine bleeding was overused, with several clinical and financial implications. One of the most difficult questions for physicians consulted by premenopausal women with metrorrhagia is to proceed by curettage and/or hysterectomy to stop metrorrhagia and/or to remove endometrial hyperstimulation. The use of progestins has also been proposed for the same purpose[20]. There is no consensus on the elective therapy to be used in these patients[20], because too many hysterectomies were performed in the past[21] and progestins may have negative effects on the cardiovascular system, lipoproteins and the liver[22,23].

Surgery may be avoided in premenopausal women. Unopposed estrogens cause endometrial hyperstimulation, leading to irregular vaginal bleeding, endometrial hyperplasia and cancer[24], and the cancer risk may persist for as long as 15 years[5,6]. In the premenopausal years endogenous estrogen/progesterone production may overstimulate the endometrium[7]. Progesterone exposure exerts an antimitotic or antiestrogenic effect in reducing DNA synthesis and nuclear estradiol receptors and exerts a secretory effect by increasing the activity of certain enzymes such as

Table 3 Abnormal endometrial growth (persistent proliferative, glandular hyperplasia and adenomatous hyperplasia) in the two groups compared at different times

	Group A						Group B					
	Baseline		180 days		360 days		baseline		180 days		360 days	
Histological	n	%	n	%	n	%	n	%	n	%	n	%
Persistent proliferation	13	31	0	0	0	0	11	25	4	10	0	0
Galndular hyperplasia	21	50	0	0	0	0	27	64	30	70	19	45
Adenomatous hyperplasia	8	19	2	5	2	5	4	10	8	20	23	55
Decidualization	0	0	40	95	21	50	0	0	0	0	0	0
Proliferation	0	0	0	0	19	45	0	0	0	0	0	0
Significance	NS		$p < 0.001$		$p < 0.001$		NS		$p < 0.001$		$p < 0.001$	

NS, not significant

17 β-estradiol and isocitric dehydrogenases[25]. Synthetic progestogens reproduce the characteristic morphological and biochemical changes of the secretory phase of the ovulatory cycle when they are used in combination with exogenous estrogens[24]. There is evidence that unopposed estrogens reduce the risk of arterial disease, the most common cause of death in postmenopausal women[26], while oral progestogens oppose favorable estrogen-induced changes in lipid and lipoprotein metabolism[22]. Furthermore, the administration of certain progestogens increases the incidence of hypertension and arterial thromboembolic disease in a dose-dependent manner[26].

The National Institutes of Health in the United States have cautioned against the widespread addition of progestogens to exogenous estrogen treatment[27]. The derivatives of 19-nortestosterone as well as progestins that possess androgenic activity increase the plasma insulin concentration (which reflects decreased sensitivity and therefore impaired glucose tolerance), and they lower the concentration of cholesterol in the high-density lipoprotein fraction of plasma. This biochemical side effect is inversely related to the incidence of cardiovascular disease in both men and women. Since the beneficial effects of long-term postmenopausal estrogen treatment in possibly reducing mortality from ischemic heart disease[28] may be cancelled by the use of these progestins, a progestin without these biochemical effects was used in our study.

Progesterone does not adversely affect plasma high-density lipoprotein cholesterol concentration and causes only minimal changes in carbohydrate metabolism[28]. Medrogestone is a progesterone derivative and its use did not affect plasma high-density lipoprotein cholesterol concentration in our study. The suppression of ovarian activity obtained with Zoladex in patients with menstrual disturbances because of unbalanced endogenous production of estrogen/progesterone was effective on the dysfunctional bleeding and reduced the endometrial overstimulation. The beneficial effects of endogenous estrogens were obtained with the use of transdermal estradiol. Patients had a significant increase in hemoglobin concentration, and adequate endometrial proliferation and differentiation was restored, thus confirming the potentially beneficial role of this therapeutic approach in preventing endometrial hyperplasia and cancer.

ACKNOWLEDGEMENTS

This work was supported by the Italian 'Consiglio Nazionale delle Ricerche' grants No.9300660 and 9202504 , and from the University of Bologna (Italy) Grant No 930212100.

References

1. Merril, J. A. (1981). Management of postmenopausal bleeding. *Clin. Obstet. Gynecol.*, **24**, 285–99

2. Gambrell, R. D. (1977). Postmenopausal bleeding. *Clin. Obstet. Gynecol.*, **4**, 129–43

3. Bulletti, C., Galassi, A., Jasonni, V. M., Martinelli, G., Tabanelli, S. and Flamigni, C. (1988). Basement membrane components in normal, hyperplastic and neoplastic endometrium. *Cancer*, **62**, 142–9

4. Bulletti, C., Jasonni, V. M., Tabanelli, S., Ciotti, P. M., Cappuccini F., Borini, A. and Flamigni, C. (1988). Increased extraction of estrogens in human endometrial hyperplasia and carcinoma. *Cancer Det. Prev.*, **13**, 123–30

5. Ziel, H. K. (1982). Estrogen's role in endometrial cancer. *Obstet. Gynecol.*, **60**, 509–15

6. Kurman, R. J. and Norris, H. J. (1982). Evaluation of criteria for distinguishing atypical endometrial hyperplasia from well-differentiated adenocarcinoma. *Cancer*, **8**, 2547–59

7. Gambrell, R.D. Jr (1986). The role of hormones in the etiology and prevention of endometrial cancer. *Clin. Obstet. Gynecol.*, **13**, 695–723

8. West, C. P. and Baird, D. T. (1987) Suppression of ovarian activity by Zoladex depot (ICI 118630), a long acting luteinizing hormone agonist analogue. *Clin Endocrinol.*, **26**, 213–20

9. Bider, D., Ben-Rafael, Z. and Shalev, J. (1989). Pituitary and ovarian suppression rate after high dosage of gonadotropin-releasing hormone agonist. *Fertil. Steril.* **51**, 578–81

10. Matta, W. H. and Shaw, R. W. (1987). Hypogonadism induced by luteinising hormone releasing hormone agonist analogues: effects on bone density in premenopausal women. *Br. Med. J.*, **294**, 1523–4

11. Thomas, A. E., McKay, D. A. and Cutlip, M. B. (1976). A monograph method for assessing body weight. *Am. J. Clin. Nutr.*, **29**, 302–4

12. Bulletti, C., Flamigni, C., Prefetto, R.A., Polli, V. and Giacomucci E. (1994). Dysfunctional uterine bleeding. In Bulletti, C., Gurpide, E. and Flamigni, C. (eds.) *The Human Endometrium*. Annals of The New York Academy of Sciences **734**, 80–90.

13. Noyes, R. W., Hertig, A. T. and Rock, J. (1950). Dating the endometrial biopsy. *Fertil. Steril.*, **1**, 3–25

14. DiSaia, P.J. and Creasman, W. T. (1984). *Clinical Gynecologic Oncology*, 2nd edn, pp. 122–33. (St Louis: CV Mosby)

15. Barsky, S. H., Rao, N. C., Restrepo, C. and Liotta, L A. (1984). Immunocytochemical enhancement of basement membrane antigens by pepsin. Applications in diagnostic pathology. *Am. J. Clin. Pathol.*, **82**, 191–4

16. Daly, D. C., Maslar, I. A. and Riddick, D. K. (1983). Prolactin production during *in vitro* decidualization of proliferative endometrium. *Am. J. Obstet. Gynecol.*, **145**, 672–8

17. Faber, M., Wewer, U. M., Berthelsen, J. G., Liotta, L. A. and Albrechtsen, R. (1986). Laminin production by human endometrial stromal cells relates to the cyclic and pathologic state of the endometrium. *Am. J. Pathol.*, **124**, 384–98

18. Siegel, G. (1956). *Nonparametric Statistics for the Behavioral Sciences.* (New York: McGraw-Hill)

19. SPSS Inc. (1985). SPSS/PC+ for IBM PC/ XMAT. (Chicago: SPSS Inc.)

20. Whitehead, M. I., Towsend, P. T., Pryse-Davies, J., Ryder, T., Lorne, G., Siddle, N. C. and King, R. J. (1982). Effects of various types and dosage of progestogens on the postmenopausal endometrium. *J. Reprod. Med.*, **27**, 539–48

21. Treloar, A. E. (1981). Menstrual cyclicity and the premenopause. *Maturitas*, **3**, 249–64

22. Hirvonen, E., Malkonen, M. and Mannien, V. (1981). Effects of different progestogens on lipoprotein during postmenopausal replacement therapy. *N. Engl. J. Med.*, **304**, 560–3

23. Gordon, E. M., Williams, S. R., Frenchek, B., Mazur, C. H. and Speroff, L. (1988). Dose dependent effects of postmenopausal estrogen/ progestin on antithrombin III and factor IX. *J. Lab. Clin. Med.*, **111**, 52–6

24. Whitehead, M.I. and Fraser, D. I. (1987). The effects of estrogens and progestogens on the endometrium. In Gambrell, D. R. (ed.) *Clinics in Obstetrics and Gynecology of North America*, vol. 14, The Menopause, pp.299–320. (Philadelphia: WB Saunders)

25. King, R. J. B., Towsend, P. T., Siddle. N. C., Whitehead, M. I. and Taylor, R. W. (1982). Regulation of estrogen and progesterone receptor levels in epithelium and stroma from pre and postmenopausal endometria. *J. Steroid Biochem.*, **16**, 21–9

26. Meade, T. W., Greenberg, G. and Thompson, S. G. (1980). Progestogens and cardiovascular reaction associated with oral contraceptives and a comparison of the safety of 50 and 30 μgr oestrogen preparations. *Br. Med. J.*, **280**, 1157–61

27. National Institutes of Health National Institute on Aging (1979). Estrogen use in postmenopausal women. *Consensus Conference on Aging*, Bethesda, 13–14 September

28. Spellacy, W. N., Buhi, W. C. and Burk, S. A. (1975). Effects of norethindrone on carbohydrate and lipid metabolism. *Obstet. Gynecol.*, **46**, 560–3

30

Precocious puberty: combined treatment with GnRH analogs and growth hormone

N. A. Bridges and C. G. D. Brook

INTRODUCTION

Gonadotropin releasing hormone (GnRH) analogs are highly effective in halting the progression of centrally mediated precocious puberty. They are free from side effects and, given in sufficient doses, rapidly suppress serum gonadotropin and sex steroid concentrations[1]. The effects are readily reversible and the resumption of normal menstrual cycles and fertility have been documented after stopping treatment[2,3]. The disadvantages of GnRH analogs are that they cannot be taken orally, and there is a period of stimulation at the start of treatment before suppression occurs.

The reason for a reduced final height in patients with precocious puberty is that the pubertal growth spurt supervenes before sufficient childhood growth has occurred. Growth hormone (GH) concentrations are similar to those seen in a normally timed puberty[4], so that the child is usually relatively tall and growing rapidly at presentation. Bone age is advanced, and both height prediction and final heights are reduced[5]. GnRH analogs have been ineffective in restoring this lost height potential, possibly because the treatment reduces sex steroid, GH and insulin-like growth factor 1 (IGF-I) concentrations[1,6] which results in a slowing of growth velocity[7].

Manipulation of puberty by using GnRH analogs in children with GH insufficiency treated with GH has resulted in increased final height regardless of the timing of the onset of puberty, either early or normal[8,9]. The addition of recombinant GH to treatment with GnRH analogs therefore offers the potential for increasing growth rate on treatment with GnRH analogs

and thus improving final height in patients with central precocious puberty.

Assessment of the effect of treatment on outcome in central precocious puberty relies on height prediction. The methods for predicting adult height are based on the growth patterns of normal children and may not be appropriate for children with abnormal growth[10,11]. Zachmann *et al.*[12] studied height prediction methods in a number of pathological conditions and demonstrated significant inaccuracies. For example, in untreated precocious puberty, Bayley–Pinneau (BP) prediction underestimated the final height of children under 11 years of age (giving an impression of increasing height prediction with age). Tanner–Whitehouse (TW) predictions, however, overestimated final height by as much as 40 cm in untreated precocious puberty[12]. Werder *et al.*[13] demonstrated an increase in height prediction with time in untreated central precocious puberty. Assessment of the long-term results of therapy for precocious puberty should, therefore, take the limitations of height prediction into account. In most studies[6,14], but not all[15], an increase in height prediction has been demonstrated during treatment with GnRH analogs, but height prediction falls after treatment ends, with subjects failing to reach their prediction at the end of treatment[16].

METHOD

A trial of the treatment involving a GnRH analog and a recombinant GH in girls with centrally mediated precocious puberty has been conducted at the Middlesex Hospital. Central precocious puberty was defined as consonant and progressive pubertal development starting before the age of 8 years, with pubertal gonadotropin concentrations. Subjects were treated with a combination of 3.6 mg of goserelin acetate as a monthly depot (Zoladex from Zeneca, Cheshire, UK) and 15–20 U/m^2/week of GH by daily subcutaneous injections (either Genotropin from Pharmacia, Stockholm, Sweden, or Norditropin from Nordisk, Gentofte, Denmark). Some subjects had received treatment with a GnRH analog alone before commencing the combination treatment.

Pelvic ultrasound scans were performed before, during and after stopping treatment. The mean time since stopping treatment was 1.4 years (range 0.3–3.9 years). Ovarian volume standard deviation scores were calculated using data from a control group[17].

RESULTS

Eight girls were treated with a GnRH analog alone before GH was added up to 3 years later. Ten girls in all were treated with the GH and GnRH analog combination from a mean age of 8.6 years (range 6.3–9.7) for 2 years.

Height predictions at the start of combined treatments were 155.0 and 166.7 cm for BP and TW respectively. Height predictions at the end of treatment were 163.5 and 169.5 cm, but final height was actually 158.2 cm.

Girls who had stopped treatment with a GnRH analog and GH had a mean ovarian volume of 6.98 ml (compared with a 50th centile volume at age 14 years of 2.52 ml for the control population) and an ovarian volume standard deviation score of +1.72, which was greater than that for girls who had been treated with a GnRH analog alone (+1.24). Ovaries with a polycystic appearance were found in 83% of scans in girls who had stopped treatment with a GnRH analog and GH[18].

DISCUSSION

Investigators have attempted to manipulate the pubertal growth spurt in a number of ways in order to alter final height. In the treatment of tall stature, the induction of puberty with sex steroids does not decrease the magnitude of the pubertal growth spurt but commences it when less childhood growth has been completed, thereby reducing adult height[19]. Treatment with somatostatin has the potential of reducing the magnitude of the pubertal growth spurt by decreasing the contribution of GH to growth[19,20]. Attempts to increase the magnitude of the pubertal spurt by the addition of GH to pubertal growth may in fact decrease the final height by accelerating pubertal development, because the action of the GH augments the action of gonadotropins[21].

In precocious puberty, holding up puberty by using a GnRH analog has little impact on final height and does not restore the loss in height that occurs in this condition. Although there may be an increase in height prediction during treatment, growth velocity is slow after stopping treatment and the increase in prediction is lost[16]. Constitutional delay of puberty does not lead to an increased final height[22,23], so it is unlikely that strategy involving the delay of normally timed puberty will result in taller women. The few data concerning this strategy support this[24,25].

A further option is to delay the pubertal growth spurt by treating with a GnRH analog and giving a GH to increase growth rate. This has not been particularly successful in normally timed puberty[26,27] and our study demonstrates that it is not successful in precocious puberty. There was an increase in height prediction over the treatment period, but slow growth velocity after stopping treatment resulted in no improvement in the final height over the initial prediction.

Ultrasound revealed that a small proportion of prepubertal children had ovaries with a polycystic appearance[17]. The prevalence increases with age and, at the end of puberty, the prevalence is similar to that seen in ultrasound studies of normal adult women (22–25%)[28]. In girls who have been treated with a combination of GnRH analog and GH, the ovarian volume during follow up after stopping treatment was large and 83% of the girls had ovaries with a polycystic appearance. There was no evidence that the ovaries decreased in size with time nor that the polycystic appearance disappeared[18]. There are no comparable data concerning the prevalence of polycystic ovaries in girls who have had untreated precocious puberty or in those who have been treated with a GnRH analog alone.

CONCLUSION

Delaying precocious puberty with a GnRH analog and increasing growth velocity with a GH should, theoretically, result in an increase in the magnitude of the pubertal growth spurt, but this was not the case: growth velocity was slow after stopping treatment. Girls who had been treated with a GnRH analog and GH did have an increased prevalence of polycystic ovaries, which may be secondary to either the treatment or to the condition itself.

References

1. Sklar, C. A., Rothenberg, S., Blumberg, D., Oberfield, S. E., Levine, L. and David, R. (1991). Suppression of the pituitary gonadal axis in children with central precocious puberty: effects on GH, IGF 1, and prolactin secretion. *J. Clin. Endocrinol. Metab.*, **73**, 734–8

2. Manasco, P. K., Pescovitz, O. H., Feullian, P. P., Hench, K. D., Barnes, K. M, Jones, J., Hill, S., Loriaux, D. L. and Cutler, G.B. (1988). Resumption of puberty after long term LHRH agonist treatment of central precocious puberty. *J. Clin. Endocrinol. Metab.*, **67**, 368–72

3. Kauli, R., Kornreich, L. and Laron, Z. (1990). Pubertal development, growth and final height in girls with sexual precocity treated with the GnRH analogue d-trp 6 LHRH. *Horm. Res.*, **33**, 11–17

4. Ross, J. L., Pescovitz, O. H., Barnes, K., Loriaux, D. L. and Cutler, G. B. (1987). Growth hormone secretory dynamics in children with precocious puberty. *J. Pediatr.*, **110**, 369–72

5. Murram, D., Dewhurst, J. and Grant, D. B. (1984). Precocious puberty: a follow up study. *Arch. Dis. Child.*, **59**, 77–8

6. Mansfield, M. J., Rudlin, C. R., Crigler, J. F., Karol, K. A., Crawford, J. D., Boepple, P. A. and Crowley, W. F. (1988). Changes in growth and serum GH and plasma SM-C levels during suppression of gonadal sex steroid secretion in girls with central precocious puberty. *J. Clin, Metab.*, **66**, 3–9

7. Manasco, P. K., Pescovitz, O. H., Hill, S. C., Jones, J., Barnes, K. M., Hench, K. D., Loriaux, D. and Cutler, G. B. (1989). Six year results of LHRH agonist treatment in children with LHRH dependent precocious puberty. *J. Pediatr.*, **15**, 105–8

8. Cara, J. F., Kreiter, M. L. and Rosenfeld, R. L. (1992). Height prognosis of children with true precocious puberty and growth hormone deficiency: effect of combination therapy with gonadotrophin releasing hormone agonist and growth hormone. *J. Pediatr.*, **120**, 709–15

9. Hibi, I., Tanaka, T., Tanae, A., Kagawa, J., Hashimoto, N., Yoshizawa, and Shizume, K. (1989). The influence of gonadal function and the effect of gonadal suppression treatment on final height in GH treated GH deficient subjects. *J. Clin. Endocrinol. Metab.*, **69**, 221–6

10. Tanner, J. M., Whitehouse, R. H., Cameron, N., Marshall, W. A., Healy, M. J. R. and Goldstein, H. (1983). *Assessment of Skeletal Maturity and Prediction of Adult Height (TW2 Method)*. (London: Harcourt Brace Jovanovitch)

11. Bayley, N. and Pinneau, S. R. (1952). Tables for predicting adult height from skeletal age: revised for use with the Greulich Pyle standard. *J. Pediatr.*, **40**, 423–41

12. Zachmann, M., Sobradillo, B., Frank, M., Frisch, H. and Prader, A. (1978). Bayley Pinneau, Roche Wainer Thissen, and Tanner height predictions in normal children and in patients with various pathologic conditions. *J. Pediatr.*, **93**, 749–55

13. Werder, E. A., Murset, G., Zachmann, M., Brook, C. G. D. and Prader, A. (1974). Treatment of precocious puberty with cyproterone acetate. *Pediatr. Res.*, **8**, 248–56

14. Oostdijk, W., Drop, S. L., Odink, R. J., Hummelink, R., Partsch, C. J. and Sippell, W. G. (1991). Long term results with a slow release gonadotrophin releasing hormone agonist in central precocious puberty. Dutch German precocious puberty study group. *Acta Paediatr. Scand.*, **372** (Suppl.), 39–45

15. Stanhope, R., Adams, J. and Brook, C. G. D. (1985). The treatment of central precocious puberty using an intranasal LHRH analogue (buserelin). *Clin. Endocrinol.*, **22**, 795–806

16. Oerter, K. E., Manasco, P., Barnes, K. M., Jones, J., Hill, S. and Cutler, G. B. (1991). Adult height in precocious puberty after long term treatment with deslorelin. *J. Clin. Endocrinol. Metab.*, **73**, 1235–40

17. Bridges, N. A., Cooke, A., Healy, M. J. R., Hindmarsh, P. C. and Brook, C. G. D. (1993). Standards for ovarian volume in childhood and puberty. *Fertil. Steril.*, **60**, 456–60

18. Bridges, N. A., Cooke, A., Healy, M. J. R., Hindmarsh, P. C. and Brook, C. G. D. (1995). Ovaries in sexual precocity. *Clin. Endocrinol.*, **42**, 135–40

19. Hindmarsh, P. C. (1992). Oestrogen therapy for girls with tall stature. *Clin. Endocrinol.*, **37**, 199–200

20. James, R. A., Chaterjee, S., White, M. C., Hall, K., Moller, N. and Kendall Taylor, P (1989). Continuous infusion of octreotide in acromegaly. *Lancet*, **ii**, 1083–7

21. Darendelier, F., Hindmarsh, P. C., Preece, M. A., Cox, L. and Brook, C. G. D. (1990). Growth hormone increases rate of pubertal maturation. *Acta Endocrinol.*, **122**, 416–20

22. Bourguignon, J. P. and The Belgian Study Group For Paediatric Endocrinology (1988). Variations in duration of pubertal growth: a mechanism compensating for differences in timing of puberty and minimising their effects on final height. *Acta Paediatr. Scand.*, **347** (Suppl.), 16–24

23. Crowne, E. C., Shalet, S. M., Wallace, W. H. B, Eminson, D. M. and Price, D. A. (1990). Final height in boys with untreated constitutional delay in growth and puberty. *Arch. Dis. Child.*, **65**, 1109–12

24. Municchi, G., Rose, S. R., Pescovitz, O. H., Barnes, K. M., Cassorla, F. G. and Cutler, G. B. (1993). Effect of deslorelin induced pubertal delay on the growth of adolescents with short stature and normally timed puberty: preliminary results. *J. Clin. Endocrinol. Metab.*, **77**, 1334–9

25. Lindner, D., Job, J. C. and Chaussain, J. L. (1993). Failure to improve height prediction in short stature pubertal adolescents by inhibiting puberty with luteinising hormone releasing hormone analogue. *Eur. J. Pediatr.*, **15**, 393–6

26. Job, J. C., Toublanc, J. C. and Landier, F. (1994). Growth of short normal children in puberty treated for 3 years with growth hormone alone or in combination with gonadotrophin releasing hormone agonist. *Horm. Res.*, **41**, 177–84

27. Saggese, G., Cesaretti, G., Barsanti, S. and Rossi, A. (1995). Combination treatment with growth hormone and gonadotrophin releasing hormone analogs in short normal girls. *J. Pediatr.*, **126**, 468–73

28. Clayton, R.N., Ogden, V., Hodgkinson, J., Worswick, L., Rodin, D. A., Dyer, S. and Meade, T. W. (1992). How common are polycystic ovaries in normal women and what is their significance for the fertility of the population. *Clin. Endocrinol.*, **37**, 127–34

31

Hormonal male contraception: suppression of spermatogenesis with GnRH antagonists and testosterone

E. Nieschlag and H. M. Behre

INTRODUCTION

Although different mechanisms of action are involved, gonadotropin releasing hormone (GnRH) agonists as well as GnRH antagonists suppress gonadotropin secretion and, in turn, testicular function. While GnRH agonists, if applied in appropriate doses, desensitize pituitary gonadotropin receptors, antagonists directly block these receptors. These effects can be used for the investigation of the physiology of pituitary–testicular interaction and the biological effects of testosterone; these effects can also be exploited in clinical medicine for the treatment of testosterone-dependent tumors. Indeed, GnRH agonists have gained a firm position in the spectrum of possibilities available for the treatment of prostate carcinoma.

Although GnRH antagonists – at least theoretically – should be the first choice in the treatment of prostate carcinoma, they have only recently entered the arena of clinical testing for this indication and are not yet available for general clinical use. The reason for this late arrival lies with the extreme difficulties chemists experienced when attempting the synthesis of potent antagonists (see Rivier and colleagues, this volume).

While pharmaceutical companies are predominantly interested in GnRH analogs for the treatment of prostate carcinoma (and for other short- and long-term applications in women, as reviewed in this volume), these compounds harbor another great potential, i.e. their application in hormonal male contraception.

PRINCIPLE OF HORMONAL MALE CONTRACEPTION

The testes have an endocrine and an exocrine function: the production of androgens and male gametes. Suppression of gamete production without affecting the endocrine function is the goal of endocrine approaches to male fertility regulation. However, since the two functions of the testes are interdependent, it has remained impossible so far to suppress spermatogenesis exclusively and reversibly without significantly affecting androgen synthesis.

Follicle stimulating hormone (FSH) and luteinizing hormone (LH)/testosterone are responsible for the maintenance of fully normal spermatogenesis[1]. If only one of the two is eliminated, spermatogenesis will be reduced, but only in quantitative terms, i.e. fewer but normal sperm will be produced and azoospermia will not be achieved. This has been demonstrated by the elimination of FSH by immunoneutralization, resulting in reduced sperm numbers but not in complete azoospermia, which – at least until quite recently – was considered to be required for an effective male method. Therefore, even if new modalities for the selective suppression of FSH should become available, it remains doubtful whether they would lead to a method for male contraception unless they were to affect sperm function as well as sperm production[2].

In order to achieve azoospermia, it appears to be necessary not only to suppress FSH, but also to deplete the testes of testosterone. Since testosterone alone can maintain spermatogenesis and much lower testosterone concentrations appear to be necessary for maintenance of spermatogenesis than previously considered, the depletion of intratesticular testosterone must be quite complete. In order to maintain androgenicity, including libido, potency, male sex characteristics, psychotropic effects, protein anabolism, bone structure and hematopoiesis, testosterone levels in the general circulation have to be replaced while the testes themselves are depleted of testosterone.

This leads to the general principle of endocrine regulation of male fertility, namely the suppression of FSH and LH, resulting in a depletion of intratesticular testosterone and cessation of spermatogenesis, while peripheral testosterone is substituted by an androgen preparation.

TESTOSTERONE ALONE FOR MALE CONTRACEPTION

According to the principle outlined above, testosterone should be the first choice for hormonal male contraception, since it not only suppresses pituitary LH and FSH secretion, but also replaces testosterone in the general circulation.

Consequently, a number of clinical trials based on testosterone application have been performed in the past. However, it is only recently that the first efficacy studies for hormonal male contraception using testosterone injections have been completed under the auspices of the World Health Oganization (WHO)[3,4].

Several hundred couples participated in these worldwide multicenter trials and a total of 506 volunteers completed the efficacy phases of these trials. The studies clearly demonstrated that the efficacy of testosterone injections in terms of preventing pregnancies was astonishingly high when azoospermia was reached, resulting in a Pearl index of 0–0.8. However, only 75% of the men attained azoospermia (68% in Caucasian and 86% in Asian men). In those couples in which the volunteers' sperm counts were suppressed only below 3 million/ml (and not to azoospermia), a relatively high pregnancy rate and a Pearl index of as high as 8.1 resulted, as illustrated in Figure 1. It should also be noted that, in addition to the necessity of weekly testosterone enanthate

Men with azoospermia
(230.1 exposure years)

Men with sperm concentration
> 0 and < 3 million/ml
(49.5 exposure years)

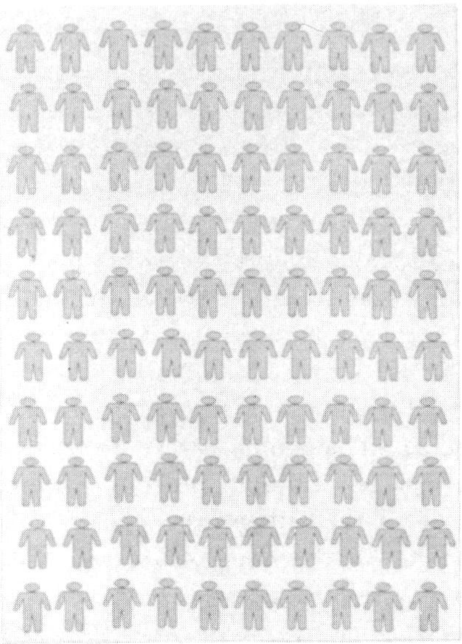

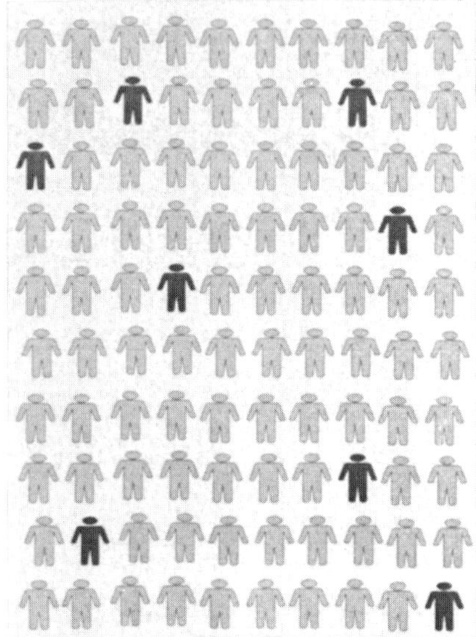

Pearl index: 0 (0.0–1.6)

Pearl index: 8.1 (2.2–20.7)

Figure 1 Pearl index (95% confidence limits) in men with azoospermia compared to men with sperm concentrations below 3 million/ml but without azoospermia in the second WHO efficacy trial of male contraception

injections, it took an average of 4 months to achieve azoospermia.

Thus, although the WHO studies can be considered milestones in the development of a male contraceptive, they also demonstrated the need for (1) a faster onset of action; (2) more complete suppression of spermatogenesis; and (3) long-acting testosterone preparations. While the last demand may be achieved by new esters, such as testosterone buciclate[5], by new application modalities of known esters, such as testosterone undecanoate[6] or by traditional testosterone implants[7], the first two requirements may need the synergism of another substance to be added to the testosterone application. For this purpose, some consider gestagens to be a suitable modality, whereas others place their confidence in GnRH analogs.

TESTOSTERONE PLUS GnRH AGONISTS

Between 1979 and 1992, 12 trials using GnRH agonists mostly in combination with testosterone for hormonal male contraception were published[8-19]. Altogether 106 volunteers participated in these trials. The GnRH agonists Decapeptyl, buserelin and nafarelin were administered at daily doses of 5–500 µg/volunteer for periods of 10–30 weeks. In about 30% of men, sperm production could be suppressed below 5×10^6/ml and azoospermia occurred in 21 men, while in the remaining volunteers, the sperm number was only slightly reduced or remained unaffected. One explanation for the ineffectiveness of GnRH agonist plus androgen is the escape of FSH suppression after several weeks of GnRH agonist treatment[19,20].

Altogether, GnRH agonists in combination with testosterone did not prove useful in male contraception. At times it has been said that higher doses of the GnRH agonists should be used, but currently no further clinical studies appear to be under way.

TESTOSTERONE PLUS GnRH ANTAGONISTS

As mentioned in the introduction, it took much longer to develop GnRH antagonists suitable for clinical application than GnRH agonists.

Nevertheless, before antagonists became available for clinical testing, non-human primates served as useful models in the development of antagonists for male contraception[21].

It could first be shown in cynomolgus monkeys that GnRH antagonists and testosterone can effectively suppress spermatogenesis in primates[22]. However, in further studies it became evident that the concomitant administration of GnRH antagonists and testosterone prevented rapid and complete suppression of spermatogenesis[23], while delayed testosterone substitution led to swift and complete suppression, as evidenced by testicular histology and azoospermia[24]. The interval between GnRH antagonist and testosterone administration could be as short as, 2 weeks[25]. At variance with these results were findings by another group that achieved azoospermia even with simultaneous antagonist and testosterone application. However, the animals started with relatively low sperm counts[26]. Despite this controversy, the monkey studies had an important pacemaker function for the ensuing clinical trials.

To date, the results of five clinical trials for male contraception using GnRH antagonists have become available[27-31] and are summarized in Table 1. Overall, 35 of 40 (88%) (Caucasian) volunteers became azoospermic, in comparison to testosterone enanthate alone, which produced azoospermia in only 68% of Caucasian men within 6 months, this was a much better rate of complete suppression. It should also be noted that in the two most recent studies all 14 volunteers became azoospermic. Although the number of subjects is still small, this is a promising result. In addition – at least in the last two studies – the mean time to achieve azoospermia was shorter than with testosterone alone.

Recent studies in monkeys suggested that the suppression of spermatogenesis achieved by GnRH antagonists could be maintained after withdrawal of the antagonist by a testosterone preparation alone[32]. This finding could not be confirmed in a first human trial, since sperm reappeared under continued 19-nortestosterone treatment when the antagonist Cetrorelix was withdrawn[31]. However, the testosterone doses used in the monkeys were higher than the 19-nortestosterone doses used in the humans; this

Table 1 Overview of five clinical trials with GnRH antagonists and testosterone for male contraception

Study	Antagonist	Daily dose	Duration of antagonist administration (weeks)	Androgen substitution	Rate of azoospermia (n/n)	Azoospermia reached by week
Pavlou et al. (1991)[27]	Nal-Glu	10 mg	20	delayed TE	6/6	12
		10 mg	10	25 mg/week		
		20 mg	+10		1/2	16
Tom et al. (1992)[28]	Nal-Glu	7.5 mg	16	delayed TE 150 mg/2 weeks	7/8	10
Bagatell et al. (1993)[29]	Nal-Glu	100 µg/kg	20	simultaneous TE 200 mg/week	7/10	4–24
Pavlou et al., (1994)[30]	Nal-Glu	10 mg	20	simultaneous TE 100 mg/week	8/8	6–10
Behre et al. (1995)[31]	cetrorelix	loading dose; 10 mg/day; maintenance dose, 2 mg/day	12	delayed 19NT 400 mg initially, 200 mg maintenance	6/6	4–12
Total					35/40	

TE, testosterone enanthate; 19NT, 19-nortestosterone hexyloxyphenylproionate

difference may be of importance. The human study also revealed that much lower doses of the GnRH antagonist may be required to maintain suppression of spermatogenesis than to induce it. This principle of a high antagonist loading dose followed by a low maintenance dose[33] is described by Reissmann and colleagues in this volume. This principle will be of further importance in the development of a Cetrorelix depot preparation (Engel and associates, this volume), which should also be of advantage in future trials for hormonal male contraception. It should be emphasized that, although daily subcutaneous injections were cumbersome, Cetrorelix was tolerated well without side effects by all volunteers for the entire period of 12 weeks. The high efficacy and the lack of side effects make this an attractive candidate for further testing.

CONCLUSION

This brief summary indicates that testosterone, in combination with GnRH antagonists, represents a favorable modality for male contraception.

There are strong indications that testosterone depot preparations, such as testosterone buciclate or implants given together with GnRH antagonist depot preparations, may fulfil both requirements for a quick onset of contraceptive protection as well as for long injection intervals. However, these trials have yet to be conducted and the studies performed to date, although promising, only provide leads. From all existing evidence it can be concluded that such a combination (if appropriate antagonists were to be used) would be free of major side effects and the suppression of spermatogenesis should be fully reversible.

Sceptics may argue that the price for GnRH antagonists may preclude them from development as a male contraceptive that should be affordable and in the price range of comparable female methods. If the prices of GnRH antagonists were in the range of GnRH agonists prescribed for the treatment of prostate carcinoma, they could never become part of a male contraceptive. However, prices are dictated by many variables and production costs will decrease with greater demand. In addition, based on screenings of new compounds by binding to GnRH receptors *in vitro*, there is a chance that a cheap and perhaps orally effective GnRH antagonist may be identified. Therefore, it remains the scientists' task to demonstrate the feasibility of the combined use of testosterone and a GnRH antagonist.

ACKNOWLEDGEMENT

Our own recent studies reported here were supported by the Deutsche Forschungs-gemeinschaft (DFG), the Federal Health Ministry (Bonn) and the World Health Organization Human Reproduction Programme (Geneva).

References

1. Weinbauer, G. F. and Nieschlag, E. (1993). Hormonal control of spermatogenesis. In DeKretser, D. (ed.) *Molecular Biology of Reproduction*, pp. 99–142. (San Diego: Academic Press)

2. Nieschlag, E. (1986). Reasons for abandoning immunization against FSH as an approach to male fertility regulation. In Zatuchni, G.I., Goldsmith, A., Spieler, J. M. and Sciarra, J.J. (eds.) *Male Contraception: Advances and Future Prospects*, pp. 395–400. (Philadelphia: Harper and Row)

3. WHO Task Force on Methods for the Regulation of Male Fertility (1990). Contraceptive efficacy of testosterone-induced azoospermia in normal men. *Lancet*, **336**, 955–9

4. WHO Programme of Research, Development and Research Training in Human Reproduction (1995). *Annual Technical Report 1994*, pp. 59–60. (Geneva: WHO)

5. Behre, H. M., Baus, S., Kliesch, S., Keck, C., Simoni, M. and Nieschlag, E. (1995). Potential of testosterone buciclate for male contraception: endocrine differences between responders and non-responders. *J. Clin. Endocrinol. Metab.*, **80**, 2394–403

6. Partsch, C. J., Weinbauer, G. F., Fang, R. and Nieschlag, E. (1995). Injectable testosterone undecanoate has more favourable pharmacokinetics and pharmacodynamics than testosterone enanthate. *Eur. J. Endocrinol.*, **132**, 514–19

7. Handelsman, D. J., Conway, A. J. and Boylan, L. M. (1992). Suppression of human spermatogenesis by testosterone implants. *J. Clin. Endocrinol. Metab.* **175**,1326–32

8. Bergquist, C., Nilius, S. G., Bergh, T., Skering, G. and Wide, G. (1979). Inhibitory effects on gonadotropin secretion and gonadal function in men during chronic treatment with a potent stimulatory luteinizing hormone-releasing hormone analogue. *Acta Endocrinol.*, **91**, 610–18

9. Linde, R., Doelle, G.C., Alexander, N., Kirchner, F., Vale, F., Rivier, J. and Rabin, D. (1981). Reversible inhibition of testicular steroidogenesis and spermatogenesis by a potent gonadotropin-releasing hormone agonist in normal men. *N. Engl. J. Med.*, **305**, 663–7

10. Doelle, G. C., Alexander, A. N., Evans, R. M., Linde, R., Vale, W. and Rabin, D. (1983). Combined treatment with an LHRH agonist and testosterone in man. *J. Androl.*, **4**, 298–302

11. Rabin, D., Evans, R. M., Alexander, A. N., Doelle, G. C., Rivier, J., Vale, W. and Liddle, G. (1984). Heterogeneity of sperm density profiles following 20-week therapy with high-dose LHRH analog plus testosterone. *J. Androl.*, **5**, 176–80

12. Bhasin, S., Heber, D., Steiner, B. S., Handelsman, D. J. and Swerdloff, R. S. (1985). Hormonal effects of gonadotropin-releasing hormone (GnRH) agonist in the human male. III. Effects of long-term combined treatment with GnRH agonist and androgen. *J. Clin. Endocrinol. Metab.*, **60**, 998–1003

13. Schürmeyer, T., Knuth, U. A., Freischem, C. W., Sandow, J., Akhtar, F. B. and Nieschlag, E. (1984). Suppression of pituitary and testicular function in normal men by constant gonadotropin-releasing hormone agonist infusion. *J. Clin. Endocrinol. Metab.* **59**, 1–6

14. Michel, E., Bents, H., Akhtar, F. B., Hönigl, W., Knuth, U. A., Sandow, J. and Nieschlag, E. (1985). Failure of high-dose sustained release luteinizing hormone releasing agonist (buserelin) plus oral testosterone to suppress male fertility. *Clin. Endocrinol.*, **23**, 663–75

15. Pavlou, S. N., Interlandi, J. W., Wakefield, G., Rivier, J., Vale, W. and Rabin, D. (1986), Heterogeneity of sperm density profiles following 16-week therapy with continuous infusion of high-dose LHRH analog plus testosterone. *J. Androl.*, **7**, 228–33

16. Frick, J. and Aulitzky, W. (1986). Effects of a potent LHRH agonist on the pituitary–gonadal

axis with and without testosterone substitution. *Urol. Res.*, **14**, 261–4

17. Bouchard P. and Garcia, E. (1987). Influence of testosterone substitution on sperm suppression by LHRH agonists. *Horm. Res.*, **28**, 175–80

18. Bhasin, S., Yuan, Q.X., Steiner, B. S. and Swerdloff, R. S. (1987). Hormonal effects of gonadotropin-releasing hormone (GnRH) agonist in men. Effects of long-term treatment with GnRH agonist infusion and androgens. *J. Clin. Endocrinol. Metab.*, **65**, 568–74

19. Behre, H. M., Nashan, D., Hubert, W. and Nieschlag, E. (1992). Depot gonadotropin releasing hormone agonist blunts the androgen-induced suppression of spermatogenesis in a clinical trial of male contraception. *J. Clin. Endocrinol. Metab.*, **74**, 84–90

20. Bhasin, S., Berman, N. and Swerdloff, R. S. (1994). Follicle-stimulating hormone (FSH) escape during chronic gonadotropin-releasing hormone (GnRH) agonist and testosterone treatment. *J. Androl.*, **15**, 386–91

21. Weinbauer, G. F., Behre, H. M. and Nieschlag, E. (1993). Gonadotropin-releasing hormone analog-induced regulation of testicular function in monkeys and men. In Bouchard, P., Caraty, A., Coelingh Bennink, H. J. T. and Pavlou, S. N. (eds.) *GnRH, GnRH Analogs, Gonadotropins and Gonadal Peptides*, pp. 211–27. (Carnforth, UK: Parthenon Publishing)

22. Weinbauer, G. F., Surmann, F. J. and Nieschlag, E . (1987). Suppression of spermatogenesis in a nonhuman primate *(Macaca fascicularis)* by concomitant gonadotropin-releasing hormone antagonist and testosterone treatment. *Acta Endocrinol.*, **114**, 138–46

23. Weinbauer, G. F., Göckeler, E. and Nieschlag, E. (1988). Testosterone prevents complete suppression of spermatogenesis in the gonadotropin-releasing hormone (GnRH) antagonist-treated non-human primate *(Macaca fascicularis)*. *J. Clin. Endocrinol. Metab.*, **67**, 284–90

24. Weinbauer, G. F., Khurshid, S., Fingscheidt, U. and Nieschlag, E. (1989). Sustained inhibition of sperm production and inhibin secretion induced by a gonadotropin-releasing hormone antagonist and delayed testosterone substitution in non-human primates *(Macaca fascicularis)*. *J. Endocrinol.*, **123**, 303–10

25. Weinbauer, G. F., Behre, H. M. and Nieschlag, E. (1992). Concomitant but not delayed androgen supplementation prevents complete testicular involution in GnRH antagonist-treated nonhuman primates. *Proceedings of the 74th Annual Meeting of the Endocrine Society* (Abstr.), p. 320, San Antonio, Texas

26. Bremner, W. J., Bagatell, C. J. and Steiner, R. A. (1991). Gonadotropin-releasing hormone antagonist plus testosterone: a potential male contraceptive. *J. Clin. Endocrinol. Metab.*, **73**, 465–9

27. Pavlou, S. N., Brewer, K., Farley, M.G., Lindner, J.,Bastias, M. C., Rogers, B. J., Swift, L. L., Rivier, J. E., Vale, W. W., Conn, P. M. and Herbert, C. M. (1991). Combined administration of a gonadotropin-releasing hormone antagonist and testosterone in men induces reversible azoospermia without loss of libido. *J. Clin Endocrinol. Metab.*, **73**, 1360–9

28. Tom, L., Bhasin, S., Salameh, W. Steiner, B., Peterson, M., Sokol, R. Z., Rivier, J., Vale, W. and Swerdloff, R. S. (1992). Induction of azoospermia in normal men with combined Nal-Glu gonadotropin-releasing hormone antagonist and testosterone enanthate. *J. Clin. Endocrinol. Metab.*, **75**, 476–83

29. Bagatell, C. J., Matsumoto, A. M., Christensen, R. B., Rivier, J. E. and Bremner, W. J. (1993). Comparision of a gonadotropin-releasing hormone antagonist plus testosterone (T) versus T alone as potential male contraceptive regimens. *J. Clin. Endocrinol. Metab.*, **77**, 427–32

30. Pavlou, S. N., Herodotou, D., Curtain, M. and Minaretzis, D. (1994). Complete suppression of spermatogenesis by co-administration of a GnRH antagonist plus a physiologic dose of testosterone. *Proceedings of the 76th Meeting of American Endocrine Society.* (Abstr.), p. 1324, Anaheim, California

31. Behre, H. M., Kliesch, S., Lemcke, B. and Nieschlag, E. (1995). Suppression of spermatogenesis to azoospermia by combined administration of GnRH antagonist and 19-nortestosterone cannot be maintained by 19-nortestosterone alone in normal men. *Proceedings 77th Meeting of Endocrine Society.* (Abstr.) Washington DC

32. Weinbauer, G. F., Limberger, A., Behre, H. M. and Nieschlag, E. (1994). Can testosterone alone maintain the GnRH antagonist-induced suppression of spermatognesis in the non-human primate? *J. Endocrinol.*, **142**, 485–95

33. Behre, H. M., Kliesch, S., Pühse, G. and Nieschlag, E. (1994). Initial high doses of a GnRH antagonist followed by low maintenance doses suppress serum LH, FSH and testosterone effectively in normal men (Abstr.). *Exp. Clin. Endocrinol.*,**102**, 53

32

Hormonal male contraception using GnRH analogs: metabolic effects on lipids

W. J. Bremner and C. J. Bagatell

INTRODUCTION

Many studies over the years have shown that various hormonal contraceptive methods will dramatically and reversibly suppress sperm production in normal men, without serious known adverse effects[1]. Azoospermia is attained in 50–80% of Caucasian men (and in higher proportions in Asian men), while severe oligospermia is nearly always attained. A World Health Organization multicenter trial has shown excellent contraceptive efficacy in men from many racial and ethnic backgrounds using testosterone enanthate alone[2]. The authors have recently shown improved ability to suppress sperm production in normal men using combinations of agents such as levonorgestrel or cyproterone acetate with testosterone[3,4].

In addition to seeking improved efficacy in the suppression of spermatogenesis with newer hormonal methods, including gonadotropin releasing hormone (GnRH) analogs, it is mandatory to ensure that such regimens will exert minimal adverse effects on other organ systems. The hormonal changes produced by male hormonal contraceptives could potentially affect many physiological processes; this chapter will concentrate on circulating lipids as one example of hormonal effects. Lipids are of particular interest because of their potential role in the pathophysiology of cardiovascular disease. It is widely appreciated that premenopausal women have a lower risk for coronary artery disease (CAD) than men, and that this risk increases in women after menopause[5,6]. The effects of estrogens on plasma lipids and other factors affecting coronary risk have been studied extensively; however, contributions of androgens to coronary risk have received less attention. In this chapter we will review the effects of androgen withdrawal using GnRH analogs and of exogenous testosterone on plasma lipids.

SUPPRESSION OF ENDOGENOUS ANDROGENS IN MEN USING GnRH ANALOGS

Endogenous androgen production is markedly reduced by surgical castration or by hormonal suppression of testosterone production. Castrated men have higher levels of α-lipoproteins and lower levels of β-lipoproteins than intact men of similar ages[7]. More recently, the development of GnRH analogs has offered investigators a means to suppress androgens by less drastic means. GnRH agonists initially stimulate the pituitary secretion of follicle stimulating hormone (FSH) and luteinizing hormone (LH), but after a period of days to weeks down-regulation of the receptors occurs, and gonadotropin secretion decreases to very low levels[8]. Because testicular production of testosterone (T) is dependent on LH stimulation, hypoandrogenism ensues after a few weeks of GnRH agonist administration. GnRH antagonists also suppress gonadotropin and T secretion. However, their effect is immediate with complete T suppression occurring within a few days after the initiation of the antagonist[8].

GnRH agonists are used clinically in the management of advanced prostate cancer and other hormone-dependent conditions. Moorjani[9] reported that, in men with advanced prostate cancer, administration of GnRH agonist together with an anti-androgen resulted in a significant increase in high-density lipoprotein (HDL) cholesterol, but no change in very low-density lipoprotein (VLDL) or low-density lipoprotein (LDL) cholesterol. They later reported[10] that men who underwent orchiectomy for their disease showed no change in HDL cholesterol, while apoprotein B levels increased. They speculated that the more complete suppression of estradiol levels in the men who had an orchiectomy accounted for the disparity in the lipid levels in the two groups.

The studies mentioned above were conducted in older men with a coexisting illness, and the results therefore might not be applicable to the male population in general. However, other studies, using healthy men as subjects, also suggest that suppression of endogenous androgens results in increased HDL cholesterol. Goldberg et al.[11] reported that in volunteers receiving GnRH agonist with no androgen replacement, T levels fell profoundly during the 7–10 week treatment period. At the same time, HDL cholesterol, apoprotein AI and apoprotein B levels increased, with no change in plasma triglycerides. All parameters returned to the baseline levels after drug administration ended. A second group of men in this study received the agonist plus partial T replacement. In these men, T levels were maintained at approximately one-half the baseline level. Modest increases in HDL cholesterol were noted towards the end of the treatment period; during the recovery period, HDL levels returned to baseline. More recently, Byerley and co-workers used a GnRH agonist to suppress androgens in normal men and then administered T at doses resulting in serum T levels at the low and high ends of the normal male range[12]. Under this paradigm plasma lipids were similar in the two groups of subjects, despite their differing T levels. These data suggest that the relationship between serum T levels and plasma HDL is not a linear one. That is, there may be a threshold below which serum T levels must fall in order to effect an increase in plasma HDL cholesterol.

The authors have used the GnRH antagonist, Nal-Glu, to study testosterone's effects on lipoproteins in healthy young men[13]. Initially, the authors studied 15 healthy young men. During the 6-week treatment period, each man received either:

(1) Nal-Glu each day subcutaneously plus sesame oil placebo each week intramuscularly (Nal-Glu alone);

(2) Nal-Glu each day subcutaneously plus T enanthate (100 mg/week intramuscularly); or

(3) Placebo (subcutaneous and intramuscular injections).

Serum T and estradiol (E_2) levels in men receiving Nal-Glu alone fell significantly within 3 days after the experimental regimen began; they reached the castrate range after 1–2 weeks and remained suppressed during the rest of the treatment period. In these men, the mean HDL cholesterol concentrations increased by 26% during the treatment period ($p < 0.05$) (Figure 1). Mean levels of HDL_2 and HDL_3 cholesterol increased by 63% and 17%, respectively, during the treatment period ($p < 0.05$), and mean apoprotein AI concentration increased by 17% ($p < 0.05$) (Figure 2). In contrast, there were no significant changes in plasma lipids in the other treatment groups, although there was a slight decrease in HDL cholesterol in men who received Nal-Glu with T replacement.

The authors later studied additional men in each of the treatment groups (for a total of nine or 10 men per group); their results were very similar. The authors also found that administration of Nal-Glu together with T (50 mg/week) resulted in no change in plasma lipoproteins. Pavlou et al.[14] reported that administration of Nal-Glu together with subphysiological T replacement (25 mg/week intramuscularly) resulted in an increase in HDL cholesterol of approximately 25% after 20 weeks of drug administration.

The authors have also demonstrated that the small amount of circulating E_2 in men is important in maintaining HDL levels, particularly the HDL_2 subfraction, in normal men[15]. Using the same approach as described above, the authors administered Nal-Glu together with T enanthate (100 mg/week intramuscularly), to healthy men for 6 weeks.

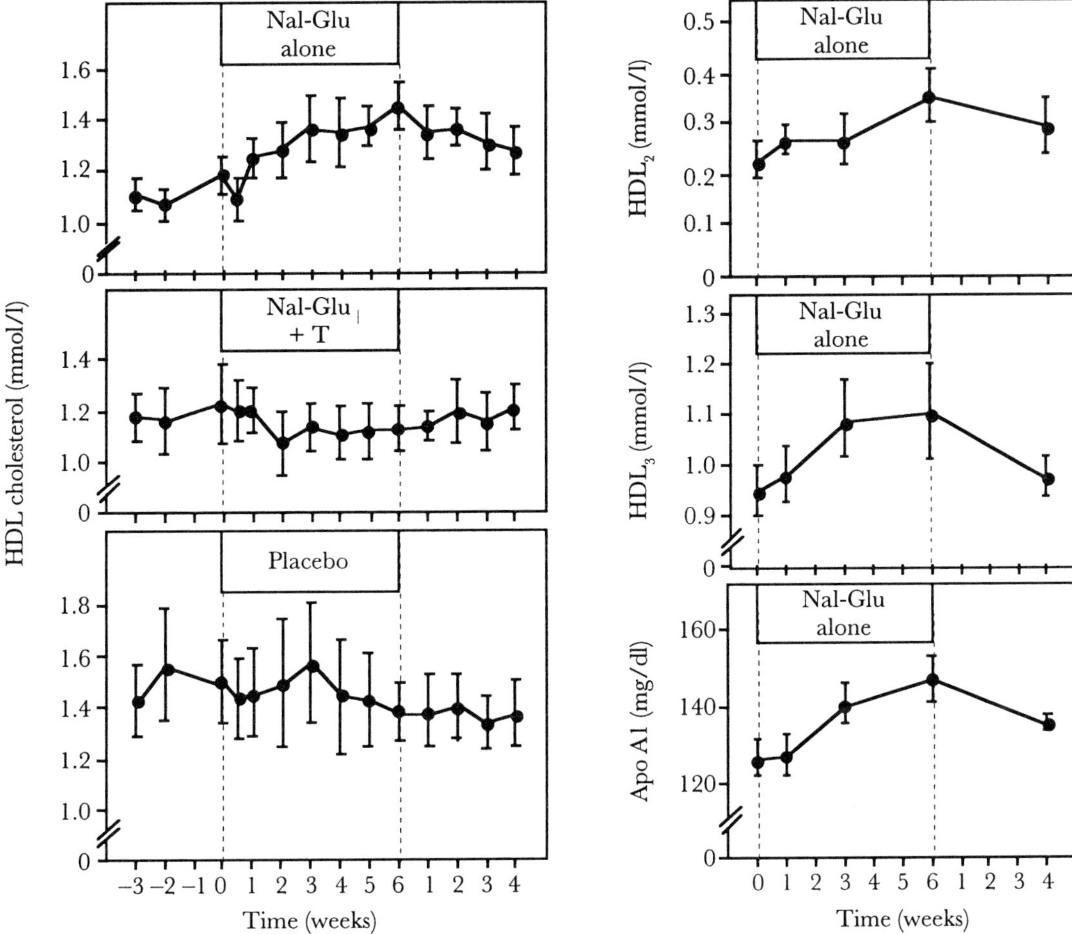

Figure 1 High-density lipoprotein (HDL) cholesterol levels (mean ± SE) during baseline, treatment and post-treatment periods. Top: Nal-Glu 75 µg/kg body weight subcutabeously per week caused hypogonadism and resulted in increased HDL levels. Middle: Nal-Glu 75 µg/Kg body weight subcutaneously per week plus testosterone (T) 100 mg intramuscularly per week when the T deficiency caused by Nal-Glu was corrected with exogenous T, HDL levels did not rise. Bottom: placebo control ($n = 5$ in each group). Nal-Glu, an antagonist of gonadotropin releasing hormone. From Bagatell, C. J., Knopp, R. H., Vale, W. W. *et al.* (1992). Physiologic levels of testosterone suppress HDL cholesterol levels in normal men. *Ann. Int. Med.*, **116**, 967–73[13]. Reproduced with permission of the American College of Physicians

Figure 2 High-density lipoprotein (HDL)-2 and -3 cholesterol and apoprotein A1 (Apo A1) levels (mean ± SE) during the baseline, treatment and post-treatment periods in men receiving Nal-Glu (an antagonist of gonadotropin releasing hormone) alone ($n = 5$). The hypogonadism induced during Nal-Glu administration led to increases in HDL_2, HDL_3 and Apo A1. Reproduced with permission from Bagatell *et al.* (1992)[13]. Full copyright information is given in Figure 1

Another group of men received Nal-Glu together with the same dosage of T; in addition, they were given testolactone orally. Testolactone is an aromatase inhibitor and inhibits the enzymatic conversion of T to E_2 in peripheral tissues. Therefore, the men who received Teslac had normal T levels but markedly suppressed E_2 levels. After 6 weeks of treatment plasma HDL, particularly the HDL_2 subfraction, was suppressed significantly in men who received Teslac, whereas these parameters were not suppressed significantly in the other men (Figure 3).

Could the physiological regulation of HDL cholesterol by androgens contribute to the

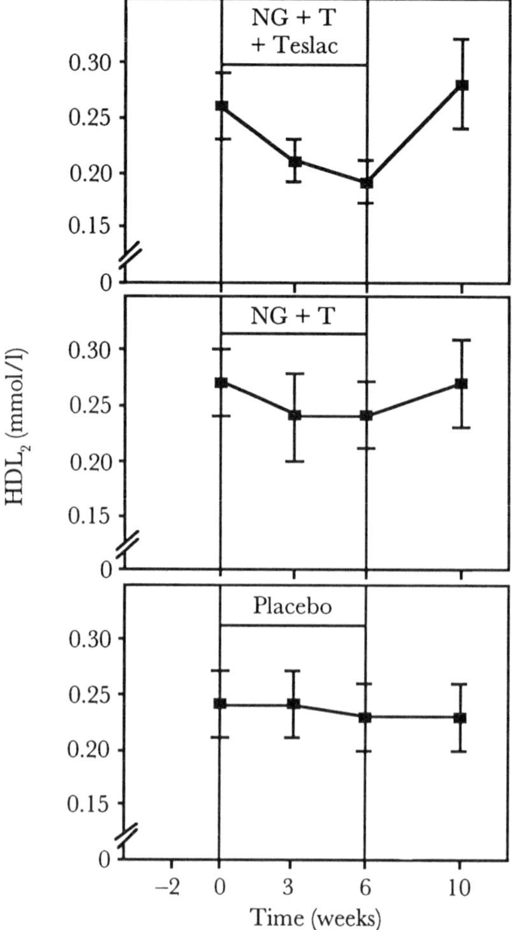

Figure 3 High-density lipoprotein (HDL)-2 cholesterol levels during the study in men receiving Nal-Glu (an antagonist of gonadotropin releasing hormone) plus T plus Teslac (top panel; $n = 10$), Nal-Glu plus T (middle panel; $n = 10$), or placebo (bottom panel; $n = 9$). From Bagatell, C. J., Knopp, R. H. and Bremner, W. J. (1994). Physiological levels of estradiol stimulate plasma density lipoprotein cholesterol levels in normal men. *J. Clin. Endocrinol. Metab.*, **78**, 855–61[15]. Reproduced with permission of the Endocrine Society

difference in the incidence of coronary artery disease between men and premenopausal women? The magnitude of increase in HDL cholesterol induced by androgen deficiency is similar to the gender difference in HDL cholesterol levels between men and premenopausal women. In the Lipid Research Clinics prevalence study[16] HDL cholesterol levels at the 50th percentile were 22%

(0.26 mmol/l) higher in women aged 30–34 years than in men of the same age. In other studies[17,18] risk for coronary disease decreased by 2–3% for each 0.026 mmol/l increment in HDL cholesterol. As noted above, there is a strong inverse relationship between plasma levels of HDL cholesterol and risk of coronary artery disease in epidemiological studies. It is therefore quite possible that suppression of HDL cholesterol induced by physiological levels of androgens contributes to the known increased risk of coronary disease in men. A GnRH analog plus low-dose T regimen could cause a small decrease in the normally circulating levels of T in men that might be beneficial in terms of cardiac risk. This could be a positive health benefit for this form of hormonal male contraception.

EFFECTS OF EXOGENOUS TESTOSTERONE

In addition to their use as replacement therapy in hypogonadism androgens, particularly T, are being explored as potential hormonal male contraceptive agents, alone[2,19,20] or in combination with other hormonal agents[14,19,21,22]. In order to be acceptable to a large number of men, a potential regimen must be highly effective, reversible, and it must also have no adverse effects on other physiological processes. Therefore, the metabolic effects of supplemental androgens are of considerable importance in this area. In addition, anabolic steroids are being used by large numbers of athletes, from high-school age to the professional level. The lipid effects of exogenous androgens are, therefore, also important clinically.

The effects of exogenous androgens on plasma lipids vary considerably with type of androgen administered (aromatizable or non-aromatizable) and with the route of administration (oral versus parenteral). The lipid responses to both T esters and alkylated androgens have been examined under a variety of experimental paradigms.

Three different groups of researchers[23–25] administered T enanthate (200–280 mg/week intramuscularly) to normal men for 3–6-week periods. Friedl *et al.*[23] reported that plasma HDL levels decreased by approximately 5%, but LDL levels did not change. Thompson *et al.*[24] and Zmuda *et al.*[25] reported decreases in plasma HDL of 9% and 16% respectively ($p < 0.05$ in each case). In the former study, LDL cholesterol levels decreased by 16% ($p < 0.05$), with no change in plasma triglycerides.

The authors have administered T enanthate (200 mg/week intramuscularly) to healthy men for 20 weeks[26]. They found that HDL cholesterol levels decreased significantly within the first 4 weeks of treatment. This suppression persisted until the period of T administration was completed (Figure 4); mean plasma HDL levels were 13% lower than baseline at the end of the treatment period. Apoprotein AI and the HDL_2 and HDL_3 subfractions were also significantly suppressed during T treatment; however, LDL cholesterol and triglycerides did not change. The decrease in plasma HDL cholesterol is maintained throughout periods of T administration lasting as long as 1 year[4].

Although the reasons for the variability of HDL suppression under differing paradigms are unclear, it seems that the duration of treatment is not a major contributing factor. However, the subjects' baseline HDL levels may affect the degree of HDL suppression seen during T administration. In the authors' study and in the study of Zmuda *et al.*[25], baseline levels were somewhat higher than in the studies of Friedl *et al.*[23] and Thompson *et al.*[24], and the degree of HDL suppression was also somewhat greater. The mechanisms underlying this effect are not known.

HDL levels are clearly suppressed by the regimen of T alone used most commonly in male contraceptive trials (T enanthate 200 mg/ week intramuscularly). These results suggest that the addition of other agents, such as GnRH analogs, which allow use of a lower dose of T, will be important in avoiding potentially adverse effects of T.

SUMMARY AND CONCLUSIONS

Androgens are physiological regulators of plasma lipoproteins, particularly exerting a suppressive effect on the HDL fraction. Their effects are

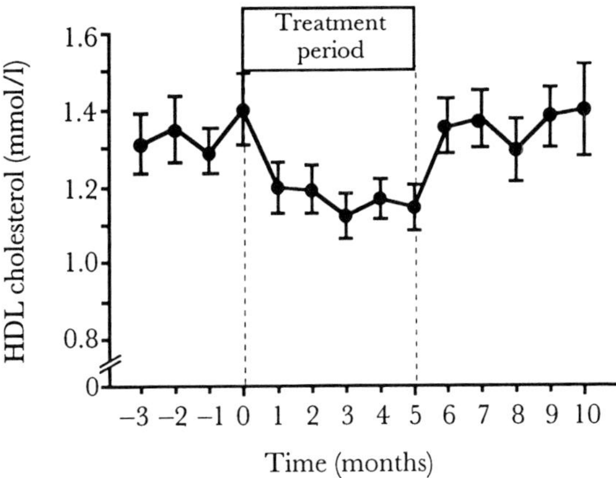

Figure 4 Plasma high-density lipoprotein (HDL) cholesterol levels in the subjects during the course of the study ($n = 19$ until month 7; $n = 8$–15 thereafter). All data points during the treatment period (testosterone enanthate, 200 mg intramuscularly per week) were significantly decreased ($p < 0.05$) compared with the baseline and post-treatment values. From Bagatell, C. J., Heiman, J. R., Matsumoto, A. *et al.* (1994). Metabolic effects of high-dose, exogenous testosterone (T) in normal men. *J. Clin. Endocrinol. Metab.*, **79**, 561–7[27]. Reproduced with permission of the Endocrine Society

modulated by the structure of each compound as well as by the route of administration. In males, both endogenous and exogenous androgens have a suppressive effect on plasma HDL cholesterol, with little effect on plasma LDL or triglyceride levels. Oral and non-aromatizable androgens have a greater suppressive effect on HDL, particularly HDL_2, than do aromatizable androgens. The E_2 formed as a result of aromatization leads to increased HDL levels in men.

The data the authors have reviewed suggest that endogenous androgens may contribute to the increased risk of cardiovascular disease in men, especially in comparison to premenopausal women. The data also suggest that the use of androgenic hormones may induce changes in plasma lipids that potentially alter risk factors for coronary artery disease. Regimens that include androgens should be evaluated carefully for their effects on plasma lipoproteins, and agents which have the fewest adverse effects on plasma lipoproteins should be used preferentially in most settings.

GnRH analogs as applied to contraceptive development have the potential to be used in addition to androgens in suppressing gonadotropin and sperm production, thereby allowing lower doses of androgens. Lower doses of androgens will decrease the potential for adverse effects and could even lead to a beneficial effect on cardiovascular health if HDL levels rise in the course of hormonal contraception.

ACKNOWLEDGEMENTS

This work was supported by the Contraceptive Research and Development Program of the Agency for International Development, NIH grant HD 12629, Department of Veterans Affairs Medical Research funds and the Andrew W. Mellon Foundation. Portions of this chapter are reprinted from Bagatell C. J. and Bremner W. J. (1995)[26,27].

References

1. Cummings, D. E. and Bremner, W. J. (1994). Prospects for new hormonal male contraceptives. *Clin. Endocrinol. Metab. North Am.*, **23**, 893–922

2. World Health Organization Task Force on Male Fertility (1990). Contraceptive efficacy of testosterone-induced azoospermia in normal men. *Lancet*, **336**, 955–9

3. Bebb, R. A., Anawalt, B. D., Christensen, R. B., Paulsen, C. A., Bremner, W. J. and Matsumoto, A. M. (1995). A promising male contraceptive approach: combined administration of testosterone and levonorgestrel. *J. Clin. Endocrinol. Metab.*, in press

4. Meriggiola, M. C., Valdiserri, A., Pavani, A., Capelli, M., Paulsen, C. A., Bremner, W. J. and Flamigni, C. (1995). A combined regimen of cyproterone acetate (CPA) and testosterone enanthate (TE) as a potentially highly effective male contraceptive: effects on spermatogenesis and hormones. In *Program and Abstracts of the 77th Annual Meeting of the Endocrine Society*, Washington, DC, p. 85

5. Castelli, W. P. (1984). Epidemiology of coronary heart disease: the Framingham study. *Am. J. Med.*, **76A**, 4–12

6. Knopp, R. H. (1988). The effects of postmenopausal estrogen therapy on the incidence of arteriosclerotic vascular disease in women. *Obstet. Gynecol.*, **72**, 295–305

7. Furman, R.H., Howard, R.P. and Imagawa, R. (1956). Serum lipid and lipoprotein concentrations in castrate and noncastrate male subjects. *Circulation*, **14**, 490

8. Karten, M.J. and Rivier, J.E. (1986). Gonadotropin releasing hormone analog design. Structure function studies toward the development of agonists and antagonists: rationale and perspective. *Endocr. Rev.*, **7**, 44–66

9. Moorjani, S., Dupont, A., Labrie, F., Lupien, P. J., Brun, D., Gagne, C., Giguere, M. and B'elanger, A. (1987). Increase in plasma high-density lipoprotein concentration following complete androgen blockage in men with prostatic carcinoma. *Metabolism*, **36**, 244–50

10. Moorjani, S., Dupont, A., Labrie, F., Lupien, P. J., Gagne, C., Brun, D., Giguere, M., B'elanger, A. and Cusan, L. (1988). Changes in plasma lipoproteins during various androgen suppression therapies in men with prostatic carcinoma: effects or orchiectomy, estrogen and combination treatment with luteinizing hormone-releasing hormone agonist and flutamide. *J. Clin. Endocrinol. Metab.*, **66**, 614–21

11. Goldberg, R. B., Rabin, D., Alexander, A., Doelle, N. and Getz, G. S. (1985). Suppression of plasma testosterone leads to an increase in serum total and high density lipoprotein cholesterol and apoproteins A1 and AII. *J. Clin. Endocrinol. Metab.*, **60**, 203–7

12. Byerley, L., Lee, W.N., Swerdloff, R.S., Buena, F., Nair, S.K., Buchanan, T.A., Goldberg, R., Steiner, B. and Bhasin, S. (1993). Effect of modulating serum testosterone levels in the normal male range on protein, carbohydrate, and lipid metabolism in men: implications for testosterone replacement therapy. *Endocr. J.*, **1**, 253–62

13. Bagatell, C.J., Knopp, R. H., Vale, W. W., Rivier, J. E. and Bremner, W. J. (1992). Physiologic levels of testosterone suppress HDL cholesterol levels in normal men. *Ann. Int. Med.*, **116**, 967–73

14. Pavlou, S. N., Brewer, K., Farley, M. G., Lindner, J., Bastias, C., Rogers, B. J., Swift, L. L., Rivier, J. E., Vale, W. W., Conn, P. M. and Herbert, C. M. (1991). Combined administration of a gonadotropin releasing hormone antagonist and

testosterone in men induces reversible azoospermia without loss of libido. *J. Clin. Endocrinol. Metab.*, **73**, 1360–9

15. Bagatell, C. J., Knopp, R. H. and Bremner, W. J. (1994). Physiological levels of estradiol stimulate plasma high density lipoprotein$_2$ cholesterol levels in normal men. *J. Clin. Endocrinol. Metab.*, **78**, 855–61

16. Lipid Research Clinics (1980). *Population Studies Data Book: the Prevalence Study*, Vol. 1. (Department of Health and Human Services)

17. Manninen, V., Elo, M. O., Frick, M. H., Haapa, K., Heinonen, O. P., Heinsalmi, P., Helo, P., Huttanen, J. K., Kaitanieme, P., Koskinen, P. *et al.* (1988). Lipid alterations and the decline in the incidence of coronary heart disease in the Helsinki Heart Study. *J. Am. Med. Assoc.*, **260**, 641–50

18. Gordon, D. L., Probstfield, J. L. and Garrsion, R. J. (1989). High-density lipoprotein cholesterol and cardiovascular disease: four prospective American studies. *Circulation*, **79**, 8–15

19. Paulsen, C. A., Bremner, W. J. and Leonard, J. M. (1982). Male contraception: clinical trials, In Mishell, D. R. (ed.) *Advances in Fertility Research*, pp. 157–70. (New York: Raven Press)

20. Matsumoto, A. (1990). Effects of chronic testosterone administration in normal men: safety and efficacy of high-dosage testosterone and parallel dose-dependent suppression of luteinizing hormone, follicle-stimulating hormone, and sperm production. *J. Clin. Endocrinol. Metab.*, **70**, 282–7

21. Bagatell, C. J., Matsumoto, A. M., Christensen, R. B., Rivier, J. E. and Bremner, W. J. (1993). Comparison of a gonadotropin releasing hormone antagonist plus testosterone (T) versus T alone as potential male contraceptive regimens. *J. Clin. Endocrinol. Metab.*, **77**, 427–32

22. Tom, L., Bhasin, S., Salameh, W., Steimer, B. S., Peterson, M., Sokol, R. Z. *et al.* (1992). Induction of azoospermia in normal men with combined Nal-Glu gonadotropin releasing hormone antagonist and testosterone enanthate. *J. Clin. Endocrinol. Metab.*, **75**, 476–83

23. Friedl, K. E., Hannan, C. J., Jones, R. E., Kettler, T. M. and Plymate, S. R. (1990). High-density lipoprotein is not decreased if an aromatizable androgen is administered. *Metabolism*, 39, 69–77

24. Thompson, P. D., Cullinane, E. M., Sady, S. P., Chevenevert, C., Saritelli, A. L., Sady, M. A. and Herbert, P. N. (1989). Contrasting effects of testosterone and stanozolol on serum lipoprotein levels. *J. Am. Med. Assoc.*, **261**, 1165–8

25. Zmuda, J. N., Fahrenbach, M. C., Younkin, B. T., Bausserman, L. L., Terry, R. B., Catlin, D. H. and Thompson, P. D. (1993). The effect of testosterone aromatization on high-density lipoprotein cholesterol level and post-heparin lipolytic activity. *Metabolism*, **42**, 446–50

26. Bagatell, C. J. and Bremner, W. J. (1995). Androgen effects on lipids: experimental effects of decreased and increased androgen levels. In Bhasin, S. (ed.) *Pharmacology, Biology and Clinical Applications of Androgens.* (New York: Wiley)

27. Bagatell, C. J., Heiman, J. R., Matsumoto, A., Rivier, J. E. and Bremner, W. J. (1994). Metabolic and behavioral effects of high dose, exogenous testosterone (T) in normal men. *J. Clin. Endocrinol. Metab.*, **79**, 561–7